Ultrasonography in Ophthalmology 12

Documenta Ophthalmologica Proceedings Series

VOLUME 53

Ultrasonography in Ophthalmology 12

Proceedings of the 12th SIDUO Congress, Iguazú Falls, Argentina, 1988

Edited by
Roberto Sampaolesi

Department of Ophthalmology, University of Buenos Aires, Argentina

KLUWER ACADEMIC PUBLISHERS

DORDRECHT / BOSTON / LONDON

Library of Congress Cataloging-in-Publication Data

SIDUO Congress (12th : 1988 : Iguazú Falls, Argentina)
   Ultrasonography in ophthalmology 12 : proceedings of the 12th
SIDUO Congress, Iguazú Falls, Argentina, 1988 / edited by Roberto
Sampaolesi.
      p.   cm. -- (Documenta ophthalmologica. Proceedings series :
53)

   1. Ultrasonics in ophthalmology--Congresses.   2. Eye--Diseases and
defects--Diagnosis--Congresses.   I. Sampaolesi, Roberto.
II. Title. III. Series: Documenta ophthalmologica. Proceedings
series ; v. 53.
   [DNLM: 1. Eye Diseases--diagnosis--congresses. 2. Ultrasonic
Diagnosis--congresses.   W3 DO637 v. 53 / WW 143 S569 1988u]
RE79.U4S5 1988
617.7'1543--dc20
DNLM/DLC
for Library of Congress   90-4472

ISBN-13: 978-94-010-6758-4   e-ISBN-13: 978-94-009-0601-3
DOI: 10.1007/978-94-009-0601-3

Published by Kluwer Academic Publishers,
P.O. Box 17, 3300 AA Dordrecht, The Netherlands.

Kluwer Academic Publishers incorporates
the publishing programmes of
Martinus Nijhoff, Dr W. Junk, D. Reidel and MTP Press.

Sold and distributed in the U.S.A. and Canada
by Kluwer Academic Publishers,
101 Philip Drive, Norwell, MA 02061, U.S.A.

In all other countries, sold and distributed
by Kluwer Academic Publishers Group,
P.O. Box 322, 3300 AH Dordrecht, The Netherlands.

Printed on acid-free paper

Table of contents

PART THREE.   VITREORETINAL DISEASES

PART FIVE.   OTHER OCULAR PATHOLOGY

PART SIX.   PHYSICS AND TECHNIQUES

Preface

The 12th Congress of SIDUO took place in Iguazú Falls, Argentina, where participants could enjoy the scenery of the magnificent Falls.

The organization was sponsored by the University Department of Ophthalmology, Buenos Aires; the University Department of Ophthalmology, El Salvador; SAUMB (Socieded Argentina de Ultrasonografia en Medecina y Biología) and CLEO (Club Latinoamericano de Ecografia Oftalmológica).

The Honorary President was Professor Horacio Soriano from Buenos Aires.

The local organizing committee consisted of the following persons:

President   : Roberto Sampaolesi
Vice President   : Atilio Lombardi
Scientific Secretary: Eduardo Mayorga
Treasurers   : Guillermo Iribarren
                     Abelardo Cavatorta

We are particularly grateful to Doctor J S Hillmann, Professor K C Ossoinig and Doctor J M Thijssen, who have helped with their counsel and advice. I would also like to thank our congress secretaries Graciela Massonat and Cristina Taegl for their enormous help in organizing SIDUO XII.

To Doctor Javier Cassiraghi and Doctor Walter de Gregory our thanks for their outstanding help in organizing the scientific sessions.

Thanks are due to the commercial exhibitors and most of all to our sponsors: Laboratorios Pfoertner Cornealent and Biophysic Medical. Our special thanks to Doctor Tomás Pfoertner for his great administrative expertise and counsel and to Christine Warren from Biophysic for her help in financing these proceedings.

The 12th SIDUO thanks for their generous support: Pupilent Plastic Lens Argentina, Grafica SA and Laboratorio Optico Santamarina.

In this volume of the Documenta Ophthalmologica Proceedings Series the topics of sessions at the congress have been maintained. The abstracts of the lectures for which no manuscript was received for publication have not been included in this volume. The reader is referred to the abstract book for a complete overview of the abstracts.

R. Sampaolesi

PART ONE

The orbit

1. Ultrasonically-guided biopsy in orbital tumors

HIDEO TORII, ETSUO CHIHARA, TADASHI HAYASHIDA
and ATSUSHI SAWADA

Summary

In general ultrasonically-guided biopsy can be done more safely and accurately than that by the blind method. In ophthalmology ultrasonically-guided biopsy has not been common, due to orbital specific structure and limited manipulation of the B-mode probe.

A specific phantom was made, which consisted of a human skull specimen, commercial plain rubber balloons filled with gelatin gel, largely meshed sponge and spherical gelatin gel. The ultrasonic equipment we used was Ophthascan S.

Using the phantoms, the technique of ultrasonically-guided orbital biopsy was studied and its safety and accuracy were proved.

Introduction

Though we are able to know the characteristics of the solid or cystic tumors by the ultrasonic examination, it is impossible to decide the final diagnosis of the tumors perfectly. As a means of a new approach, a method combining ultrasonic examination with biopsy has been performed. Ultrasonically-guided biopsy is commonly used in the field of general surgery, but not in ophthalmology, due to specific structure of the orbit and limited manipulation of the B-mode probe. Using the phantom we especially made, the technique of the ultrasonically-guided orbital biopsy was studied and its safety and accuracy were proved.

Materials and methods

Ultrasonic scanning equipment Ophthascan S (Biophisic Medical s.a.) was

Department of Ophthalmology, Miyazaki Medical College, Miyazaki, Japan

R. Sampaolesi (ed.), Ultrasonography in Ophthalmology 12, 3–14.

used, which offers the standardized A-mode scan with B-mode. The B-mode probe (BM3) has the following characteristics:

1. mechanical sector scanning with a waterbath,
2. scanning angle is 40°,
3. sweep speed is 5 images per second,
4. frequency of the transducer is 10MHz.

The B-probe has so small a surface of 21 mm in diameter that we can manipulate easily either in the longitudinal or transverse section in scanning the whole orbit. The orbital phantom is composed of the human skull specimen, a commercial plain rubber balloon of 24 mm in diameter filled with gelatin gel, largely meshed sponge and spherical gelatin gel. In the first step we covered the orbital wall of the human skull specimen with largely meshed sponge of 5–10 mm in thickness for orbital fat and other supporting tissues, in which a commercial plain rubber balloon of 24 mm in diameter filled with gelatin gel for the eye ball was plugged. As the next step we enveloped the surface of the orbital cavity with a sheet of surgical drape, and the phantom of the normal orbital structure was accomplished (Fig. 1). In the present experiment, other orbital tissues, extraocular muscles, optic nerve, nerves and vessels were all neglected.

In the study of orbital tumors we used the spherical or hemispherical gelatin gel as an orbital cystic tumor, which was made by the following

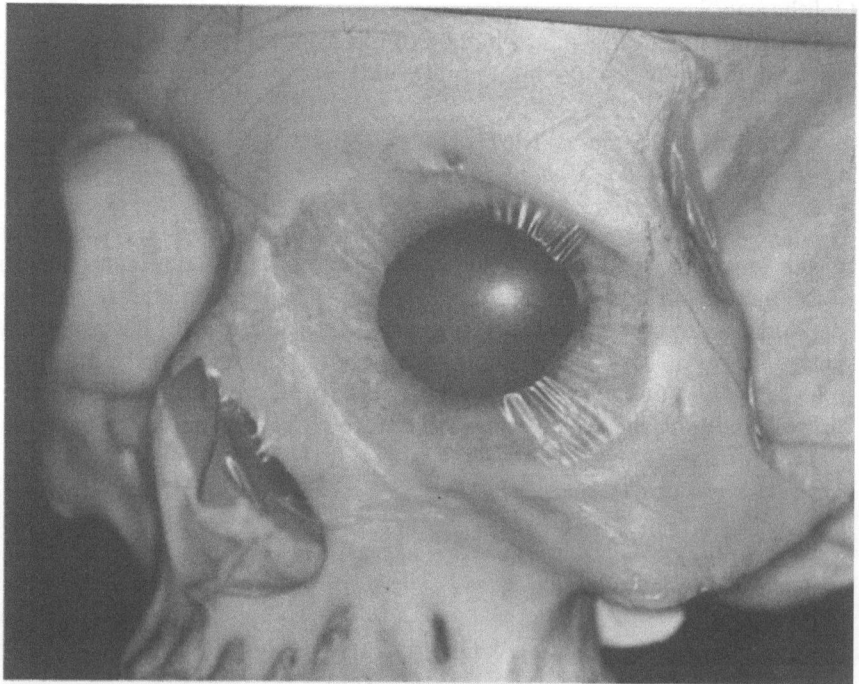

Fig. 1. The normal orbital phantom.

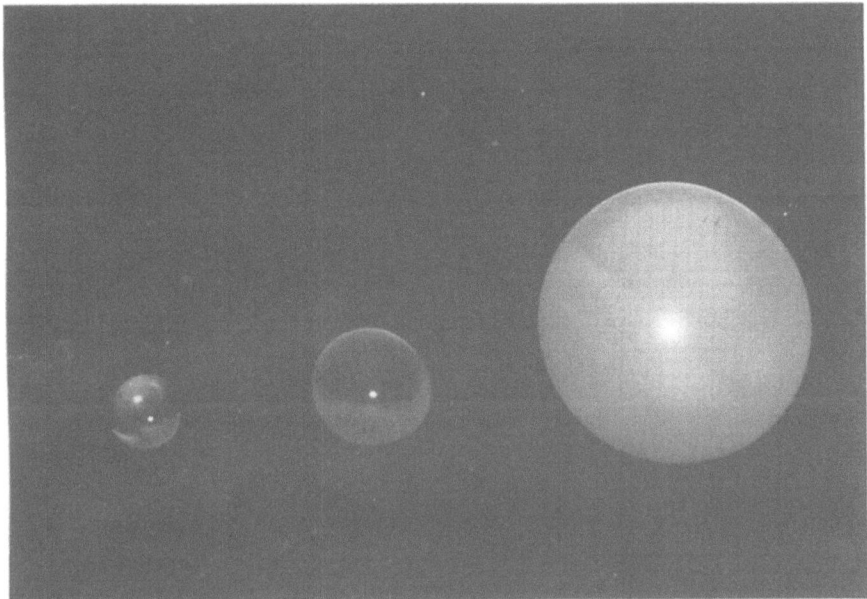

Fig. 2. The spherical gelatin gel, of 24 mm in diameter covered with a commercial plain rubber balloon (right), 10 mm in diameter (center), 5 mm in diameter (left).

method. Commercial gelatin powder of 5 g. weight dissolved in 50 mL of hot distillated water, was poured into the balloon of 5 mm or 10 mm in diameter (Fig. 2). The sound velocity of the gelatin gel used, is 1507 m/sec at 20°C (Ide 1985), which is between fresh water (1480 m/sec) and vitreous (1532 m/sec). These small spherical or hemispherical gelatin gel were buried into the posterior part of the orbital cavity or into the anterior part of the periorbital region. After that as in normal orbital phantom, a surgical drape was used to envelope the surface of the orbital cavity. We immersed the phantom into the waterbath up to the rim of the orbital cavity, and ultrasonically-guided needle aspiration was done.

As a biopsy needle the Hakko Sonoguide Biopsy needle 'SONOPSY-C1' of 0.8 mm in diameter was used. 'SONOPSY-C1' consists of the inner needle, the overcoating needle and the cylinder with the plunger. The length of the overcoating needle is 17 cm, and the inner needle is 1.5 mm longer that the overcoating needle. The tip of the overcoating needle is obliquely cut and very sharp. On the contrary the tip of the inner needle is of a circular cone shape (Fig. 3). They produced high reflectivity in the echogram. In ultrasonically-guided needle biopsy for the posterior orbital mass, we bent the straight needle thus imitating a retrobulbar anesthetic needle.

The technique of the ultrasonically-guided needle biopsy of the orbital tumor was as follows:
1. display of the target lesion.
2. insert the biopsy needle parallel to the major axis of the B-mode probe.

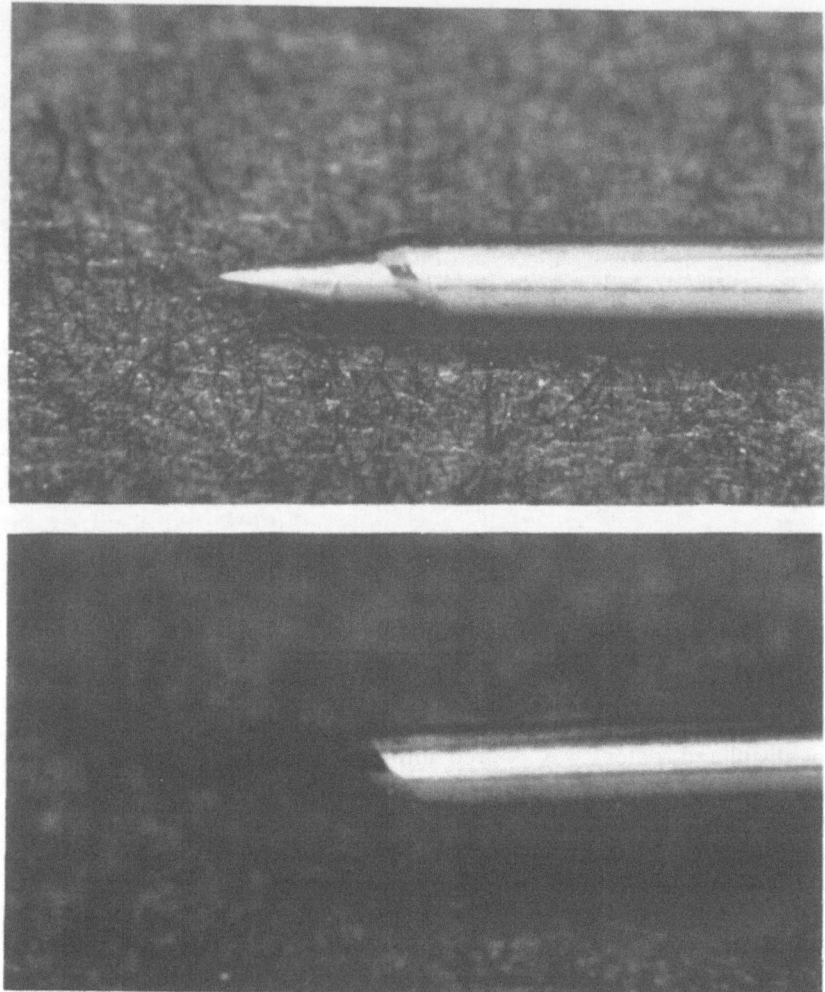

Fig.·3. The tip of the biopsy needle. The inner needle tip is of the circular cone shape (upper), and the overcoating needle is obliquely cut and very sharp (lower).

3. confirm the echo of the tip of the biopsy needle.
4. pull up the plunger of the cylinder after the tip of the needle reaches the target lesion.
5. aspirate the fragment of the gelatin gel into the overcoating needle.

Results

Figure 4 shows the B-mode echograms of the human left eye, arranged clockwise. B-scanning is done along the long face of the probe. The inscription engraved in the probe body is used as a tactile mark, correspond-

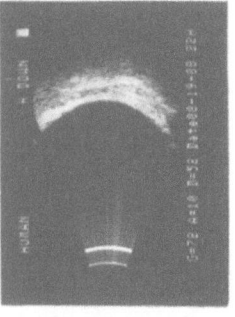

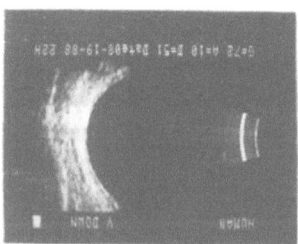

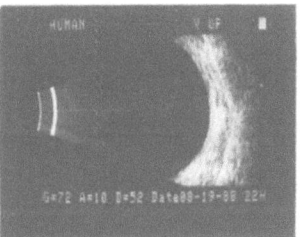

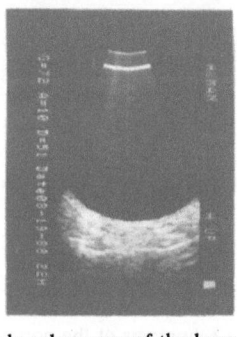

Fig. 4. Clockwise arranged B-mode echograms of the human left eye.

ing to the top of the screen. In the left eye, the probe was applied horizontally at the 6 o'clock position on the lid and the opposite orbital tissue was then examined by the technique for a transocular examination. At the time, the tactile mark of the probe was nasally aimed. Similarly the probe applied horizontally at 12 o'clock scaned the 6 o'clock orbital tissues. The probe was also applied vertically at 3 and 9 o'clock. The probe was to be moved in the clockwise direction. Behind echo-free area representing the vitreous cavity the posterior ocular wall and the orbital tissue are displayed as the delineated high reflective image and the jagged high reflective image. When the ultrasound beam is perpendicular to the orbital wall, the wall is displayed as an interrupted line behind the orbital echoes.

Figure 5 shows the clockwise arranged echograms of the normal orbital phantom of the left. Though the ultrasound beam is less attenuated due to absence of the lid in the phantom, the echograms of the phantom are similar to those of the human, but the orbital wall is more delineated than the human orbital wall. In the phantom, echoes of the extraocular muscles and optic nerve are not displayed.

1. Phantom of posterior orbital tumor

We set the small spherical gelatin gel of 5 or 10 mm in diameter in the posterior orbit, which corresponded to the space in the muscle cone in the

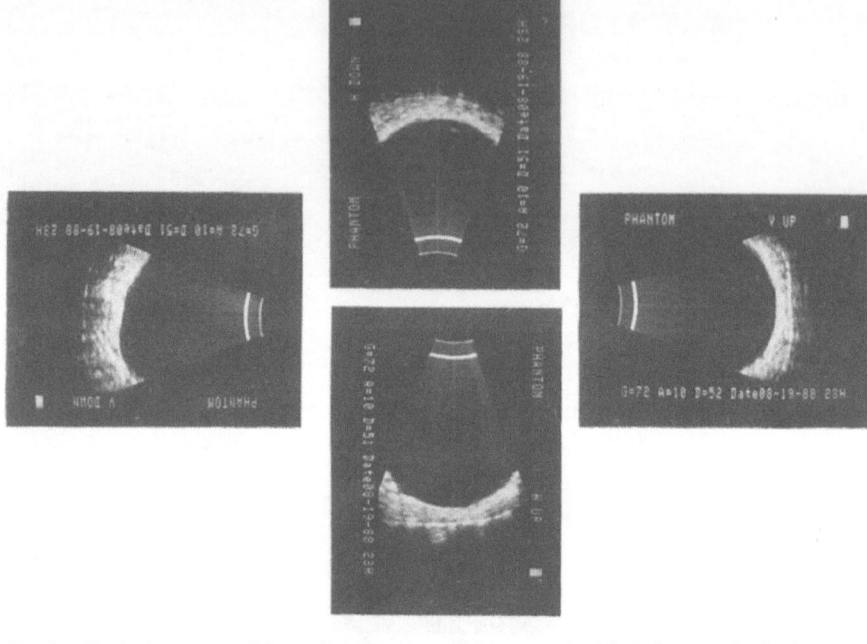

Fig. 5. Clockwise arranged B-mode echograms of the normal orbital phantom in the lett.

human. Figure 6 shows echograms of the posterior orbital mass of 10 mm in diameter in the phantom, which are simultaneous images with B and cross-vector A-mode. The upper is in eye display and the lower is in orbit display. The round echo-free lesion of the gelation gel substituted for a cystic tumor is displayed in the strong echoes of the largely meshed sponge behind the echo-free area representing the eye ball of gelatin gel.

Figure 7 shows echograms of the same case. We inserted the curved biopsy needle from the temporal side of the orbit along the orbital wall, parallel to the major axis of the B-mode probe. In this case, the probe was applied horizontally, and the top of the screen corresponded to the temporal side of the globe and orbit. While we fixed the B-mode probe to display the mass lesion, we advanced the biopsy needle posteriorly slowly so as to display the tip of the needle as a moving high reflective echo in the top of the screen. Then we penetrated the cystic lesion under ultrasonic guidance. The successful rate of the biopsy of the posterior orbital mass was about 90% in cases of 5 mm in diameter gelatin gel ball. In the residual 10% cases we ruptured the balloon for the eye ball. In cases of cystic mass of 10 mm in diameter, the rate is over 90%.

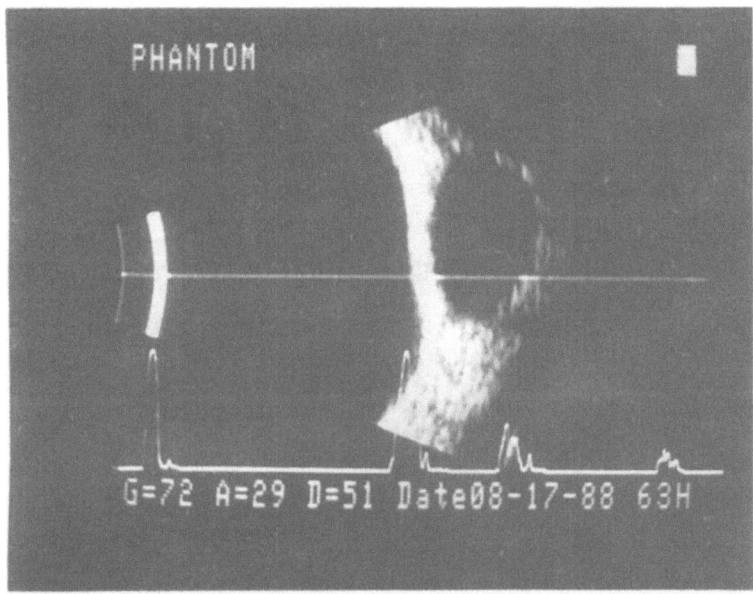

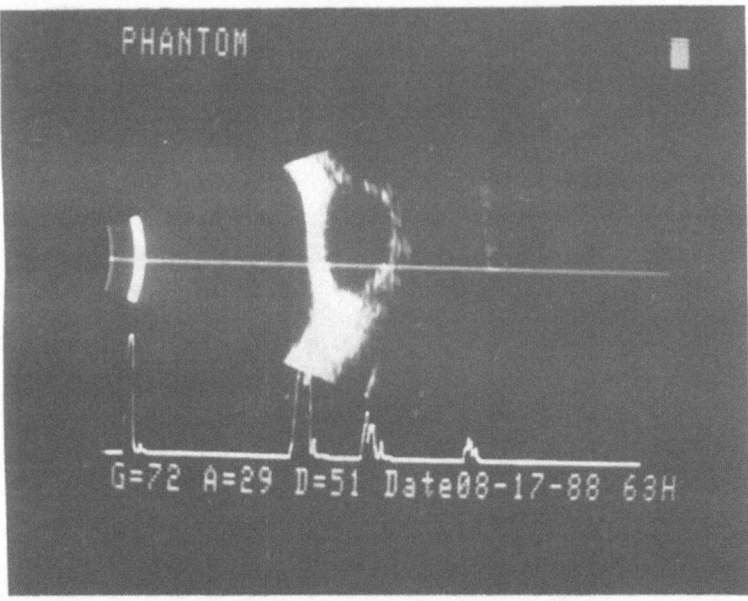

Fig. 6. B- and cross-vector A-mode echograms of a posterior mass of 10 mm in diameter in the phantom, in eye display (upper), and in orbit display (lower).

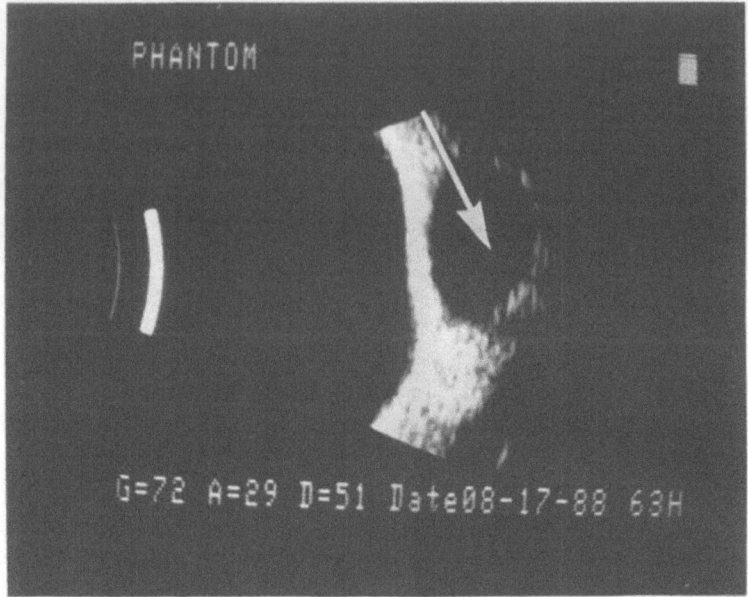

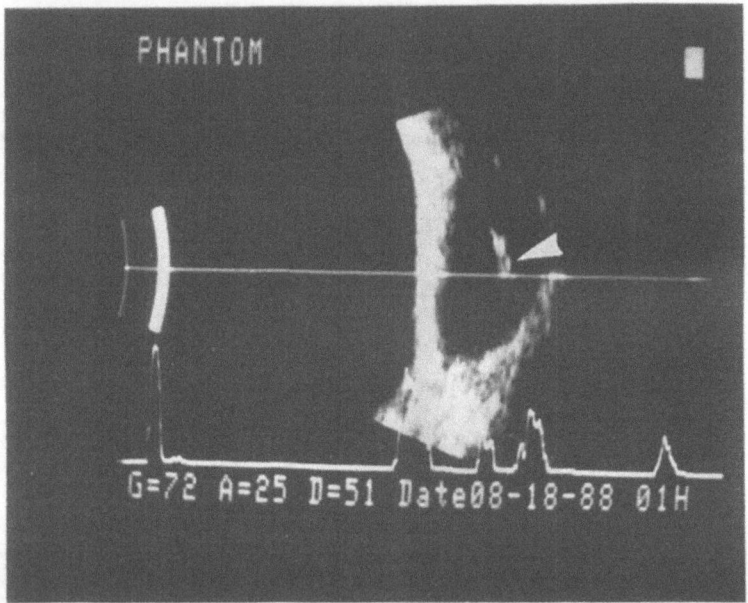

Fig. 7. Echograms of the case as in Fig. 6. The white arrow shows the course of the biopsy needle (upper). The white arrowhead indicates the tip of the biopsy needle (lower).

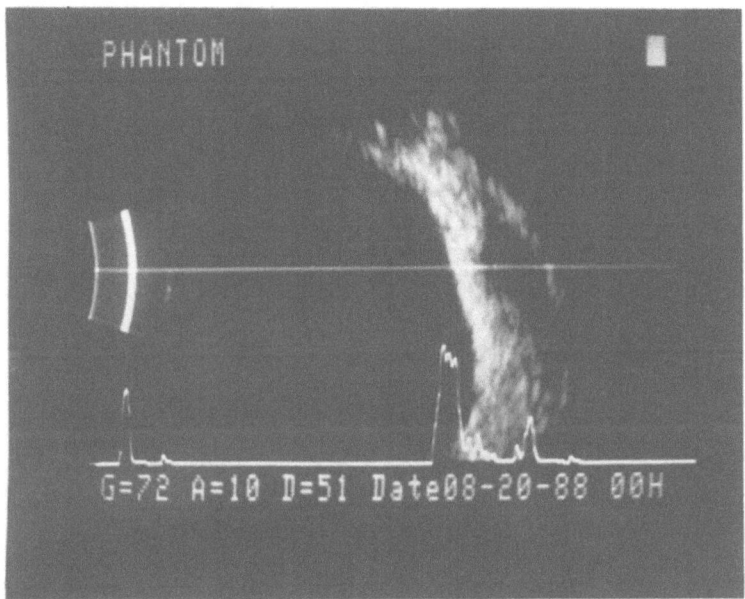

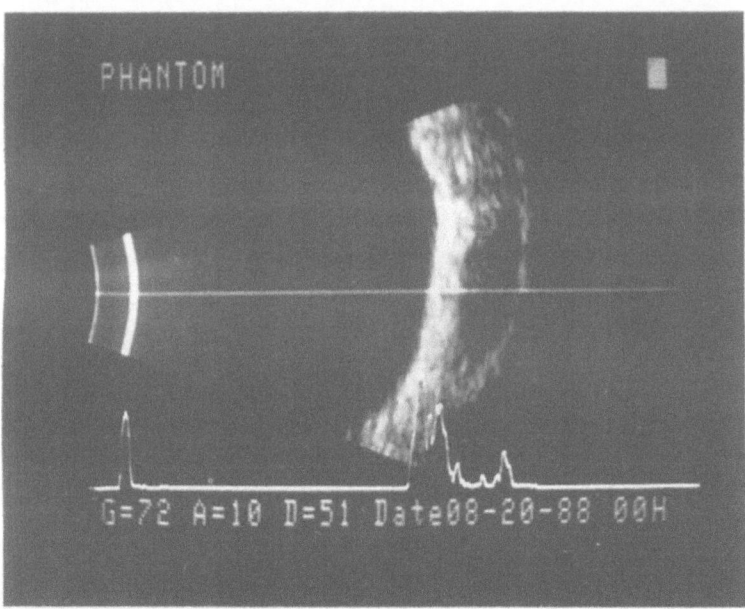

Fig. 8. B- and cross-vector A-mode echograms of a cystic mass phantom located in the superotemporal quadrant in longitudinal section (upper), and in transverse section (lower).

12

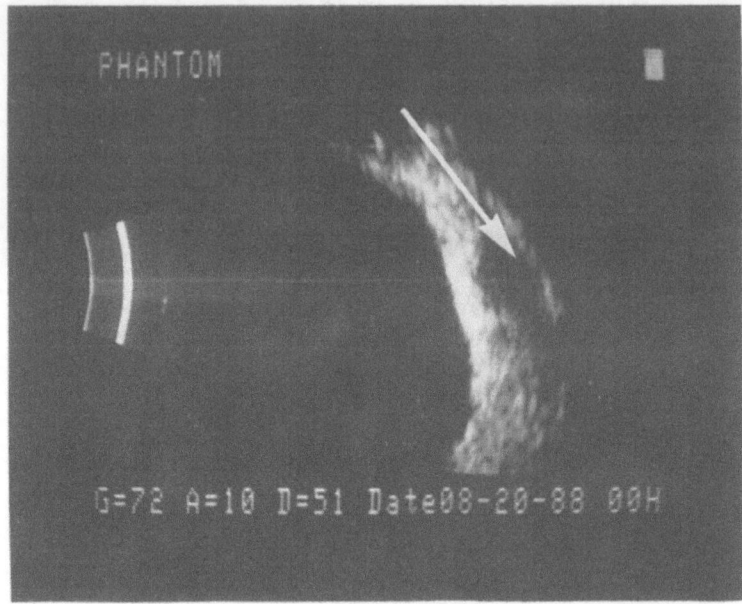

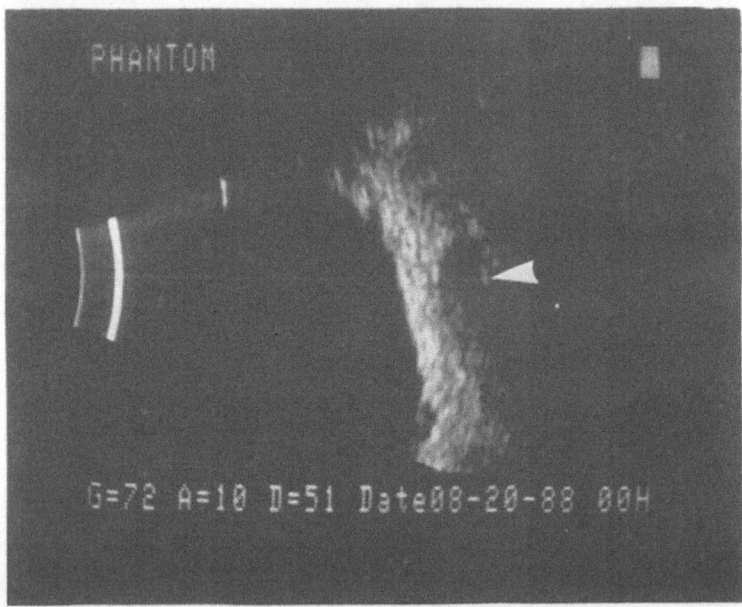

Fig. 9. Echograms of the case as in Fig. 8. The white arrow shows the course of the biopsy needle (upper). The white arrowhead indicates the tip of the biopsy needle (lower).

2. Phantom of anterior orbital tumor

We buried the hemispherical gel of 10 mm in diameter, attached to the orbital wall, anterior to the equator of the eye balloon. Figure 8 shows echograms of a cystic mass phantom located in the superotemporal quadrant for a lacrimal gland tumor. In that phantom we inserted the straight needle at the supertemporal edge of the orbital wall and moved it posteriorly along the orbital wall until the tip of the needle was displayed at the top of the screen and pushed it further slowly under ultrasonic guidance. After confirming the echo of the needle tip in the cystic lesion, we pull up the plunger to aspirate gelatin gel fragments (Fig. 9). In the same way we performed the ultrasonically-guided biopsy for a hemispherical cystic mass of gelatin gel, located in the supernasal, inferonasal or inferotemporal quadrant. The rate of success was almost 100%.

Discussion

Berlyne (1961) first reported the usefulness of the ultrasonically-guided biopsy by carrying out the renal biopsy under ultrasonic A-mode guidance. The transducer, the needle and the method on percutaneous ultrasonically-guided biopsy have been remarkably improved and developed since his report (Holm et al., 1972; Rasmussen et al., 1972; Hancke et al., 1975). In ophthalmology Spoor et al. (1980), Skalka (1981), and Kennerdell et al. (1985) have reported the clinical fine needle biopsy of orbital lesions under B-mode ultrasonic guidance. They all accepted the ultrasonically-guided aspiration needle biopsy as a very useful method. The ultrasonically-guided biopsy has the following advantages.
1. It makes not only echographic diagnosis but also histopathological diagnosis.
2. It is possible in the case of small lesion within 10 mm in diameter.
3. It is more reliable and safer than the former blind method.
4. It can be done in the outpatient clinic.
5. It does not require the x-ray, the dark room and the use of a contrast medium.

In other medical fields this kind of biopsy has been used commonly, but in ophthalmology it has not been used because of the orbital specific structure and limited manipulation of the B-scan probe. The B-mode probe equipped in Ophthascan S is small enough to manipulate in the longitudinal and transverse section of the echographic examination. The Handling of this probe in the longitudinal section, which is important in ultrasonically-guided biopsy, is easier than that of the old B-mode model probes. In this study we

14

developed a specific phantom of the orbit, and operated the ultrasonically-guided aspiration needle biopsy for orbital mass. As the results, in the phantom of the posterior orbital tumor of 5 and 10 mm in diameter, the rate of success was almost 90% and over 90%, respectively. In the phantom of the anterior orbital mass, we could operate the biopsy of the hemispherical mass of 10 mm in diameter at the success rate of almost 100%. We are sure of the safety and accuracy of this technique in ophthalmology. The Biopsy needle used in this experiment is somewhat long for use during the biopsy of orbital lesions. It requires some technical skill to insert the biopsy needle parallel to the long axis of the B-mode probe.

In the future the needle is expected to be shortened to 8 cm in length, and it is necessary to develop the special attachment to this probe. Using the special attachment and shortened needle will surely rise the rate of success in the ultrasonically-guided biopsy of smaller orbital mass within 5 mm diameter.

Acknowledgement

This study was supported in part by a grant-in-aid for scientific research (62771379) from the Japanese Ministry of Education.

References

Berlyne G M. 1961. Ultrasonics in renal biopsy. Lancet 1: 750.
Holm H H, Kristensen J K, Rasmussen S N, Northeved A, Barlebo H. 1972. Ultrasound as a guide in percutaneous puncture technique. Ultrasonics 10: 83.
Hancke S, Holm H H, Koch F. 1975. Ultrasonically guided percutaneous fine needle biopsy of the pancreas, Swrg. Gynec & Obst. 140: 361.
Ide M. 1985. Study on phantom for B-mode ultrasonic diagnostic equipment. JSUM Proceeding 36: 435.
Kennerdell J S, Slamovits T L, Kekker A, Johnson B L. 1985. Orbital fine needle aspiration biopsy. Am J Ophthalmol 99: 547–551.
Rasmusssen S N, Holm H H, Krinsensen J K, Barleb H. 1972. Ultrasonically-guided liver biopsy. Brit Med J 2: 500.
Spoor T C, Kennerdell J S, Dekker A E, Johnson B L, Rehkopf P G. 1980. Orbital fine needle aspiration biopsy with B-scan guidance. Am J Ophthalmol 89: 274.
Skalka H W. 1981. Ultrasonography and percutaneous orbital aspiration. Docum Ophthal Proc Ser 29: 375.

2. Echodriven fine needle aspiration biopsy in orbital tumor diagnosis

C. TAMBURRELLI*, F. FOCOSI* and A. FABIANO**

Summary

Twenty-nine patients with suspected orbital tumors were evaluated with Standardized Ophthalmic Echography. On the basis of echographic findings, 18 of this group were selected for a further study by means of fine needle biopsy. The remaining 11 patients were excluded because echographic examination detected a pathology where fine needle biopsy would be useless (Graves disease, Posterior Scleritis) or even extremely dangerous (A-V fistulas). All the cases underwent fine needle biopsy aspiration under echographic control. Echographic evaluation was divided in two phases: the first before the introduction of the needle in order to find by A- and B-scan the best location for puncture, the depth of the center of the lesion from the cutaneous plane and also, on the basis of Standardized A-scan tissue recognition, the chance for obtaining enough material from aspiration.

The second phase was performed during the aspiration by monitoring with a bimanual technique all the locations and advancement of the needle inside the orbit, thus preventing any risk of damage for structures contiguous to the tumor. The data obtained with Standardized Echography, before and during aspiration can greatly improve the results of fine needle aspiration and can prevent highly dramatic consequences such as eyeball perforation, optic nerve damage or even excessive penetration of the needle and passage through Superior Orbital Fissure.

Introduction

First report on Fine Needle Aspiration Biopsy to diagnose Orbital Neoplasms in exophthalmos appeared in the literature in 1975 (Schybers) [10].

* Department of Ophthalmology.
** Department of Pathology.
 Catholic University of Rome, Rome, Italy

R. Sampaolesi (ed.), Ultrasonography in Ophthalmology 12, 15–25.
© *1990. Kluwer Academic Publishers, Dordrecht*

Later on Kennerdell et al. published [9] large series where FNAB had an 80% positive identification rate for several orbital tumors [4, 5, 6]. Different result, only 50% accuracy, was found by other authors (Krohel et al.) [7]. Two major reasons were responsible for the negative results, the first one is the erroneous placement of the needle at the time of the aspiration (in front, beyond or beside the lesion) and a second reason depended on the histologic charactheristic of the tumor specially if the lesions were highly fibrous with sparse or extremely cohesive cell populations. Standardized Echography can be very helpful for reducing negative results by directing the needle during the biopsy and because Standardized A-scan evaluation gives information about the internal structure of the tumor [8, 9]. Echography also can be extremely useful and almost imperative, in preventing serious complications.

Don Liu in his original work, carried out a survey among several surgeons with a total of 152 patients and he found that the most serious complications occured when FNAB was performed by ophthalmologists not familiar with the complex anatomy and pathology of the orbit. There were three deaths. Not everyone of these patients has had either Computed Tomography or Echography performed before or during the procedure [2].

Echography should be strictly included in the protocol as it is a very useful technique and orbital surgeons familiar with Standardized Echography of the orbit or ophthalmologist with subspecialisation in echography are the only physicians that should perform this procedure. It is our purpose to describe echographic findings obtained during FANB and our technique to localize and to guide the needle and report our results.

Materials and methods

Twenty-nine patients with a diagnosis of orbital tumor were examined. All patients had a thorough ophthalmic examination, which included CT scan and Standardized Echography. After this examination patients were selected for further study by FNAB.

We excluded patients with any type of A-V fistulas, and all patients with muscles or Tenon's capsule inflamation, but two patients with chronic lacrimal gland inflamation of unknown etiology were included. We decided not to perform FNAB on patients with an echographic sign of cystic wall or thickened capsule [1, 8, 9]. Therefore we excluded patients with diagnosis of Dermoid Cyst, Cavernous Hemangioma and Benign Mixed Tumor of Lacrimal Gland. We prefered not to take a biopsy from these lesions to prevent any spillage of irritating or proliferating material into the orbit.

Eighteen patients were selected to undergo FNAB. Those patients were studied, before aspiration, with A- and B-scan obtaining the following information; First of all location and size of the tumor, mostly done with A-Scan in a paraocular approach, indicating clockwise the meridian corresponding to the limits of the lesion (e.g. OD: 9:00 to 12:30). Between these

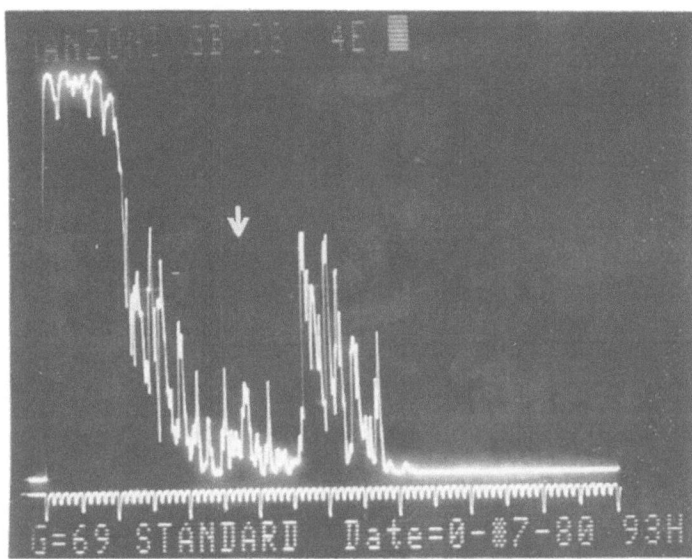

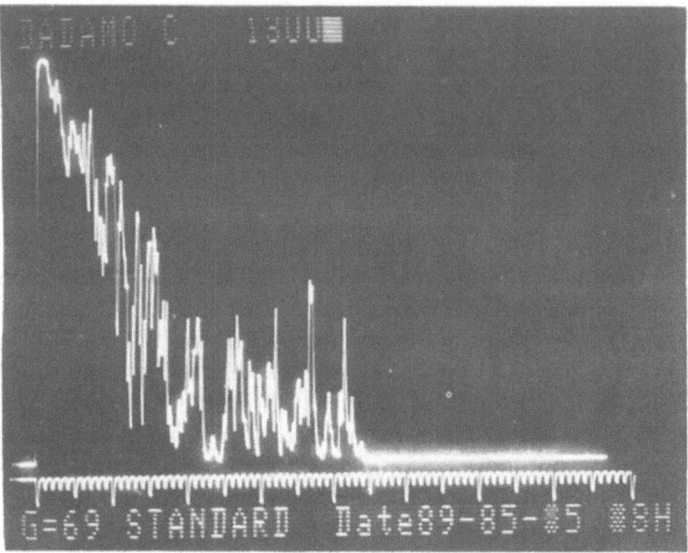

Fig. 1. Paraocular A-scan from two different lesions, obtained placing the probe on the meridian where was displayed the widest pattern of the tumor. At the top a Schwannoma which measured 27.5 mm on the meridian 4.00, OS. The arrow points at the distance from the cutaneous plane which corresponds to the best location for biopsy. In this case the distance was 18.5 mm. At the bottom a paraocular A-scan from an Adenoid Cystic Carcinoma of the lacrimal gland. Last spike on the right measured 37.2 mm at 1.30 meridian OS. In this case the needle was not pushed beyond 20 mm from cutaneous surface.

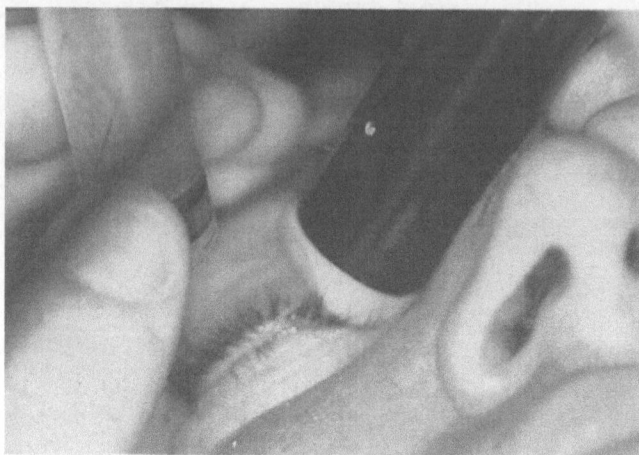

Fig. 2. The left hand holds the syringe while the right scans with the B-scan probe the entire meridian from anterior to posterior to localize the needle. In this case a transverse section of the 11.00 meridian OD has been performed.

two limits we tried to find the meridian corresponding to the deepest extension of the tumor from the cutaneous plane, represented by the widest pattern of the tumor in the paraocular approach. At this meridian we measured two points: one corresponding to the distance from the tip of the probe to the last spike of the tumor pattern, and another midway between these two, corresponding to the center of the lesion, which ideally is the best location for biopsy, Fig. 1.

The meridian found by this technique is appropriate to perform the puncture. We prefer not to mark a this point while keeping with a finger the same pressure exerted with a probe, because cutaneous tissue may slide over the lesion, thereby shifting the mark and changing the point.

It is very useful to place the syringe exactly in the same direction as the A-scan probe to display the widest pattern in the paraocular approach. We push the needle for two or three milimeters underneath the cutaneous plane and then we stop briefly the pressure, meanwhile we place on the opposite meridian the B-scan probe scanning with a transverse section the entire meridian where the needle was placed. At this point we keep with one hand the probe and with the other the syringe (Fig. 2).

We start pushing the needle again into the tumor trying to display the strong echo signals from the metallic tip of the needle. The visualization of this signal is not easily accomplished, as a matter of fact, we need in turn to angle the probe from anterior to posterior sections of the meridian trying to find the strong signal of the needle and once we have displayed this signal we push gently the syringe holding the B-scan probe immobile so we can see the movements looking directly at the screen thus confirming that the echos seen are produced by [9] reflection from the needle. The procedure described

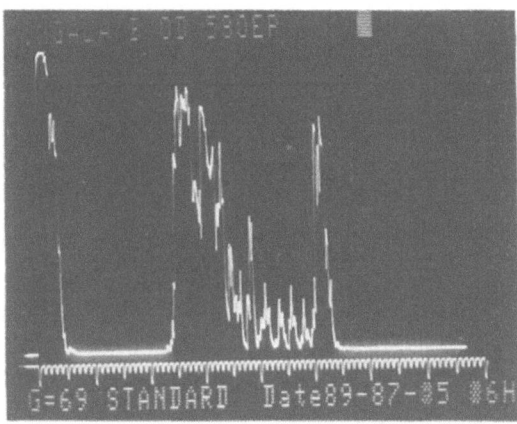

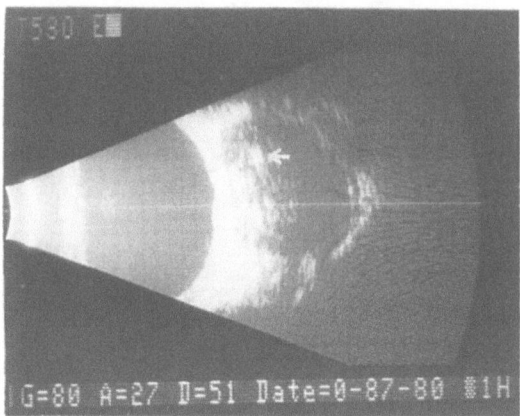

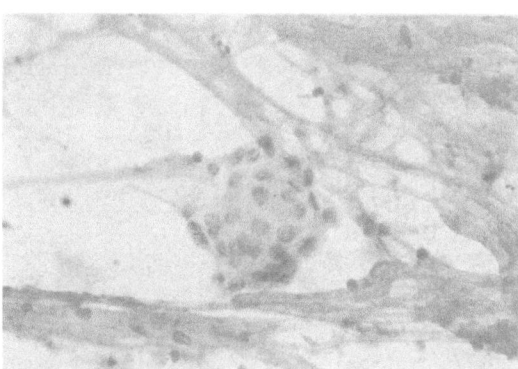

Fig. 3. Top: Standardized A-scan. Regularly structured and low reflective lesion. Middle: B-scan transverse section. The arrow points at the needle inside the tumor, clearly visible, with an accurate amplification setting. Bottom: Cytologic aspirate. Cells with regular nuclei and tipically growing in pavingstone clusters and whorls, indicating a meningioma.

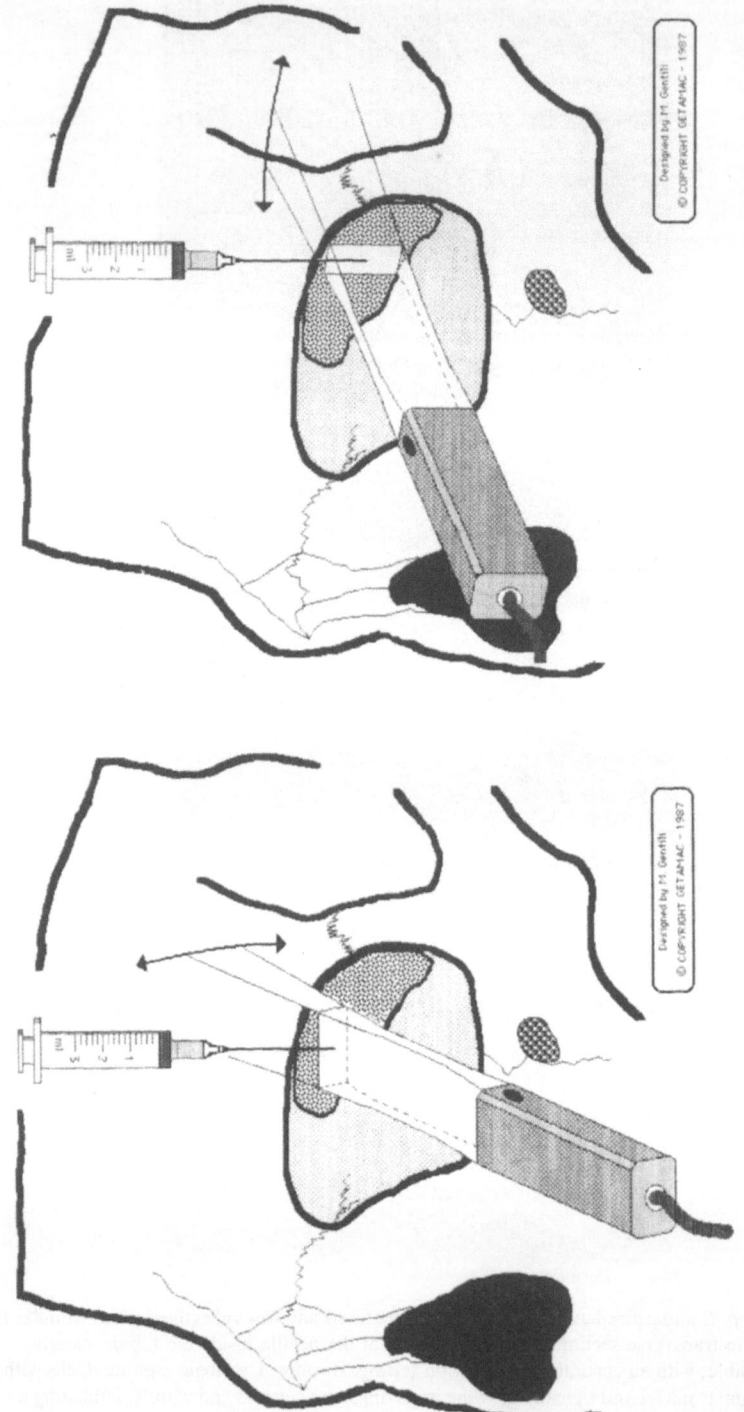

Fig. 4. Schematic drawings showing a transverse scanning on the left and a longitudinal on the right, both along the 1.30 meridian OS. To localize the needle we start with a transverse section then rotate the probe over 90 degrees to perform a longitudinal scanning. We begin with a transverse scanning, because it is easier to find the needle with this approach than with a longitudinal.

is very useful when examining irregularly structured or highly reflective lesions, where strong echoes from the tumor may be confused with echoes from the needle. On the other hand it is easier to localize the needle in low- or very low-reflective lesions, Fig. 3. Once we have localized the needle inside the tumor we hold the syringe immobile and rotate over 90 degrees the B-scan probe, while aligning the scanning plane parallel to the meridian, thus performing a longitudinal section of the meridian (Fig. 4). Theoretically, this section should display a long section of the needle but this is rarely obtained, because it is very difficult to exactly align the scanning plane parallel to the axis of the needle. When it did occur the probe was in a position midway between transverse and longitudinal, corresponding to an oblique section of the meridian.

Results

Twenty-nine consecutive patients with unilateral exophtalmos have been evaluated with Standardized Echography and with CT scan. Eighteen patients out of this group were selected for further evaluation by means of FNAB.

Table 1 lists cases that underwent FNAB in comparison with echographic diagnosis, internal reflectivity, difficulty to identify the needle and finally histologic diagnosis.

We obtained three negative aspirations and 15 positive. Negative results were obtained in two cases from highly reflective lesions and in one from a medium reflective tumor.

Among 15 positive aspirations there were:
8 low to very low reflective lesions
2 medium to low,
2 highly reflective and 3 irregularly structured.

We could localize the needle inside the tumor in all the examined lesions. However we found different degrees of difficulty in displaying the needle. Difficult cases occurred mainly in highly reflective and in irregularly structured lesions. For these patients echo signals from the needle showed not a clear difference in reflectivity with the surrounding structures and the identification of the needle was based mainly on the movements made by the syringe. Three cases had negative results despite the correct localization, we did not collect any cell for examination. Histology diagnosed in two cases a Chronic Dacryoadenitis, with massive connective proliferation, and the remaining case was diagnosed as a Schwannoma. Chronic Dacryoadenitis presented, on Standardized A-scan evaluation, an irregular structure and high reflectivity; Schwannoma showed a regular structure and a medium reflectivity.

We had only a minor complication performing FNAB on an highly vascular meningioma with a consequent lid hematoma which resolved in a

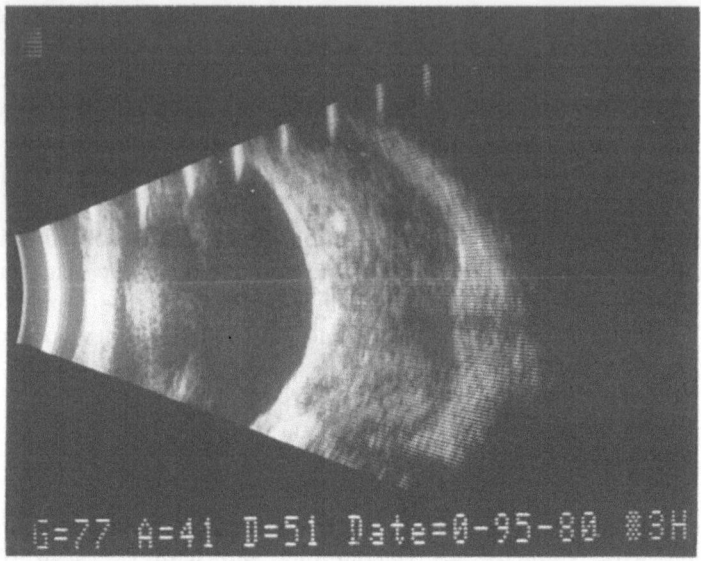

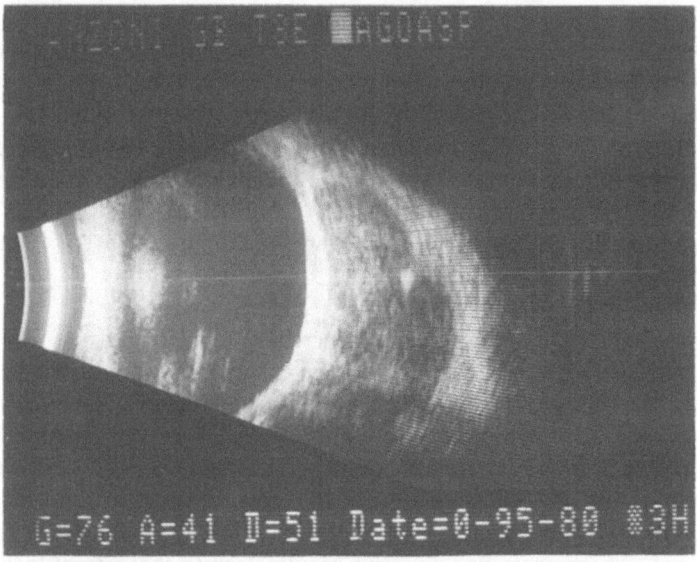

Fig. 5. Transverse scanning along 3:00 meridian OS. At the top the needle appears as an highly reflective roundish spot inside the low reflective tumor. In this case it was too close to the posterior borders of the tumor, we were not sure that the tip was really inside the lesion. The needle was withdrawn slithly and placed (bottom) in a position midway the globe and the posterior border of the tumor.

week. In all patients where the echo signal from the needle was clearly visible because of the low reflectivity of the tumor, it was depicted as a small roundish and strong echo when the scanning plane was perpendicular to the axis of the needle (Fig. 5). A highly reflective line, was displayed when the scanning plane was parallel to the axis of the needle (Fig. 6). We have never obtained reverberation signals.

Table 1. Comparison of histologic, cytologic and echographic diagnosis; the difficulty to localize the needle and the reflectivity (obtained with a Standardized A-scan) of the examined lesions are listed as well.

Histology	Difficulty	Echo diagnosis	Reflectivity	Cytology
1 Adenoid cystic carcinoma of lacrimal gland	++	Adenoid cystyc carcinoma	High (V-H)	Carcinoma
2 " "	" "	" "	" "	" "
3 Lymphoma	+	Lymphoma/Pseudotumor	Low-Very Low	Atypic Lymphoid cells
4 " "	" "	" "	" "	" "
5 " "	" "	" "	" "	" "
6 Inflammatory Pseudotumor	+	Lymphoma/Pseudotumor	Low-Very Low	Lymphhoid Hyperplasia
7 " "	" "	" "	" "	" "
8 Chronic Dacryoadenitis	+++	Chronic Dacryoadenitis	High (V-H)	Negative
9 " "	" "	" "	" "	" "
10 Meningioma	+	Hemangiopericytoma	Low	Meningioma
11 Neurinoma	+	Scwhannoma/Neurinoma	Medium	Spindle cells
12 " "	" "	" "	" "	" "
13 Breast Mets	++	Orbital Malignancy	Irregular	Carcinoma
14 " "	" "	" "	" "	" "
15 Rabdomyosarcoma	++	Lymphoma/Sarcoma	Low	Atypical Mesenchimal Cells
16 Prostatic Carcinoma	++	Orbital Malignancy	Irregular	Carcinoma
17 Cordoma	+	Sinus Carcinoma	Low	Mesenchimal Tumor
18 Schwannoma	+	Neurogenic Tumor	Medium	Negative

Conclusion

FNAB is still a controversial procedure, this technique evoked mixed opinions from different authors. However it is not our purpose to formulate another one, but simply we want to stress a few aspects on the combined

24

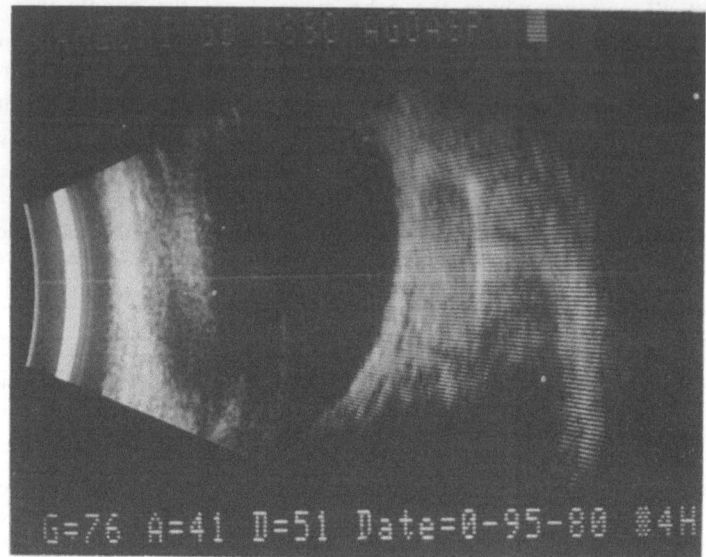

Fig. 6. Longitudinal section along the 3:30 meridian OS. The needle presented as a long highly reflective line which enters the tumor from above and ends into the lesion.

and consecutive use of FNAB and Echography. Although every ophthalmologist is familiar with retrobulbar puncture, clearly different is the situation when there is a pathology. This is the reason why Echography has to inform in advance whether it is advisable to perform FNAB. In this regard Standardized Echography plays a better role than CT Scan because it permits to obtain more precise information on the borders of the lesion such as a cystic wall or a thick capsule and on the internal structure.

The exact location of the mass, the identification of the needle during the procedure and the precise data regarding the distance of the center of the lesion from the cutaneous surface, make FNAB much more safe and harmless when performed under echographic control. In our experience only in one case FNAB diagnosed a lesion that was misdiagnosed by Echography, but on the other hand we presented three negative results where echography formulated the correct diagnosis. FNAB did not add any real improvement in diagnostic accuracy of Standardized Echography.

Eighteen cases represent a small group of patients, therefore, it is not possible to indicate a clear relationship between the internal reflectivity and the chances of collecting cells to be examined. We never got a negative aspiration from low to very low reflective lesions and, on the other hand, there were no low to very low reflective lesions in the group of negative biopsy.

Finally, we want to stress that precise indication for FNAB together with the consecutive and combined use of Standardized Echography allowed us to prevent any major complication. In this regard it is our opinion that opthalmologists familiar with Standardized Echography can perform FNAB with less complications and more positive aspiration results.

References

[1] Blodi F, Ossoinig K C. 1982. Modern diagnosis of orbital tumors. In: Symposium on Diseases and Surgery of the Lids Lacrimal Apparatus and Orbit. St. Louis: C V Mosby, pp. 129–149.
[2] Don Liu 1985. Complication of fine needle biopsy of the orbit. Ophthalmology 92: 1768–1771.
[3] Dubois P J, Kennerdell J S, Rosenbaum A E, Dekker A, Johnson B R, Swink C A. 1979. Computed tomographic localization for fine needle aspiration biopsy of orbital tumors. Radiology 131: 149.
[4] Kennerdell J S, Dekker A, Johnson B L, Dubois P J. 1979. Fine-needle aspiration biopsy; its use in orbital tumors. Arch Ophthalmol 97: 1315–7.
[5] Kennerdell J S, Dekker A, Johnson B L. 1980. Orbital fine needle aspiration biopsy: the results of its use in 50 patients. Neuro-Ophthalmol 1: 117–21.
[6] Kennerdell J S, Slamovits T, Dekker A, Johnson B L. 1985. Orbital fine needle aspiration biopsy. Am J Ophthalmol 547–51.
[7] Krohel G B, Tobin D R, Chavis R M. 1985. Inaccuracy of fine needle aspiration biopsy. Ophthalmology 92: 666–670.
[8] Ossoinig K C. 1978. The role of clinical echography in modern diagnosis of periorbital and orbital lesions. In: Proc. of the 3rd Int. Symp. on Orbital Disorders, Amsterdam, 1977 (G. Bleeker, ed), pp. 496–540. Dr. W. Junk Publ., Amsterdam.
[9] Ossoinig K C, Blodi F. 1980. The role of echography in the diagnosis of orbital disorders. In: Palestra Oftalm Panamericana 4: 12–19.
[10] Schyberg E. 1975. Fine needle biopsy of orbital tumors. Acta Ophthalmol Suppl. 125: 11.
[11] Westman-Naeser S, Naeser P. 1978. Tumors of the orbit diagnosed by fine needle biopsy. Acta Ophthalmol 56: 69.

3. Echography assisted fine needle aspiration biopsy for diagnosing orbital pseudotumor and lymphoma

DANIELE DORO, EDOARDO MIDENA, PAOLO BOCCATO,*
ENRICO MANTOVANI, GIOVANNI B. MOSCHINI
and FERRUCCIO MORO

Summary

Standardized echography evidenced low reflective lesions in the anterior or mid orbit of four patients but lymphoma or inflammatory pseudotumor could not be differentiated. The results of echo-assisted fine needle aspiration biopsy (FNAB) enabled us to establish a definite diagnosis of pseudotumor or lymphoma in three out of four cases. Immunohistochemistry was required to identify the type of lymphoma in one patient. The usefulness and limits of B-scan assisted FNAB in diagnosing orbital lesions are outlined. Thus, in selected patient this low cost office procedure can furtherly improve the accuracy of standardized echography.

Echography has proved to be a useful diagnostic tool in detecting and differentiating orbital lesions [1]. While several types of lesions such as hemangioma or mucocele have distinctive acoustic hallmarks, both clinical appearance and combined echographic and CT scan examination may often be inconclusive for differentiating orbital idiopathic inflammatory pseudotumor from lymphoma [2, 3].

Establishing a correct diagnosis of an orbital disorder is obviously important for planning adequate therapy. We found that B-scan assisted fine needle aspiration biopsy (FNAB) can improve the acoustic information of ultrasound examination in different cases [4, 5].

Methods

Standardized echography with adequate techniques [6] was used to investigate all patients. Orbital echography has been performed both with the Kretztechnik 7200 MA (8 MHz A-scan probe) and the Coopervision Ultrascan Digital IV B (contact B-scan 10 MHz probe). Drawings of the echographic results have been made in order to correctly address FNAB.

University Eye Clinic of Padua, Italy
* Servizio di cit' Diagnostica 2°, Ospedale Civile, Padua, Italy

R. Sampaolesi (ed.), Ultrasonography in Ophthalmology 12, 27–36.
© *1990. Kluwer Academic Publishers, Dordrecht*

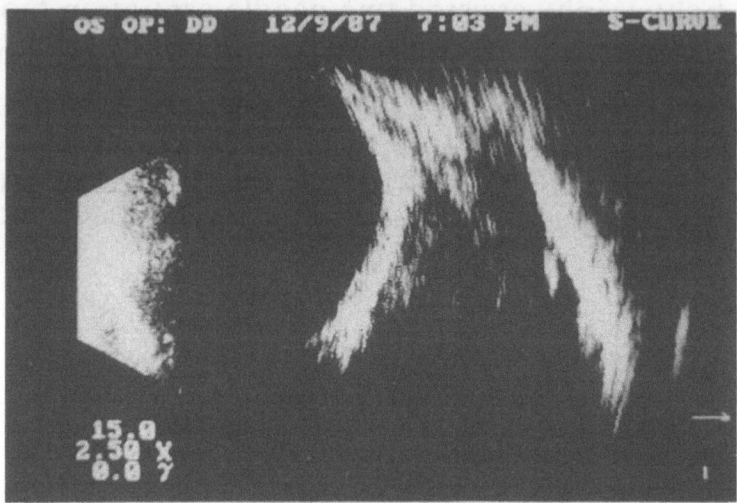

Fig. 1. Case 1. Contact B-scan echography of the left orbit: low reflective temporal mass in the anterior-mid orbit with rare medium reflective echo spikes; the lateral rectus belly is embedded in the mass.

FNAB has been performed according to the technique described by Kennerdel et al. [7] and as modified by Midena et al. [8]. A pistol grip attached to a 20 ml disposable syringe was employed. A fine butterfly disposable needle was connected whenever a palpable or anterior orbit mass lesion was detected [9]; otherwise, a 21–25 gauge 4 cm needle with obturator was used to avoid normal orbital tissue contamination during the insertion.

Contact real-time B-scan echography was performed at normal system sensitivity setting to properly identify the orbital mass; the probe was located away from the site of the needle insertion. System amplification was reduced to exactly localize the high reflective needle tip, which could be better evidenced by slight movements of the needle. After restoring a higher system sensitivity we could verify that the needle tip was within the orbital mass. After aspiration biopsy firm pressure was applied to avoid hematoma.

Cytologic smears were stained according to the Papanicolaou and May-Grünwald-Giemsa techniques. Some unstained specimens have been used for immunohistochemistry and immunological investigation when needed.

Case presentation

Case 1

A 75 year old woman had been suffering from bilateral proptosis, lid edema and marked episcleral congestion for about one year. Oral steroids had been administered without clinical improvement.

Hemathological exams including thyroid tests and organ and non-organ specific autoantibodies were negative. A history of lung and knee synovia tubercolosis was obtained. No systemic disease symptoms or signs were present, but skull X-rays revealed an empty enlarged sella.

On admission visual acuity was finger count and 20/200 in the right and left eye respectively; motility was severely restricted both horizontally and vertically and proptosis of 23 and 25 mm was recorded (Hertel); media were clear; intraocular pressure was normal; the optic disc of the right eye was temporally pale. Goldmann kinetic perimetry evidenced sectorial incongrous loss of the inferior visual field in both eyes.

CT Scan of the orbits with contrast enhancement suggested the presence of bilateral pathological tissue invading nearly the entire orbit with shifting of the retrobulbar optic nerve and compression at the apex; the optic canals were normal sized. The only distinguishable right lateral and left medial rectus muscles appeared normal.

Contact B-scan revealed a gross mass lesion in the right nasal orbit and in the left temporal orbit both extending posteriorly out of the echographic reach. In both eyes standardized A-scan echography evidenced outlined mass borders and internal regular low or very low reflective areas with rare medium reflective echo spikes; the latter characteristic was confirmed by contact B-scan evidence of internal rather irregular texture. Sound transmission through the orbital lesion was good. All rectus muscles showed normal thickness and high reflectivity except right medial and left lateral rectus which were embedded in the mass (Fig. 1). On A-scan echography the right retrobulbar optic nerve appeared thickened (8 μsec) with evidence

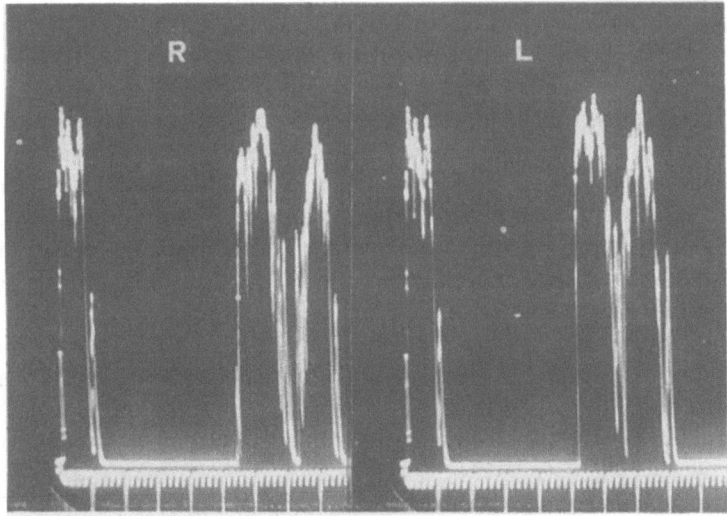

Fig. 2. Case 1. Standardized A-scan echography of the retrobulbar optic nerve. Right eye: increased width and evidence of subarachnoid fluid. Left eye: moderately increased width and perineural sheath thickening.

of subarachnoid fluid between perineural sheaths; increased width (6.25 μsec) and thickened perineural sheaths of the retrobulbar left optic nerve were observed (Fig. 2). No orbital defect or subtenonial space enlargement (T-sign) was evidenced.

Bilateral involvement, unresponsiveness to steroids, absence of tenonitis raised the reasonable suspicion of orbital lymphoma; marked inflammatory signs, enlarged muscles and compressive optic neuropathy, however, pointed towards the diagnosis of orbital pseudotumor. CT scan gave no additional diagnostic information in this case.

The material obtained from the echo-assisted FNAB showed a population of mononuclear cells with mostly lymphocytes but also centrocytes and plasma cells. Thus, FNAB was crucial for the diagnosis of inflammatory orbital pseudotumor.

Combined steroid and radiation therapy was successful in reducing the proptosis and restoring ocular motility, visual field and, partially, visual acuity (RE: 20/100, LE: 20/30 after two months).

Case 2

A 51 year old male patient complained of progressive bilateral proptosis with mild inflammatory signs and intermittent dyplopia. A pancreatic immunocyctic lymphoma, diagnosed by means of surgical biopsy eight years before, had been successfully treated with chemotherapy.

Eye examination including visual field was bilaterally normal with full visual acuity; palpable masses were present in both upper temporal orbits. General physical examination showed no evidence for sytemic disease. Skull X-rays and routine blood tests including serum electrophoresis revealed no abnormalities. CT scan was not performed.

In both eyes contact B-scan revealed kidney-shaped 1.5 × 2.0 cm mass in the anterior upper orbit extending towards the extraconal temporal middle orbit; borders were well defined, as confirmed by standardized A-scan examination. No bone defects or bulbus indentation were present. The thickness of rectus muscles was normal, however, superior rectus belly was bilaterally confused with the mass. A-scan and B-scan echography showed a regular, low or absent internal reflectivity. Sound trasmission was good; no T sign could be evidenced.

Cytologic smear obtained from B-scan assisted FNAB of both masses in the anterior orbit (Fig. 3) demonstrated limphoplasmacytoid cells; immuno-histochemistry identified positive lambda chain monoclonal B-cells (Fig. 4). The diagnosis of low grade malignancy lymphoplasmocytoid lymphoma was made.

History, clinical appearance and echographic features pointed towards a probable diagnosis of lymphoma. The results of echo guided FNAB enabled us to promptly administer chemo and radiation therapy and avoid CT and surgical biopsy.

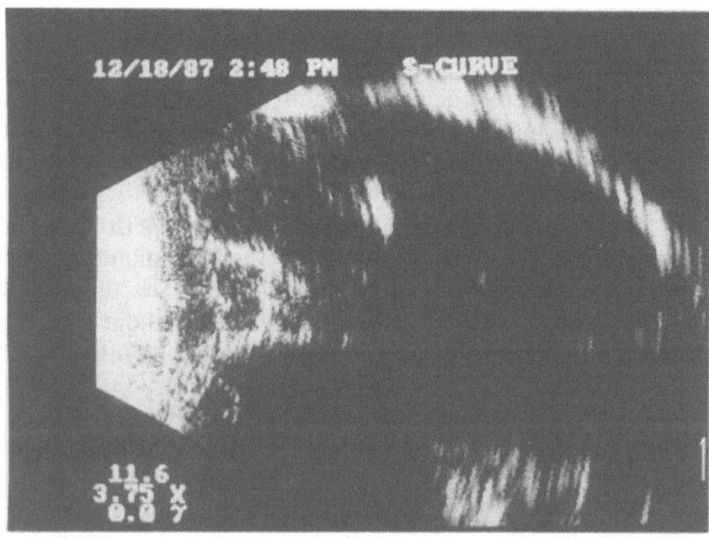

Fig. 3. Case 2. Contact B-scan guided fine needle aspiration biopsy of the left upper temporal orbit. Needle tip is well evidenced within the mass at reduced system sensitivity setting.

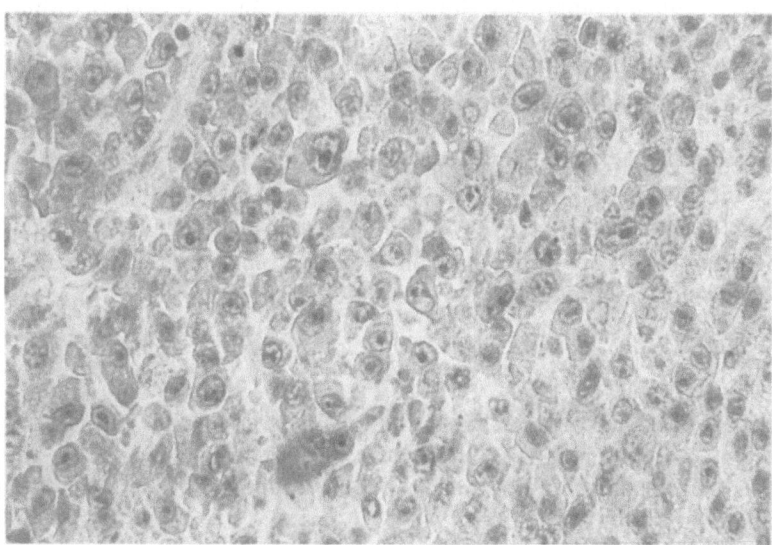

Fig. 4. Case 2. Fine needle aspiration from the left upper temporal mass: positive lambda chain monoclonal B-cells are identified by immunohistochemistry indicating the diagnosis of lymphoma.

Case 3

Marked proptosis, severe edema and neovascularization of the cornea, episcleral congestion and lid edema were the prominent features of the left fixed abducted eye of a 35-year old male patient with a ten year history of ipsilateral recurrent orbital inflammation.

Surgical biopsy of the lacrimal gland has been performed in 1977; histology showed the presence of granulomatous inflammation with fibrotic tissue. No systemic disease could be ascertained. Low dosage radiation therapy and retrobulbar steroids were administered without success shortly after the biopsy. The proptosis did not change during the following ten year span.

In April 1988 the patient complained of progressive visual loss, due to corneal involvement, and was completely reevaluated. Immunological and hematological investigations ruled out a systemic disease. Ct scan showed an orbital intraconal mass lesion which encompassed almost the entire bulbus compressing and dislocating the retrobulbar optic nerve. NMR confirmed the presence of low signal pathological orbital tissue but did not help in distinguishing between chronical inflammation and lymphoma.

Echographic examination of the left orbit revealed as huge uncompressible mass lesion in the 360 degree middle orbit. With standardized echography rectus muscle bellies were partially confused with the lesion, which showed defined borders; a good sound transmission was present. Internal texture of the lesion was irregularly distributed with higher reflectivity in proximal portions. A-scan echography showed medium reflective echoes within very low or low reflective areas of the mass (Fig. 5).

No material was obtained from orbital FNAB with B-scan guidance, even if the needle tip has been addressed to the more homogeneous areas of the mass lesion.

Thus, no conclusive information could be obtained by non-invasive means alone. A lateral orbitotomy was planned and the orbital mass was excised. Histopathological examination led to the diagnosis of sclerosing orbital pseudotumor. Acceptable reduction of proptosis but no improvement of ocular motility resulted.

Case 4

A hard painless uncompressible orbital lesion was located in the region of the right lacrimal gland of a 67 year old woman. A mass of the left submaxillary gland had been excised four years before; no details about histopathology were available.

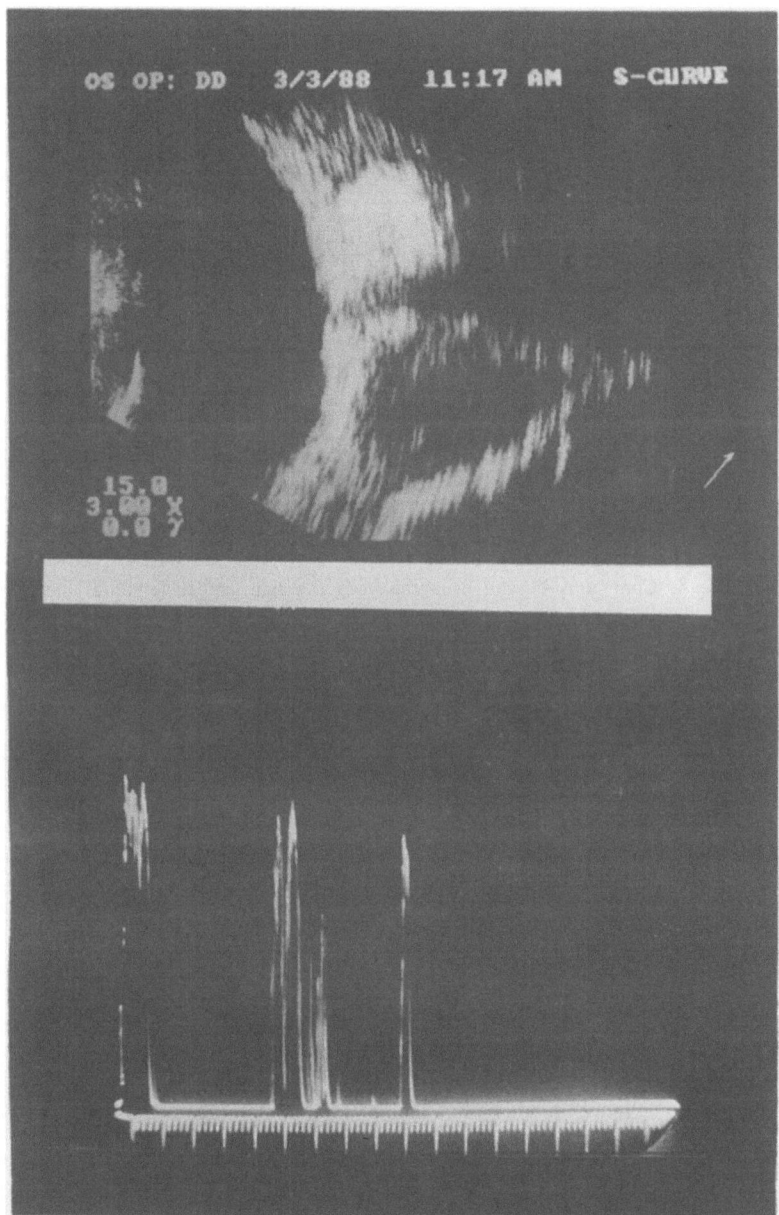

Fig. 5. Case 3. Top: contact B-scan; bottom: standardized A-scan echography of the left orbit showing low reflective mass lesion with definite borders and higher internal reflectivity in proximal portions.

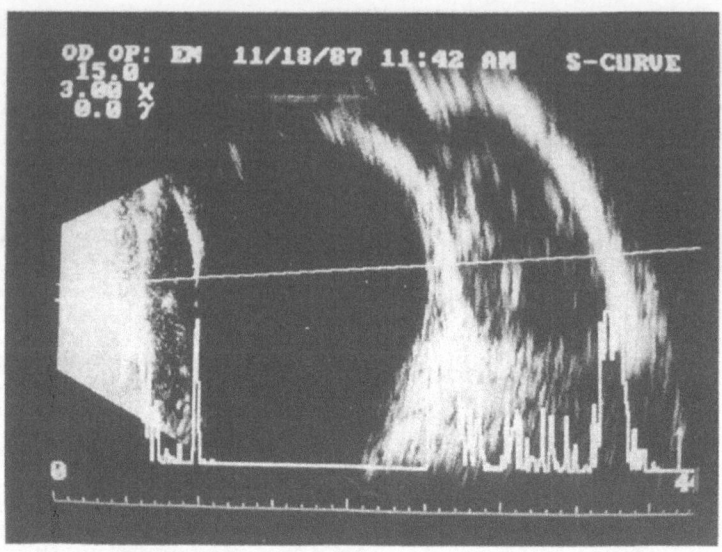

Fig. 6. Case 4. Contact A-/B-scan echography of the right upper temporal orbit: rather irregular texture of the mass lesion.

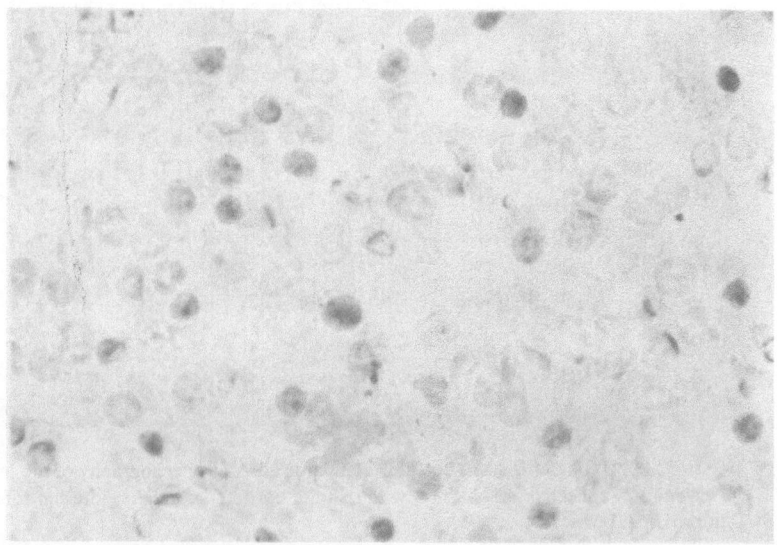

Fig. 7. Case 4. Fine needle aspiration from the right upper temporal orbit. Cytologic smear demonstrates lymphocytes and plasma cells mixed up with non-cuboidal elements, a typical picture in Sjoegren's disease.

On admission, no inflammatory orbital signs were present and the right eye was slightly dislocated downwards and nasally, but no diplopia was complained of. Ophthalmological examination including ocular motility was negative except for a pathological Schirmer I test. Routine blood tests including rheumathological evaluation were negative.

Standardized echography of the right eye showed an outlined mass lesion in the anterior (2 × 1 cm) and mid (1 × 1.5 cm) upper temporal orbit. Internal reflectivity was mostly very low (standardized A-scan) and rather irregular texture could be evidenced on B-scan examination (Fig. 6). Rectus muscles and retrobulbar optic nerve were normal.

No CT scan was performed. FNAB obtained smears demonstrated several lymphocytes and plasma cells intringled with non-cuboidal elements (Fig. 7), indicating the characteristic benign lymphoepithelial lesion of Sjögren's disease.

History and the results of echographic examination alerted us towards the diagnosis of inflammatory pseudotumor of the lacrimal gland; a lymphoma could not be ruled out on the basis of echographic examination only. FNAB was the crucial tool to correct diagnosis and treatment.

Conclusions

In our experience echography assisted orbital FNAB has proven to be a low cost office procedure and a valuable diagnostic tool.

Three out four of our cases were clearly diagnosed by echo-guided FNAB. In all three cases the orbital mass was located in anterior or mid orbit and adequate cytological smears were always obtained. FNAB of a lesion located in the posterior orbit could not have been done under B-scan but only under CT scan guidance because of the limitations of ultrasonic imaging in that area.

Negative aspiration from fibrous lesions, as in case no. 3, did not substantiate the echographic diagnostic suspicion and surgical biopsy was necessary. Thus, sclerosing pseudotumor is a condition that cannot be reliably diagnosed by non-invasive techniques.

In all our cases clear echographic differentiation between orbital idiopathic inflammatory pseudotumor and lymphoma was almost impossible; typical T-sign and echographic appearance of myositis [10, 11] were not present in our pseudotumor cases. Cytology and in one case (no. 2) immunohistochemistry of the material obtained by FNAB were necessary to establish a correct diagnosis.

Actually, it was confirmed [12] that the identification of the various orbital lymphoid infiltrates becomes more distinct when cyto-immunological techniques are added to the classical and histopathological methods of investigation [13].

However, we found echography very helpful not only in the differentiation and prediction of the histological pattern of major orbital tumors in the anterior and middle orbit areas but also in simply performing FNAB.

References

[1] Ossoinig K C. 1979. Standardized echography: basic principles, clinical applications and results. Intern. Ophthalmol. Clinics 19: 107–210.

[2] Gallenga P E, Mazzeo V, Scorrano R, Rossi A. 1981. Misinterpretation in orbital diagnosis. In: C Alvisi and CR Hill (eds) Investigative Ultrasonography: 2°: Clinical Advances, Pitman Press, Bath, pp. 312–324.

[3] Frezzotti R. 1985. Patologia, clinica e terapia delle malattie dell'orbita. LXV S.O.I. Congress (Siena), pp. 279–309 and pp. 563–593.

[4] Skalka H W, Callahan M A. 1979. Ultrasonically-aided percutaneous orbital aspiration. Ophthalmic Surg 10: 41–43.

[5] Spoor T C, Kennerdell J S, Dekker A, Johnson B L, Rehkopf P. 1980. Orbital fine needle aspiration biopsy with B-scan guidance. Am J Ophthalmol 89: 274–277.

[6] Ossoinig K C: Orbital disorders. In: M De Vlieger et al. (eds) Handbook of Clinical Ultrasound. John Wiley & Sons, New York, 881–904.

[7] Kennerdell J S, Dekker A, Johnson B L, Dubois P J. 1979. Fine needle aspiration biopsy: a report of its use in orbital tumors. Arch Ophthalmol 97: 1315–1317.

[8] Midena E, Segato T, Piermarocchi S, Boccato P. 1985. Fine needle aspiration biopsy in ophthalmology. Surv Ophthalmol 29(6): 410–422.

[9] Boccato P. 1987. Fine needle aspiration biopsy of small targets. Acta Cytol 31: 200–201.

[10] Goes F. 1987. Ultrasonographic and clinical characteristic of orbital pseudotumors. In: K C Ossoinig (ed) Ophthalmic Echography. Proceed. 10th S.I.D.U.O. Congress Martinus Nijhoff / Dr W. Junk Publ., Dordrecht. Docum. Ophthalmol. Proc. Series 48: 499–507.

[11] Ravalli L. 1987. Diagnostica orbitaria. In: V. Mazzeo (ed) L'Ecografia dell'Apparato Oculare Fogliazza, Milano pp. 281–327.

[12] Gaag Rvd, Koorneef L, van Heerde P, Vroom T H, Pegels J H, Feltkamp C A, Peeters H J F, Gillissen J P A, Bleeker G M, Feltkamp T E W. 1984. Lymphoid proliferations in the orbit: malignant or benign? Br J Ophthalmol 68: 892–900.

[13] Moro F. 1966. Les pseudotumeurs de l'orbite. Ophthalmologica 151: 349.

4. Ultrasound diagnosis of orbital histiocytofibromas

O. BERGES* and R. GUTHOFF**

Summary

Fibrous histiocytomas are not rare. The diagnosis of fibrous histiocytoma might be evoked in case of a well circumscribed, heterogenous tumor, with bony deformation and no bony erosion. New B-mode equipment with high energetic, high resolution good gray scale probes proved to be very helpful, giving as much information as Standardised A-mode. It is always possible to differentiate such a tumor from cavernous hemangioma. Unfortunately, differential diagnosis with hemangiopericytoma and peripheral nerve sheath tumors is not always possible.

Fibrous and connective tissue tumors are rare. They include fibromas, fibrosarcomas and fibrous histiocytomas (hystiocytofibromas).

Pure fibromas are extremely rare. One mainly sees angiofibromas, fibro-lipomas and fibromyosarcomas. Fibromas have to be differentiated from nodular fasciitis and from fibrosarcoma. Fibrosarcoma has been reported mostly in children, most frequently after irradiation for retinoblastoma.

Fibrous histiocytoma (histiocytofibroma, fibroxanthoma) is the most common mesenchymal orbital tumor. It was frequently misdiagnosed by the pathologists. This explains the very low frequency of the cases reported in two large series [1, 2] of orbital tumors. Nevertheless, the orbit is a site of predilection for this tumor.

They usually are benign lesions, well circumscribed and cystic myxoïd and hemorrhagic areas may also be noted. Usually hemorrhage is seen in malignant tumors. Recurrence of the lesion is linearly related to the aggressivity and the malignancy of the tumor. Microscopically, there is variable admixture of spindle-shaped fibroblast like cells and hystiocytic cells.

We report 4 cases of fibrous histiocytoma. They all happened in an adult: 3 intraconal lesions and 1 extraconal inferolateral lesion. All the lesions were well delineated. The good limitation of the anteriorly situated lesion was more difficult to appreciate.

* Fondation Rothschild, Paris, France
** Universitats Krankenhaus, Hambourg, FRG

R. Sampaolesi (ed.), Ultrasonography in Ophthalmology 12, 37–41.

38

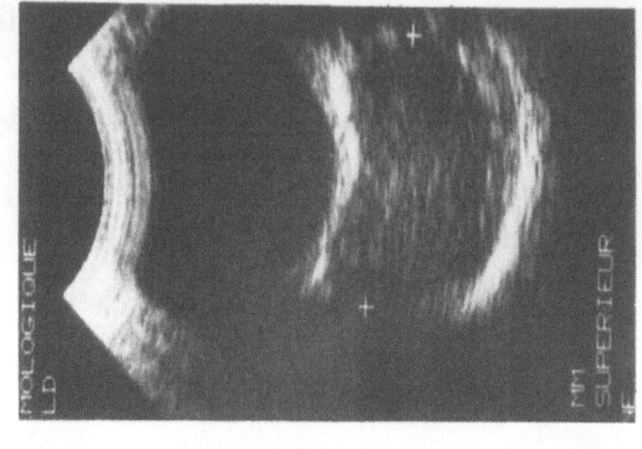
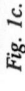

Fig. 1c.

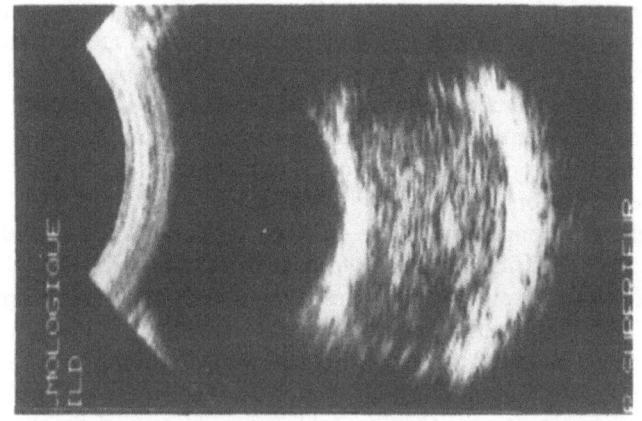

Fig. 1b.

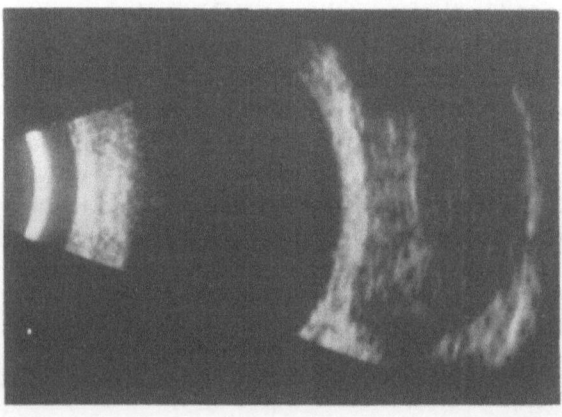

Fig. 1a.

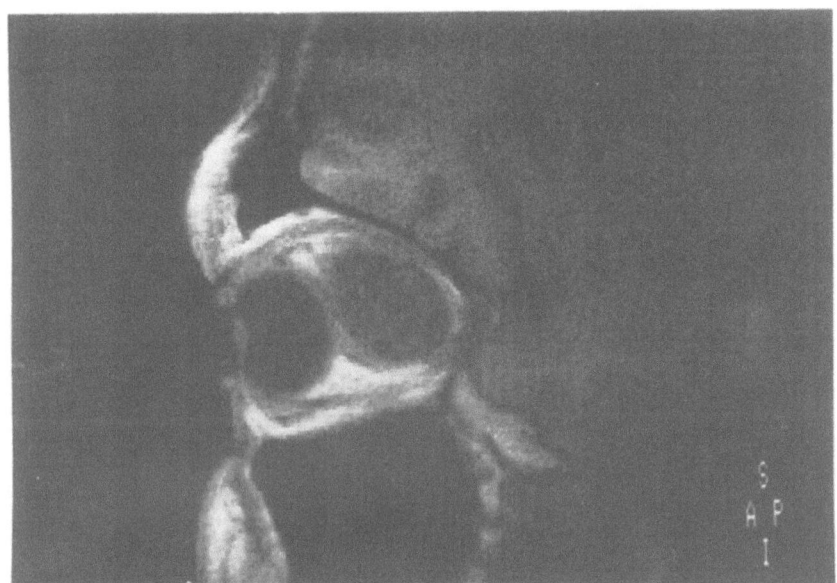

Fig. 1d.

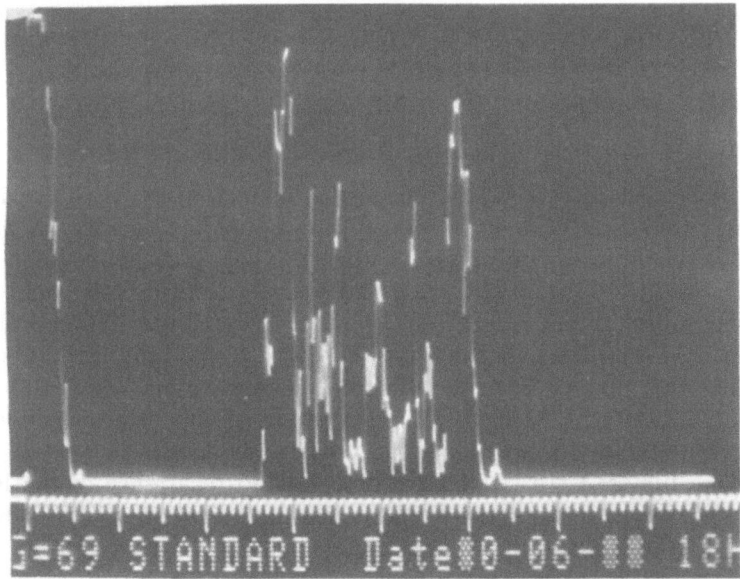

Fig. 1e.

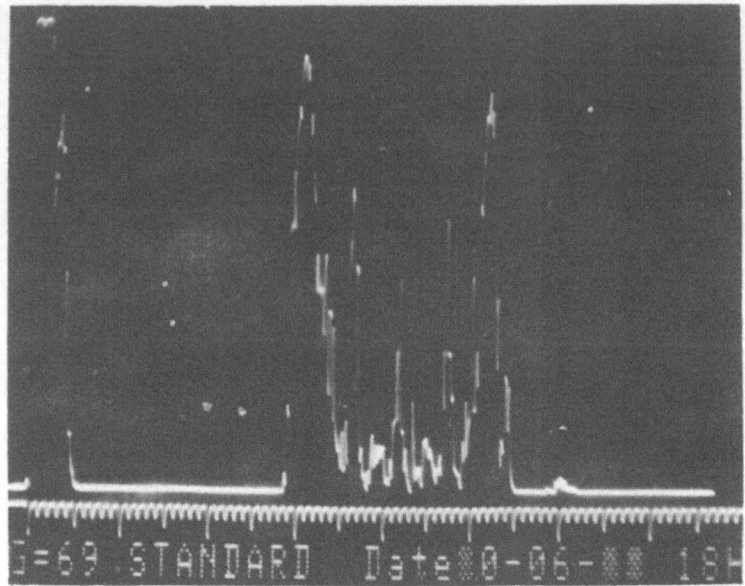

Fig. 1f.

Fig. 1. Fibrous histiocytoma in a 35 year old caucasion female. (a) Highest sensitivity setting B-mode section obtained with Ophtascan S (BM3 Probe). (b) B-mode section obtained at the same level with a CGR Sonel 400 (7,5 MHz Probe), at Tissue Sensitivity. (c) Same section as in b at high sensitivity setting. (d) Sagittal oblique MRI T1 weighted section. (e and f) Trans ocular A-scans of the lesion at Tissue Sensitivity. The lesion appears very well limited. The small myxoid pool is well noted on the high sensitivity B-mode section. The regularity of the inner structure is well approached on A-scans.

All the lesions appeared low reflective at tissue sensitivity with relatively strong attenuation. With high energetic probe at high sensitivity, all the lesions appeared heterogenous, with strands of high reflectivity. In one case high sensitivity B-mode section revealed a low reflective small pool, corresponding to a myxoïd cyst (Fig. 1). The anteriorly situated lesion, that was examined with a paraocular approach appeared to have a lower reflectivity than the other tumors. Bone deformation was present and seen on B-mode sections in two cases. There was a deformation of the posterior pole of the eyeball by the tumor in one case that proved to be locally aggressive.

All the tumors were operated. There was no recurrence of the locally aggressive, large tumor, but two recurrences of the anteriorly located lesion. The primary lesion and the recurrence were purely benign.

References

[1] Henderson J W. Orbital tumors. 2nd ed. New York. Brian C. Decken Division of Thieme Stratten.

[2] Jakobiec FA, Font RL. 1986. Fibrous and connective tissue tumors in Ophthalmic Pathology. An Atlas and Textbook. Vol. 3. 3rd Ed. Spencer WH Ed. Orbit. Chap. 12: 2459–2860. WB Saunders Com., Philadelphia, London, Toronto, Mexico City, Rio de Janeiro, Sidney, Tokyo, Hong-Kong. pp. 2568–2582.

[3] Kennedy RE. An evaluation of 820 cases. Trans arm Ophthalmol Soc. 82: 134–157.

[4] Offret G, Dhermy P, Brini A, Bec P. 1974. Anatomie pathologique de l'oeil et de ses annexes. Rapport de la Société Française d'Ophtalmologie. Masson et Cie Ed. Paris.

5. Orbital myxoma: ultrasonographic diagnosis

YANNINA BRITTO*, HORACIO SORIANO,
JACK POUJOL, JACK PANEYKO and IMELDA PIFANO

Summary

Orbital myxoma is a benign tumor, extremely rare. It virtually does not occur in children and adolescents. From the ultrasonographic standpoint, these tumors have been studied little due to their extreme rarity.

We present one case of orbital myxoma in a child, with the ultrasonographic findings. It is important to notice that the tumor in this girl began when she was 7 years old, the youngest age reported.

Myxoma is a benign tumor formed by stellate and sometimes spindle cells set in a myxoid stroma which contains mucopolysaccharid. Henderson [7] reports that probably myxoma originates in remnants of primitive or embryonic mucinous tissue which neither undergoes adult differentiation nor merges with other types of connective tissue specializing in support. A myxoma is usually found in the heart or jaws [2, 5, 6, 8]. It is a tumor of adult life which virtually does not occur in children and adolescents.

Myxoma of the orbit are extremely rare. Blegvad's survey [1] (1913–1944) collected four orbital myxomas. Interestingly, the four cases were in women of 40, 29, 29, and 25 years of age, respectively.

Dutz and Stout [3] in a review of world-wide literature report 27 myxomas in children, the majority of which originating from superficial lax tissue, callings to our attention the existence of *only one case* of orbital myxoma in a thirteen year old child which was published by Lamb [9]. This case is considered in the Dutz review as a curiosity.

No cases of myxoma were reported during the period of Henderson's survey [7] (1948–1966).

From the ultrasonographic standpoint [10, 11], these tumors have been studied little due to their extreme rarity.

The knowledge of this entity is particularly important because this lesion

* Santa Rosa de Lima Calle C, Residencias Samanta 1Y piso, 1B Caracas, Venezuela

R. Sampaolesi (ed.), Ultrasonography in Ophthalmology 12, 43–48.

which is cured by local removal may be easily confused with sarcoma and specially with botryoide type rhabdomyosarcoma.

It is the reason of this paper to present one case of recurrent orbital myxoma in a 12 year old girl and demonstrate the ultrasonographic findings.

Case report

A 12 year old girl was seen at Caracas, Venezuela University Hospital in July 1984, complaining of enlargement of her left superior eyelid and proptosis of the left eye (Figs. 1 and 2) in the last six months.

In her past history there is a removal of a tumor at the same site at age 7 which was diagnosed microscopically as rhabdomyosarcoma. The patient did not return to postoperative controls. She remained apparently ophthalmologically asymptomatic for 4 and a half years until six months prior to her hospital admission. Ophthalmological examination revealed VA OD 20/20 and OS 20/200, no refraction was performed at this time due to poor patient cooperation. Biomicroscopy showed a moderate superficial conjunctival congestion in OS, the eyeball was in exo-hypotropia with accentuated limitation of ocular movements. Both fundus examinations were normal.

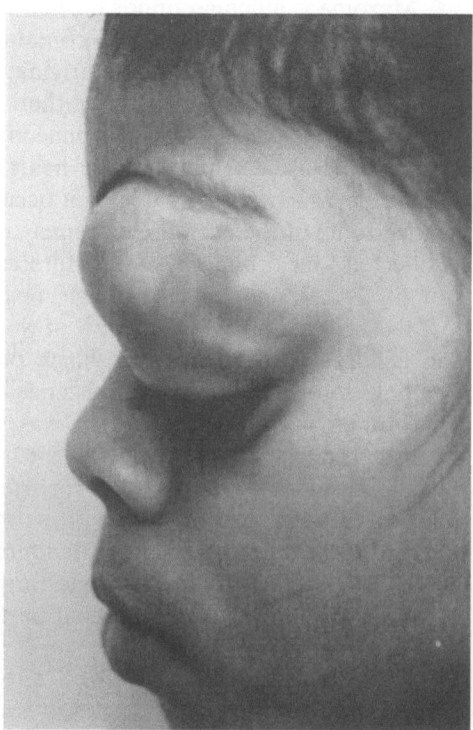

Fig. 1. Orbital myxoma. The mass protruded under the superior left eyelid and pushed it forward.

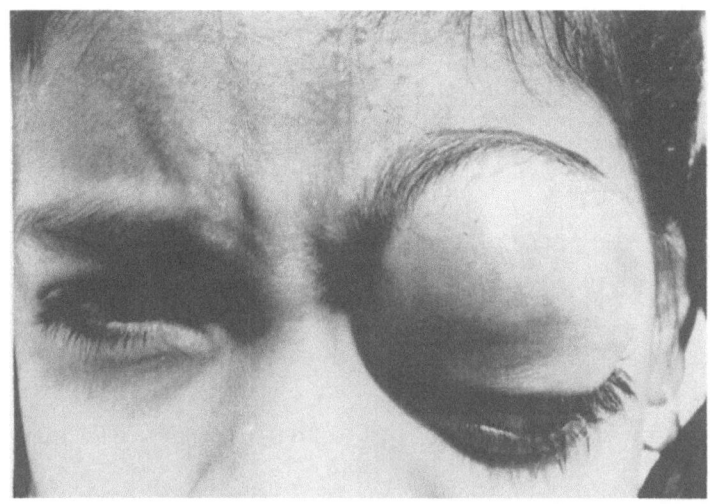

Fig. 2. The mass was rounded lobulated, soft and painless. The eyeball was in exo-hypotropia.

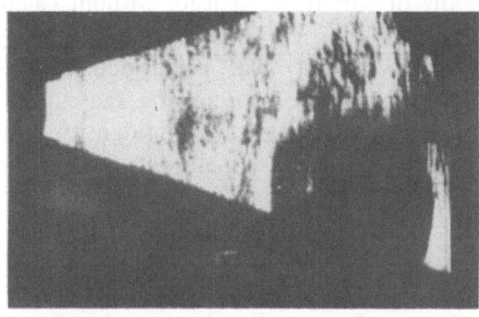

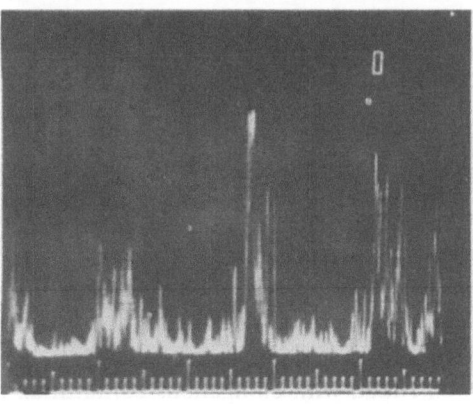

Fig. 3. Ultrasonographic evaluation.
(Top) B-scan findings.
(Bottom) A-scan findings.

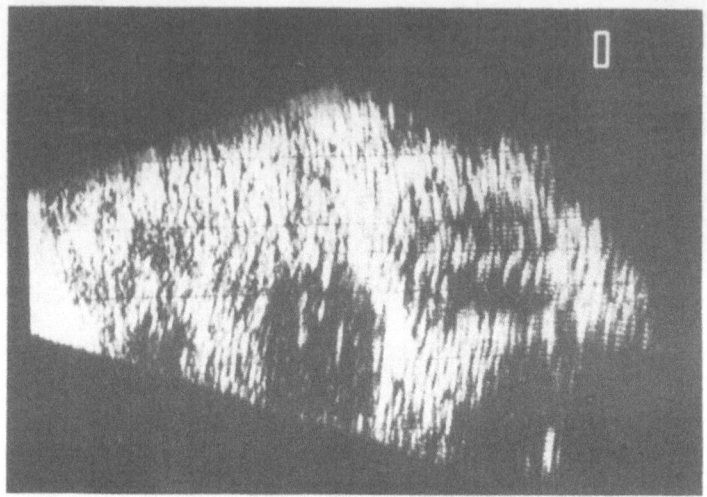

Fig. 4. B-scan (Ocuscan 400). These appearance, with the B-scan fits exactly with the histological description given by Gifford in 1931 as 'a bunch of grapes'.

The mass protruded under the superior left eyelid and pushed it forward, it was rounded, lobulated, soft, transiluminable and painless.

Orbital X-Ray reported a shadow of soft tissue density without calcifications occupying the left orbit.

Ultrasonography evaluation (Figs. 3 and 4) was performed with an Ocuscan 400 unit. B-scan showed a tumoral mass occupying the superior external quadrant of the orbit, formed by ovoid low acoustic density zones which could correspond with a liquid or gel-like material, these zones appeared circumscribed by higher reflectivity areas. The mass shows good sound transmission. The A-scan shows anechoic areas followed by medium to high reflectivity echoes which correspond to the areas described in the B-scan.

These appearances with the B-scan fit exactly with the histological description given by Gifford in 1931 [4] as 'a bunch of grapes'.

CT-Scan reported a significant increase in size of the left orbit occupied by a tumoral mass over the eyeball, which was displaced down and forward, internal orbital wall showed erosion. The probable diagnosis was tumoral mass of orbital soft tissue mesenchymal etiology.

The lesion was removed and the biopsy reported: Orbital myxoma (benign tumor).

Pathology

At lower magnification (Fig. 5) stellate myxomatose cells were observed, they had scarce cytoplasm which extended with elongations conforming the

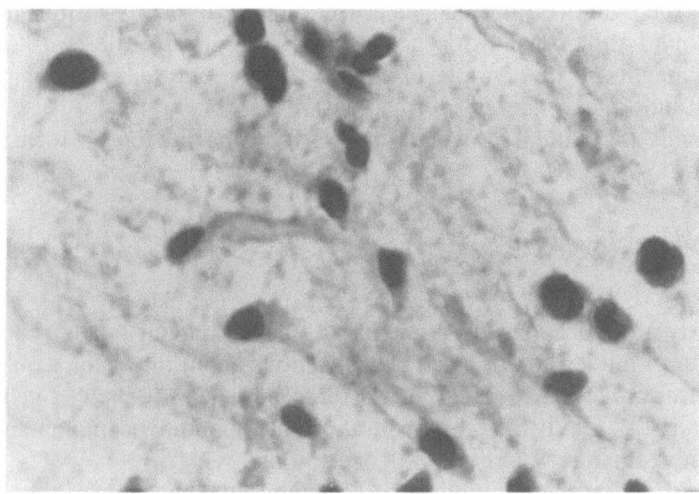

Fig. 5. At lower magnification stellate myxomatose cells, were observed. They had scarce cytoplasm which extended with elongations conforming the stellate aspects. No mitosis.

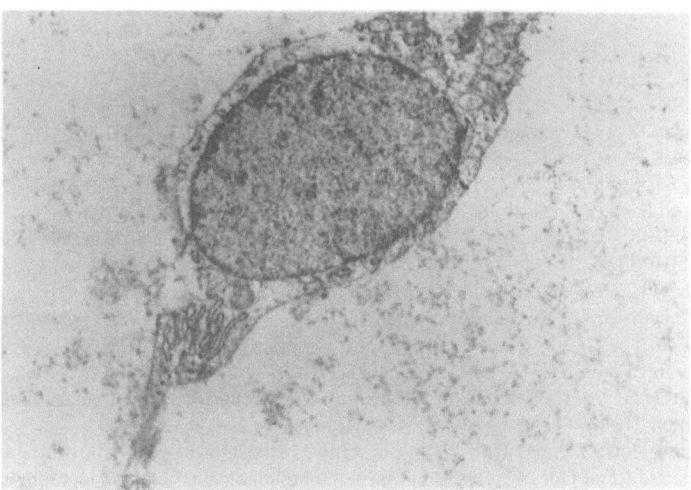

Fig. 6. Electron microscopy. The tumoral cells.

stellate aspect, small hyperchromatic oval or round nucleus, abundant amounts of myxoid intercellular material which is well distinguished by Alcian Blue staining little pleomorfism, no giant multinucleated cell nor mitosis.

Electron microscopy (Fig. 6) revealed a tumor mainly made of amorphous material of low electrondensity, the tumoral cells are isolated or in small

48

groups, the oval or round nucleus is irregular with one or various nucleolos, the cytoplasmatic organels do not tend to form groups, there are ondulated microfilaments in the cytoplasm similar to the microfilaments of the intercellular substance, they are not neoplastic.

Actually the patient is asymptomatic, there have been no recurrences of the tumor.

Comments

In this case, paradoxically time was on the patient's side, the clinical behavior of the lesion proposed new questions about the lesion's malignancy. The ultrasonographic evaluation was determinant as it showed echographic characteristics totally different from those of rhabdomyosarcoma and similar to the myxomatose tumors in other locations.

We arrived at the final diagnosis of orbital myxoma which is considered a rarity at this location and age group.

It is important to notice that the tumor in this patient began when she was 7 years old, the youngest age reported.

References

[1] Blegvad O. 1944. Myxoma of the orbit. Acta Ophthalmol 22: 131–140.
[2] Bruce K W, Royer R Q. 1952. Central fibromyxoma of maxilla. Oral Surg 5: 1277–1281.
[3] Dutz W, Stout A P. 1961. The myxoma in childhood. Cancer 14: 629–635.
[4] Gifford S R. 1931. Myxoma of the orbit. Arch Ophthalmol 5: 445–448.
[5] Greenfield S D, Friedman O. 1951. Myxoma of maxillary sinus. New York State J Med 51: 1319–1320.
[6] Harbert F, Gerry R G. 1949. Myxoma of maxilla. Oral Surg 2: 1414–1421.
[7] Henderson J W. 1973. Orbital tumors ed 10. Philadelphia, W. B. Saunders Co. pp. 198–200.
[8] Hovnanian A P. 1953. Myxoma of maxilla, report of 2 cases. Oral Surg 6: 927–936.
[9] Lamb H D. 1928. Myxoma of orbit, with case report and anatomical findings. Arch Ophthal 57: 425–429.
[10] Ossoinig K C, Till P. 1975. A 10-year study of clinical echography in orbital disease. In: Francois, J and Goes F (eds) Bibliotheca Ophthalmologica: Ultrasonography in Ophthalmology (Proc. of SIDUO V, Ghent, Belgium, 1973, 83: pp. 236–244.
[11] Poujol J. 1975. A-Scan ultrasound: Accuracy of diagnosis in orbital disease. In: Bleeker G M, Garston J B (eds) Modern Problems in Ophthalmology: Orbital Disorders. (Proc. of the 2nd International Symposium on Orbital Disorders, Amsterdam 1973, 14: 250–253.
[13] Stout A P. 1948. Myxoma tumor of primitive mesenchyme. Ann Surg 127: 706–719.

6. Pre-operative and post-operative echographic results on patients undergoing optic nerve sheath decompression

KATHY A. LYCZKOWSKI, THOMAS C. SPOOR, DIAN-XIONG SHI
and JOHN M. RAMOCKI

Summary

Thirteen patients (20 eyes) were diagnosed with pseudotumor cerebri and subsequently underwent an optic nerve sheath decompression. In addition to improvement in visual function, an ultrasound examination demonstrated a significant change in the size of the optic nerve immediately posterior to the globe post-operatively. The posterior nerve measurements did not significantly change. These findings are useful in determining the possible mechanisms involved in optic nerve decompression.

Introduction

Thirteen patients (20 eyes) were examined at the Kresge Eye Institute between July, 1986 and March, 1988; All patients were diagnosed as having pseudotumor cerebri. Patients diagnosed as having pseudotumor cerebri exhibited symptoms of increased intracranial pressure (ICP) and papilledema. The patients had an ICP greater than 300 mm of H_2O upon lumbar puncture. CSF examinations, including cytology, were negative. Neurological examinations were normal, excepting one patient with a bilateral abducens palsy. Computed tomography was normal except for enlarged optic nerves, venous sinus thrombosis was ruled out by computed tomography. Patients underwent echographic examination to determine optic nerve sheath distention. All patients tested positive on ultrasound for increased subarachnoid fluid. Goldmann and automated perimetry were used to determine the extent of visual field loss.

When progressive visual field loss occurred, patients underwent optic nerve sheath decompression (ONSD) via transconjunctival medial orbitotomy. Optic nerve sheath decompression (ONSD) was performed on 20 eyes. The globe is retracted laterally, the optic nerve sheath is identified,

Kresge Eye Institute, Detroit, Michigan, USA

R. Sampaolesi (ed.), Ultrasonography in Ophthalmology 12, 49–53.

surrounded by fat, ciliary vessels, and nerves. Once the optic sheath is identified, the overlying ciliary vessels and nerves are dissected free from the nerve sheath and retracted to expose an area for incision. A very superficial 2 mm longitudinal incision is made with a Superblade into an area of optic nerve sheath cleared of overlying vessels. There is often a mild oozing of clear cerebrospinal fluid; a dramatic spurt of CSF is the exception. Dissection is continued using a blunt nerve hook to lyse subarachnoid trabeculations between the optic nerve and its overlying sheath. Additional CSF flow is often encountered during this procedure. A section 3.5 mm long and 1.5 mm wide (or as wide a nerve sheath window as possible) is then excised with scissors.

Materials and methods

Ultrasound examinations were performed using the CooperVision Ultrascan Digital 'B' System and standardized echography was performed using a Kretztechnik 7200 ma unit. Both units had been serviced and calibrated prior to the study and calibrated by the technologist prior to each examination [6]. The Digital 'B' System was serviced and maintained by Cooper Vision.

Ultrasound examinations were performed prior to an optic nerve sheath decompression. The pre-operative examination was performed an average of 4.2 days prior to surgery in 18 out of 20 cases. Of these cases, 13 eyes were examined within 3 days of surgery.

Standardized echography was repeated post-operatively at one week (average 7.6 days) in 12 cases; at one month (average 26.4 days) in 10 cases; at 2 months (average 69.8 days) for 10 cases; and at 6 months (average 189.4 days) in 8 cases.

Posterior optic nerve measurements (7–12 mm behind the globe) were taken pre- and post-operatively in all cases. Thirty degree tests were performed pre- and post-operatively on 18 eyes. The thirty degree tests involved measuring the optic nerve diameter with the eye in primary gaze and remeasuring the nerve after shifting the eye approximately 30° temporally from the primary gaze position as described by Byrne and Glaser [3] The 30° test is used to identify an increase of subarachnoid fluid. Thirteen cases had anterior (approximately 1–4 mm behind the globe) optic nerve diameter measurements taken in addition to the posterior nerve diameter measurements and 30° tests.

Results

The effects of ONSD upon the distended optic nerve sheath are described in Table 1 and graphically demonstrated in Figure 1. The anterior optic nerve

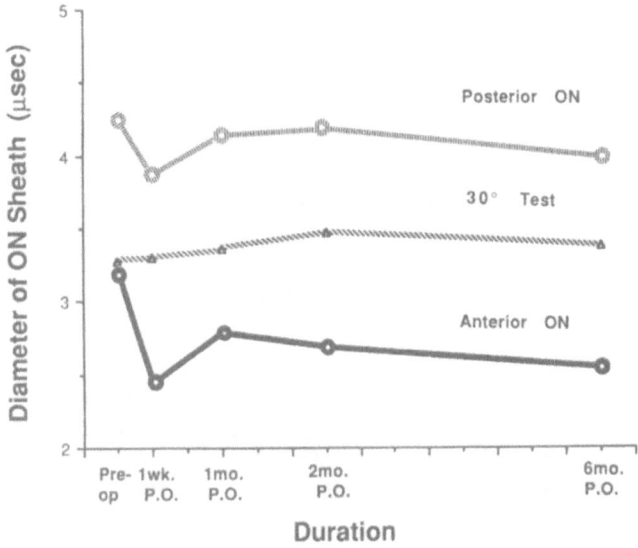

Fig. 1. Diameter of optic nerve sheath *vs* duration. Pre-operative and post-operative means for anterior, posterior and 30 degree dural sheath diameters.

measurements demonstrated a significant change post-operatively (p value < 0.01). The overall results for the posterior optic nerve diameter and 30° tests did not demonstrate a significant change when examined pre- and post-operatively (p value > 0.05) (Table 1). Visual function improved after surgery in all cases.

The anterior optic nerve size decreased significantly (p value = 0.002) after an ONSD (Table 1). The mean for the 13 nerves measured pre-

Table 1. Pre-operative and post-operative echographic results on optic nerve dural sheath diameters.

Duration	Echographic outside diameter of dural sheath of optic nerve (Mean in sec ± SEM)		
	Anterior portion (n = 13)	Posterior portion (n = 20)	30° test (n = 18)
1 Week before surgery	3.20 ± 0.16	4.23 ± 0.16	3.28 ± 0.15
1 Week after surgery	2.46 ± 0.08	3.89 ± 0.12	3.30 ± 0.19
1 Month after surgery	2.79 ± 0.10	4.15 ± 0.20	3.36 ± 0.25
2 Months after surgery	2.69 ± 0.13	4.19 ± 0.21	3.47 ± 0.14
6 Months after surgery	2.55 ± 0.12	4.00 ± 0.14	3.39 ± 0.11
	P = 0.002*	P = 0.612*	P = 0.957*
	P < 0.001**		

* One way analysis of variance.
** Two way analysis of variance.

operatively was 3.20 microseconds (μsec) with a standard error of 0.16. For the cases measured at one week post-operatively, the mean for the anterior optic nerve diameter was 2.46 (μsec with a standard error of 0.08. The anterior measurements remained significantly lower (one month, 2 months, and 6 months post-operatively) than the pre-operative measurements.

The posterior optic nerve and 30° test measurements did not follow the same trend as the anterior measurements. The pre-operative means for the posterior measurements and 30° tests were 4.23 μsec (standard error of 0.16) and 3.305 μsec (standard error of 0.15) respectively. All patients were tested positively for increased subarachnoid fluid. Post-operatively, there was no significant change for the posterior nerve measurements (p value = 0.612) or 30° tests (p value = 0.957).

Two of the 20 cases examined revealed a bilateral decrease in optic nerve diameter following a unilateral ONSD. The first patient demonstrated a decrease of 1.60 μsec in the unoperated eye within a month of the surgical procedure. The other case demonstrated a change of 1.23 μsec in the unoperated eye.

Discussion

Two possible mechanisms explain why ONSD may reduce papilledema and improve visual function. The first hypothesis states that a permanent fistula is created during ONSD [5]. This open fistula allows fluid to be continuously drained from the sheaths into orbital fat, thus protecting the lamina cribrosa and visual function. The other mechanism involves a closing of the fistula with fibrosing occurring at this point [1, 2]. When intracranial pressure increases; the fluid is blocked by the fibrosis protecting the optic nerve head from the effect of increased intracranial pressure.

The echographic findings support fistulization as the mechanism protecting the optic nerve at the lamina cribrosa. The size of the anterior nerve was reduced significantly post-operatively. This portion of the nerve remained smaller at 6 months post-operatively. The post-operative size of the posterior nerve remained statistically equivalent to the pre-operative size. The findings from the 30 degree tests also remained essentially unchanged. An increase in the posterior optic nerve sheath diameter and an increase in subarachnoid fluid would be expected if fibrosis at the more anterior operation site were the protective mechanism. The unchanged posterior diameter and 30 degree test support slow filtration of CSF as the protective mechanism.

The optic nerve measurements determined in this study were found to be lower than the normal and abnormal values determined by Hupp et al. [4]. The Kretztechnik unit used for the study had been standardized prior to the study. A normal series was developed. The mean, based on 25 eyes, for anterior optic nerve measurement from the normal series was found to be

Table 2. Echographic outside diameter of dural sheath of optic nerve – normal series.

	Count	Mean		Std. dev.	Std. error
		(sec)	(mm)	(sec)	(sec)
Anterior portion	25	2.15	1.67	0.31	0.06
Posterior portion	25	2.93	2.27	0.39	0.08

2.15 μsec (standard error of 0.06) or 1.67 mm and 2.93 μsec (standard error of 0.08) or 2.27 mm for the posterior optic nerve. The normal series was also found to be lower (Table 2). Therefore, any error in the measurements was consistent and the results were reproducible.

The results from this study support Keltner's fistulization theory [5] as the mechanism for optic nerve sheath decompression and that the anterior portion of the optic nerve remained significantly smaller post-operatively. The results also demonstrate that papilledema was reduced or prevented and visual function returned and remained good for patients undergoing thprocedure.

References

[1] Davidson S I. 1969. A surgical approach to plerocephalic disc edema. Trans Ophthalmol Soc UK 89: 669–90.
[2] Davidson S I. 1972. The surgical relief of papilledema. In: Cant J S (ed) The Optic Nerve. London, Henry Kimpton. pp. 174–179.
[3] Frazier-Byrne S, Glaser J S. 1983. Orbital tissue differentiation with standardized echography. American Academy of Ophthalmology 90: 1070–90.
[4] Hupp S, Glaser J S, Frazier-Byrne S, Glaser J S. 1987. Optic nerve sheath decompression, review of 17 cases. Arch Ophthalmol 105: 386–9.
[5] Keltner J, Albert D M, Lubow M et al. 1977. Optic nerve sheath decompression. Arch Ophthalmol 95: 97–104.
[6] Ossoinig K C. 1983. How to obtain maximum measuring accuracies wi h standardized A-scan. Hillman J C, Le May M M (eds) Ophthalmic Ultrasonography. The Netherlands, Dr. W. Junk Publishers.

7. Evaluation of the subarachnoidal space — comparisons between ultrasound and high resolution NMR-techniques

R. GUTHOFF, G. TRIEBEL, W. SCHROEDER, CH. ONKEN
and F. ABRAMO

Summary

In patients with enlargement of the dural diameter of the optic nerve A- and B-scan ultrasonograms compared with coronal sections of high resolution NMR-images using a specially designed surface coils. According to preliminary results subarachnoidal space widening can be differentiated with both techniques, but the true nature and its chemical and physical properties still remain uncertain preoperatively. Tumors such as meningeomas, gliomas as well as various reasons of disc edema are analyzed.

Introduction

Diagnostic ultrasound was the first method to identify the orbital part of the optic nerve. Basic works have been done by Ossoinig and Schroeder. Schroeders' experimental works published in 1979 have shown that a swollen subarachnoidal space surrounding the optic nerve can only be identified when 3 triple echos are achieved. As indicated in his experiments the empty dural sheets are responsable for double spike peaks the denuded nerve itself generates one single spikes on each surface.

The technique frequently used in Hamburg is applied during maximal abduction of the globe where sound waves are able to hit the optical nerve structures as perpendicular as possible (Fig. 1). In spindle shaped tumors like gliomas the thickening of the nerve could easyly be found in A-scan ultrasound, but the specific spape of the tumor simultaneously displaying the papille edema can only be imaged in sectional B-scanning (Schroeder, 1978).

Technology has improved considerably since the early days of ultrasound, B-scan imaging techniques have shown to be as effective in identifying

Universitäts-Augenklinik Hamburg, Hamburg, FRG

R. Sampaolesi (ed.), Ultrasonography in Ophthalmology 12, 55–62.

56

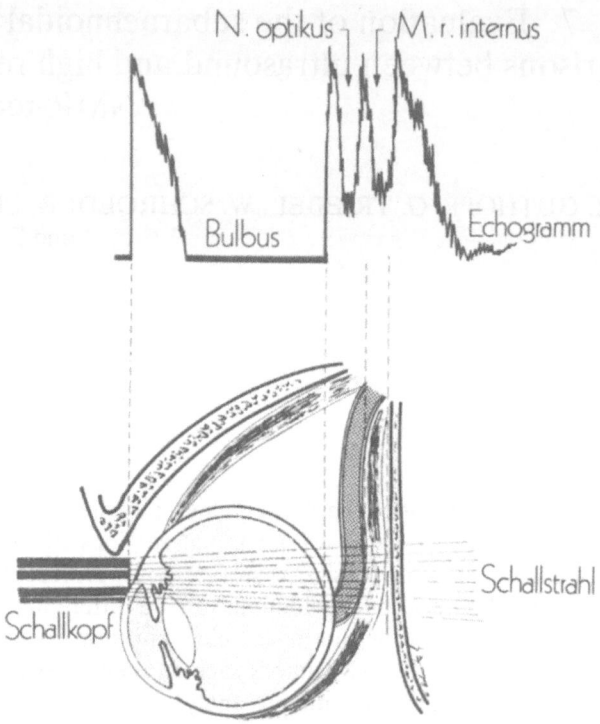

Fig. 1. Schematic drawing of sound beem geometry measuring the dural diameter of the optic nerve in maximal abduction of the globe. (With kind permission of the author) Schroeder W. 1976. Schallaufzeitmessungen im distalen Schnervenquerschnitt. Klin Mbl Augenheilk, Enke–Verlag Stuttgart, 169: 743.

acoustical interfaces such as optical nerve sheets and the axional cylinder (Guthoff, 1985).

In vitro examinations of human optic nerves have demonstrated B-scan capability of differentiating nerve sheets from axional cylinder especially in the physiologically enlarged most distal part of the nerve. For clinical examinations small B-scan transusers have proven to be sensitive instruments in identifying and measuring optic nerve thickening (Fig. 2). It was only since 1984 that NMR-imaging techniques have reached a standard mainly due to the application of specially design surface coils that made differentiation of optic nerve structures possible.

Material and methods

During the last 2 years we were able to examine 13 patients (Table 1) with optic nerve problems simultaneously with ultrasound, CT-scan and NMR. The ultrasonographical examinations were performed using a Cooper Digital

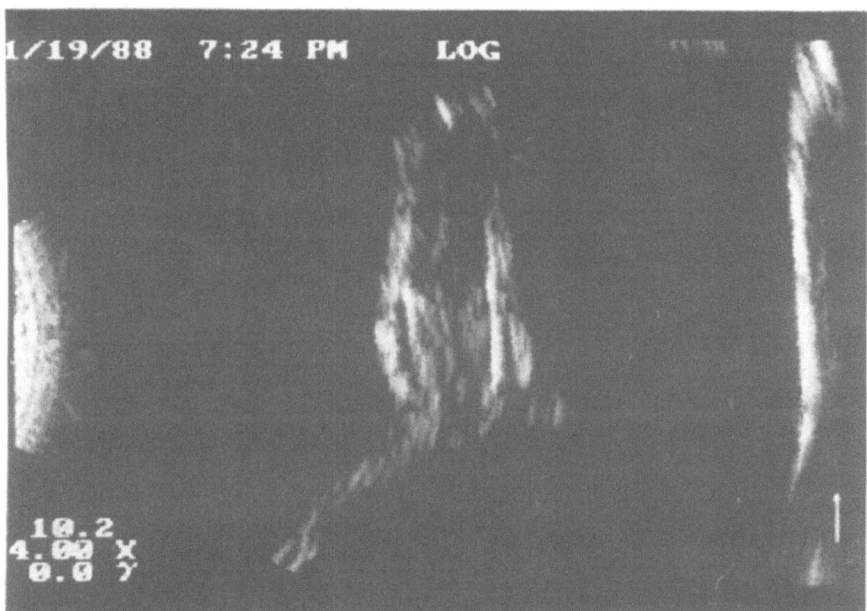

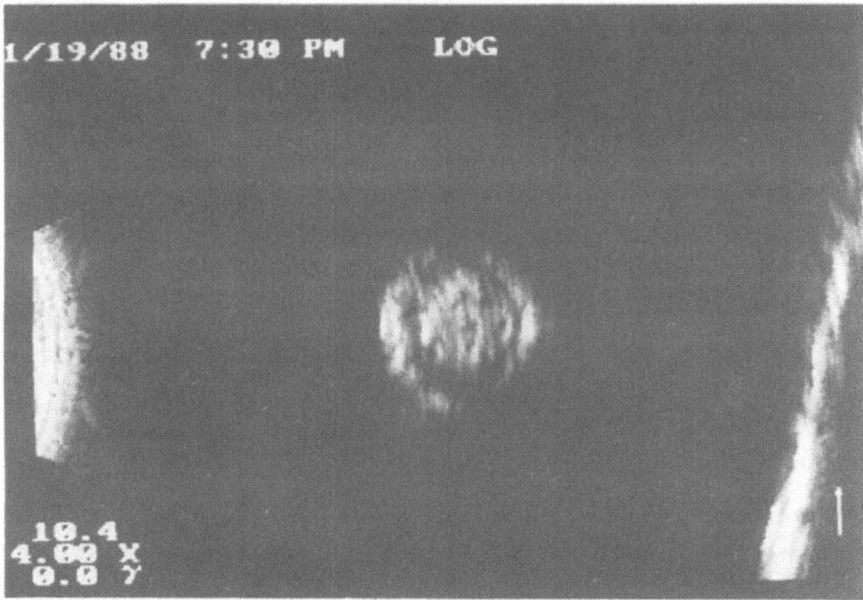

Fig. 2b.

Fig. 2. In vitro imaging of the distal optic nerve distal optic nerve using immersion technique and contact B-scan-Probe (Digital-B Cooper Vision). (a) Longitudinal section through optic nerve including dural sheets and adjacent sclera. (b) Frontal section through distal part of optic nerve, differentiation between optical nerve sheets, subarachnoidal space and axonal nerve seems to be slightly possible.

Table 1. Clinical findings in 13 patients (19 orbits) with suspected widening of subarachnoidal space in the orbit.

Diagnosis	No. of pat.	Orbits	Optic disc Swollen	Atrophic	Normal	ECHO Subarachn. space: Outlined +		NMR Subarachn. space: Outlined +	–
Graves dis.	4	8	2	1	5	8			
Meningeoma (spenoidal)	1	1			1	1			1
Pseudotumor cerebri	2	4	4			2	2	4	
Optic nerve glioma	2	2	1	1		1	1	2	
Orbital lymphangioma	1	1	1					1	1
Disc swelling unknown orig.	2	2	2			1	1	2	
	13	19	11	3	5	13	6	17	2

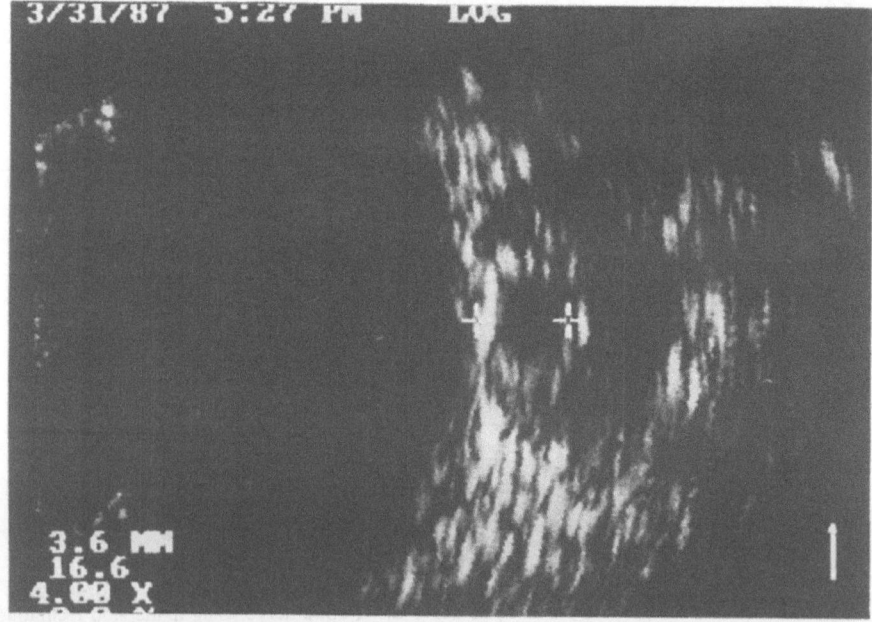

Fig. 3. Enlargement of optic nerve, dural diameter and a marked separation of optic nerve sheets and nerve structures itself. According to B-Scan measurements there was a normal axial cylinder of 3,4 mm in diameter and an extensively widened subarachnoidal space with a total diameter of 8,1 mm.

B unit, NMR-imaging was performed with a Siemens Magnetom and a Phillips Gyroscan. There had been 4 patients with Grave's disease, 1 meningeoma arising from the sinoid bone, 2 patients with pseudotumor cerebri, 2 optic nerve glioma, 1 serous orbital cyst, 1 extensive orbital lymphangioma and 2 patients with swelling of unknown origin until now. To summarize our findings, the arachnoidal space could be identified using ultrasonography in 13 out of 19 cases applying NMR-imaging techniques in 17 out of 19 examinations. Two patients should be presented in detail.

Patient No. 1

A 53 year old male patient presented with a 3 months history of blurred vision on the left eye. On examination we found a visual acuity of 100% on the right eye and 40% on the left eye. There was a mild swelling of the left disc all other ophthalmological findings, including motility and Hertel readings were normal. Visual evoced potentials showed normal latencies with slightly misconfigurated readings concerning the left optic nerve.

On routine ultrasonographical examination there was an extensive enlargement of both optic nerves and a marked separation of optical nerve

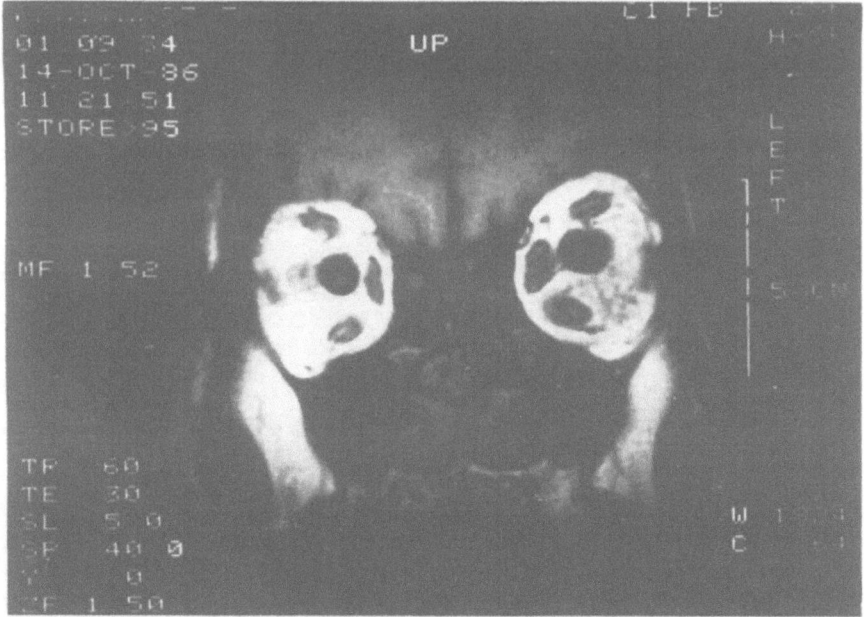

Fig. 4. T1-weighted image through the orbit of a patient with immune thyreopathy (see also Fig. 3).
Both optic nerves are highly enlarged, a separation between nerve cylinder and subarachnoidal space is possible.

sheets and the nerve structures itself. According to B-scan measurements there was a normal axial cylinder of 3,4 mm in diameter and an extensively widened subarachnoidal space with a total diameter of 8.1 mm (Fig. 3).

CT-scans revealed also a marked thickening of the optical nerve sheets which due to an oblique positioning of the patient is only visible on the left side. NMR-imaging in T1-weighted pictures did not give additional information. T2-weighted images, however, showed a considerable variation in signal intensity between the nerve fibres and the swollen subarachnoidal space which showed a signal behaviour similar to that of the vitreous cavity. On coronal sections the marked swelling of the external eye muscles were clearly outlined (Fig. 4).

Patient No. 2

There was a 20 year old male patient with known Recklinghausen disease. On examination we found no light perception on the right eye and full vision on the left eye. Ophthalmoscopically unilateral optic atrophy was present. No vascular anomalies like cilioretinal shunt vessels were found (Fig. 5). B-scan ultrasonography showed a marked swelling of the optic nerve surrounded by an extensive widening of the subarachnoidal space.

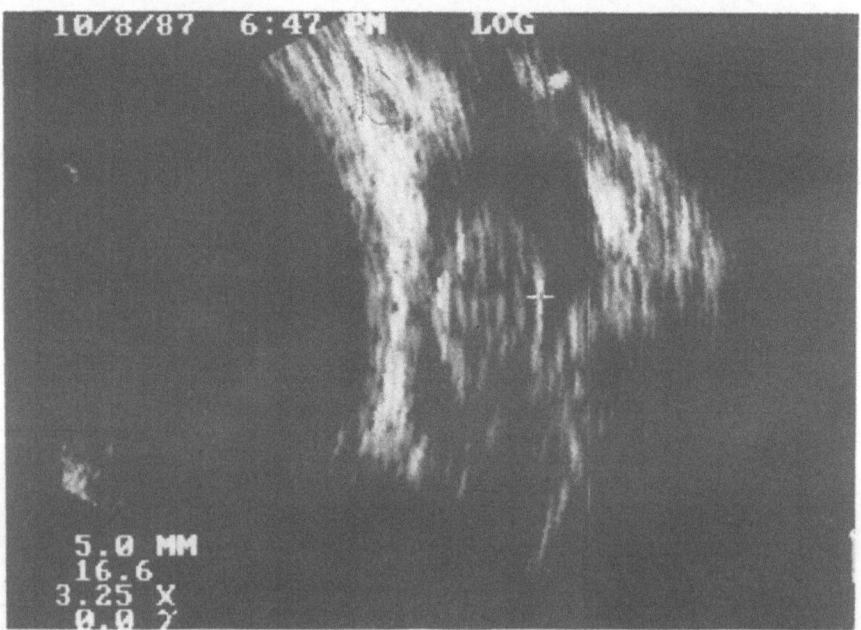

Fig. 5. B-scan Ultrasonography of a patient with unilateral blindness in Recklinghausen's disease. Marked swelling of optic nerve surrounded by an extensive widening of subarachnoidal space.

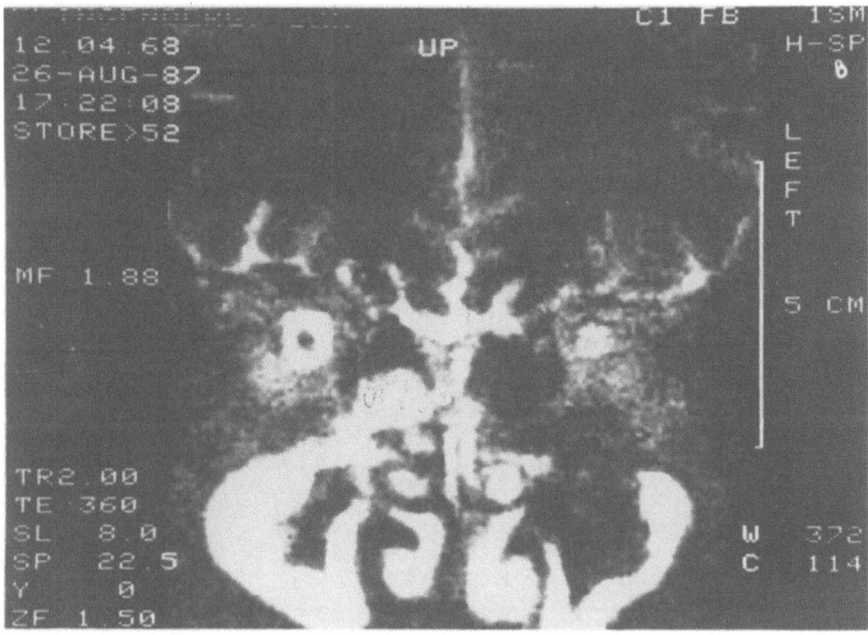

Fig. 6. T2-weighted image demonstrating extensive widening of subarachnoidal space with a signal behaviour comparable with that of subarachnoidal fluid elsewhere in the brain.

These findings could be reconfirmed with NMR where in unilateral widening of subarachnoidal space with a signal behaviour comparible with that of the subarachnoidal fluid elsewhere in the brain or the vitreous cavity was present (Fig. 6).

To summarize our results identification of widened subarachnoidal space is possible with modern ultrasound as well as by NMR techniques. In our series NMR showed to be slightly more sensitive especially when surface coils were applied. Differentiation between axonal structures and Fluid accumulation, and the identifying of the true nature of disc swelling, still remains difficult. The true nature of disc swelling mainly differentiation between axonal structures and fluid accumulation still remains difficult. Findings first published by Skalka (1980) where Grave's ophthalmopathy may be able to widen the subarachnoidal space and the orbital optic nerve is reconfirmed using digitized B scan equipment and NMR-technology.

References

Ossoinig K C. 1976. Echography of the eye. In: P H Arger (Hrgs) Regiology of the Orbit. Wiley & Sons, New York.

Schroeder W. 1979. Ultraschalldiagnostik des Sehnerven. Habilitationsschrift, vorgelegt dem Fachbereich Medizin der Universität Hamburg.

Schroeder W. 1976. Schallaufzeitmessung im distalen Sehnervquerschnitt. Klin Mbl Augenheilk 169: 743.

Schroeder W. 1978. Topographische Orbitadiagnostik mit der Knotakt-B-Bild-Echographie. Klin Mbl Augenheilk 172: 12.

Skalka H W. 1981. Ultrasonography of the Optic Nerve. Neuroophthal 1: 261.

8. Lesions of the lacrimal fossa: a retrospective echographic study

G. CENNAMO, F. TRANFA and G. BONAVOLONTĂ

Summary

The authors present a retrospective echographic study on 140 patients with lacrimal fossa lesions, performed at the Institute of Ophthalmology — 2nd Medical School — University of Naples.

The results show the quantitative echography the most reliable criterium for a correct diagnosis. In particular the study of sound attenuation (angle K) is indispensable for the final evaluation.

Introduction

Lesions of the lacrimal fossa and of the lacrimal gland represent one of the most interesting and at the same time most challenging diagnostic topic of orbital disease. In this paper we try to evaluate the role of echography in the diagnosis of lacrimal fossa lesions. The differential diagnosis may involve the lacrimal gland (dacryops, dacryoadenitis, lymphoma, pseudolymphoma, benign mixed tumor, adenoid cystic carcinoma) or some other diseases (dermoid cysts, cavernous hemangioma and schwannoma in atypical location).

The search for a precise differential diagnosis of the type of lesion is not only an academic exercise but it is very important in the choice of the correct surgical approach [1, 2]. Four different approaches to the orbit are used in these situations: lateral osteoplastic, anterior subperiostal, anterior transeptal and transconjunctival orbitotomy.

Lateral osteoplastic orbitotomy is indicated when the removal of the entire mass, without damaging the capsule of the lesion, is required.

The anterior subperiosteal approach is performed in cases of dermoid cyst; these lesions, infact, usually are firmly attached to the periosteum.

Institute of Ophthalmology, 2nd Medical School, University of Naples, Italy

R. Sampaolesi (ed.), Ultrasonography in Ophthalmology 12, 63–78.
© *1990. Kluwer Academic Publishers, Dordrecht*

Anterior transeptal orbitotomy is required in cases of small lesions or when it is necessary a biopsy sample from the orbital portion of the lacrimal gland as in case of dacryoadenitis, lymphomatous or metastatic lesions. This approach reduces the spread of metastatic cells preserving the integrity of the periosteal barrier.

The transconjunctival approach is only performed for a biopsy in diseases of the palpebral portion of the lacrimal gland (lymphoma, pseudolymphoma, dacryoadenitis) or in cases of dacryops.

Thus standardized echography is crucial in the choice of the surgical approach.

Materials and methods

We studied 140 patients, we have observed in the last 12 years, with lesions of the lacrimal fossa. All patients were examined using standardized echography [5, 8]. A retrospective study of the echographic patterns obtained from each disease was carried out with a comparison of the acoustic criteria previously described in literature for each disease.

Table 1.

	Examined cases	Cases histo-logically verified	Echography results		
			Correct	False (−)	False (+)
Lymphomas	26	17	23	3	1
Pseudolymphomas	2	2	0	2	0
Dacryoadenitis	71	22	63	8	2
Benign mixed tumors	14	14	13	1	5
Adenoid cystic carcinomas	8	8	8	0	4
Dacryops	4	4	4	0	0
Dermoid cysts	10	7	9	1	2
Cavernous hemangiomas	3	3	3	0	2
Schwannomas	2	2	0	2	0

The patients were classified according to their disease as described in Table 1. We have to point out that a pathological report was obtained in many cases, with the exception of some cases of lymphoma, dacryoadenitis and dermoid cyst. Lymphoma is considered a systemic disease and for this reason the diagnosis was proved by findings of the same kind of lesion in other parts of the body. In many cases of dacryoadenitis however the diagnosis was proved by improvement with steroid therapy whereas, in 2 cases of dermoid cyst, the clinical course and CT scan proved the echographic diagnosis.

Table 2. Benign mixed tumor.

Quantitative echography
Regular heterogeneous internal structure
High reflectivity (80–95%)
Medium sound attenuation (K = 45°)

Kinetic echography
No detectable blood flow
Immobile
Hard or partially soft

Topographic echography
Well outlined, encapsulated
Roundish→oval shape
Location in lacrimal fossa

Table 3. Cavernous hemangioma.

Quantitative echography
Regular heterogeneous internal structure
High reflectivity (80–95%)
Medium sound attenuation (K = 45°)

Kinetic echography
No detectable blood flow
Often immobile
Hard with delayed compressibility

Topographic echography
Well outlined, encapsulated
Roundish—oval shape
Rarely located in lacrimal fossa

Table 4. Dermoid cyst.

Quantitative echography
Irregular internal structure
Irregular reflectivity
Irregular sound attenuation

Kinetic echography
No detectable blood flow
Immobile
Partially soft

Topographic cyst
Well outlined, encapsulated
Roundish—oval shape
Rarely located in lacrimal fossa

Table 5. Schwannoma.

Quantitative echography
Regular homogeneous internal structure
Low reflectivity (5–20%)
Weak sound attenuation (K < 30°)

Kinetic echography
No detectable blood flow
Immobile
Hard

Topographic echography
Well outlined, encapsulated
Roundish—oval shape
Rarely located in lacrimal fossa

Discussion

From our data we can point out that quantitative echography was of great importance in the differential diagnosis of this kind of lesions and in particular in the study of sound attenuation (angle K) [7]. Less important information are obtained studying the reflectivity and the internal structure.

In kinetic echography the study of the consistency of the lesion gives complementary information [6].

We observed that the acoustic criteria of the encapsulated lesions (benign mixed tumor, cavernous hemangioma and in some cases of dermoid cyst) were similar (if not identical). Quantitative echography, in fact, reveals a regular and heterogeneous internal structure: high and long peaks alternate with low and short peaks; high reflectivity is shown in the first 10 microseconds; a medium sound attenuation is present with an angle k of about 45 degrees. Only kinetic echography, and paticularly the study of the consist-

66

ency, may refer to a particular type of disease: in fact whereas pleomorphous adenoma is not compressible, the dermoid cyst is moderately compressible, the cavernous hemangioma however has a delayed compressibility with a prolonged pressure ranging from 30 to 60 seconds (Tables 2, 3, 4, Figs. 1–8) [6].

Table 6. Lymphoma.

Quantitative echography
Regular homogeneous internal structure
Low reflectivity (5–20%)
Weak sound attenuation (K < 30°)

Kinetic echography
No detectable blood flow
Immobile
Hard

Topographic echography
Well outlined, encapsulated
Roundish — oval shape
Often located in lacrimal fossa with thickness of fellow lacrimal gland

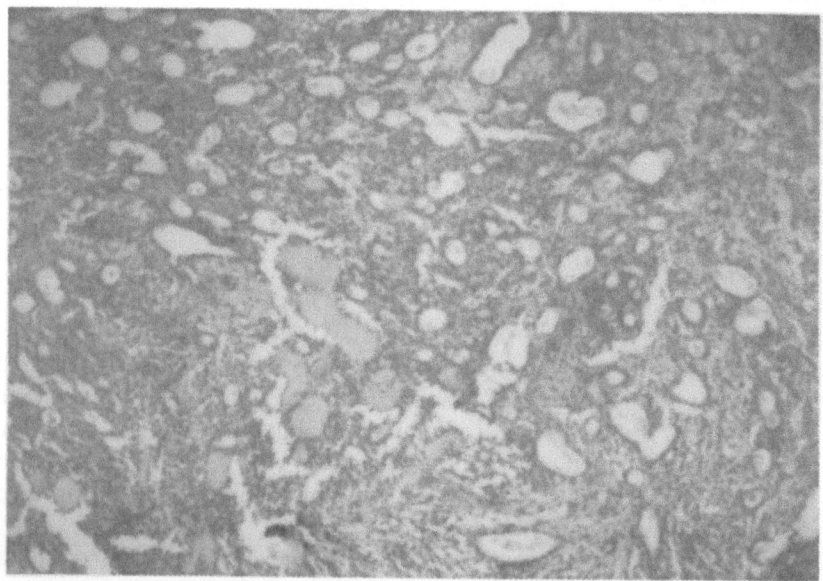

Fig. 1. Benign mixed tumor of the lacrimal gland having cystoid spaces (H & E ×40).

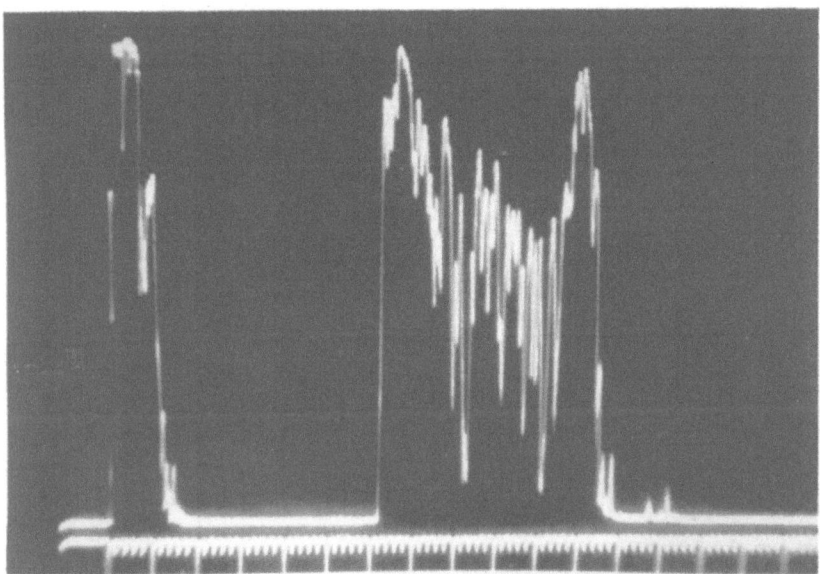

Fig. 2. Standardized A-scan echography: Benign mixed tumor.

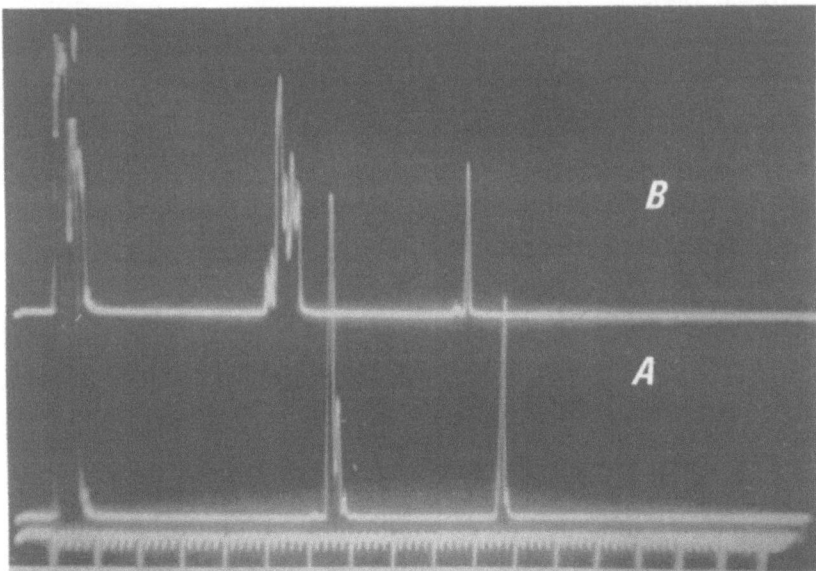

Fig. 3. The kinetic echography shows the absence of compressibility of the lesion:
   (A) Lesion before compression test;
   (B) Lesion during compression test.

68

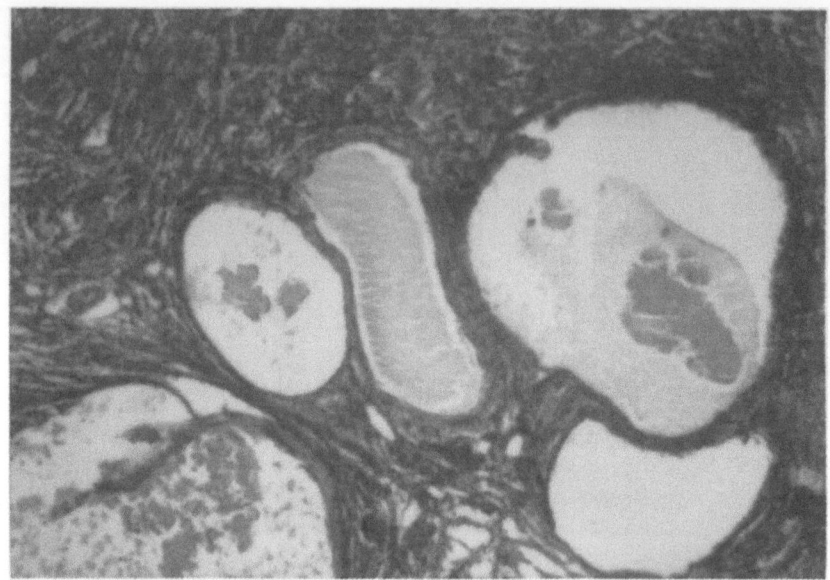

Fig. 4. Cavernous hemangioma: widely dilated vascular spaces are filled with red blood cells (H & E ×100).

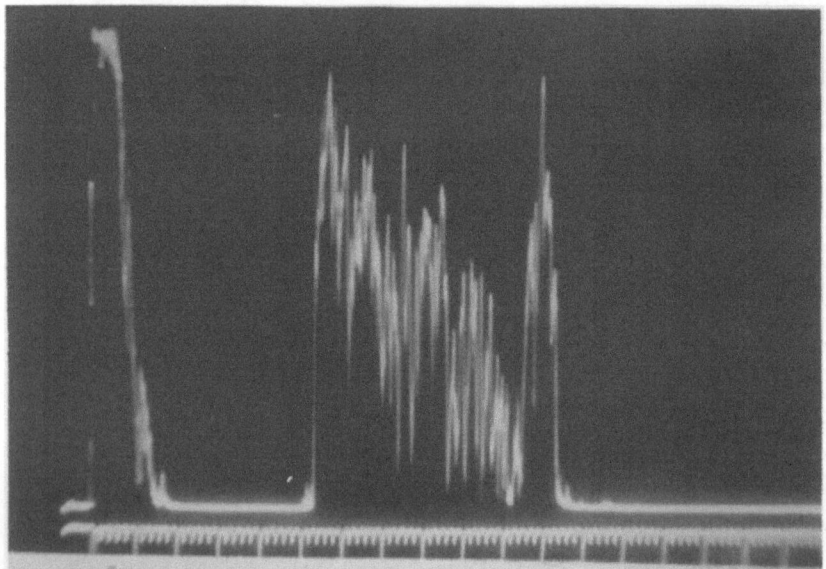

Fig. 5. Standardized A-scan echography: Cavernous hemangioma.

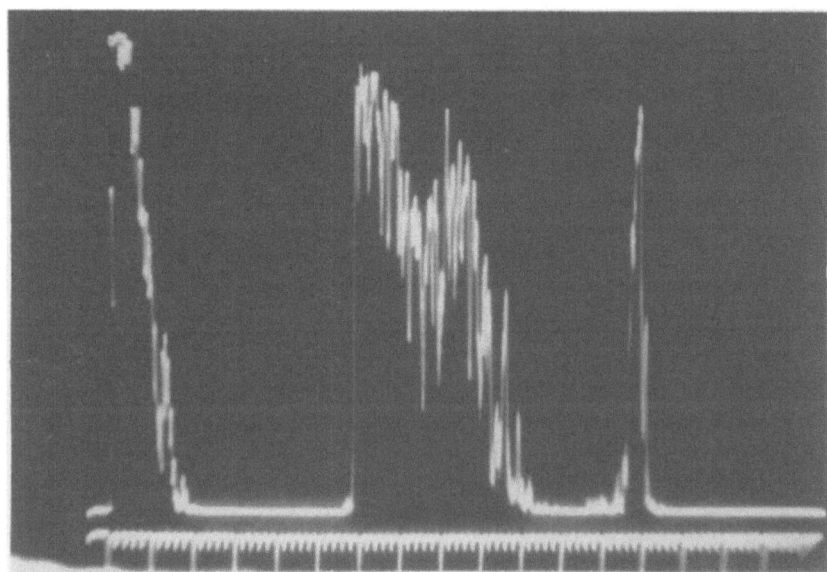

Fig. 6.

Fig. 7.

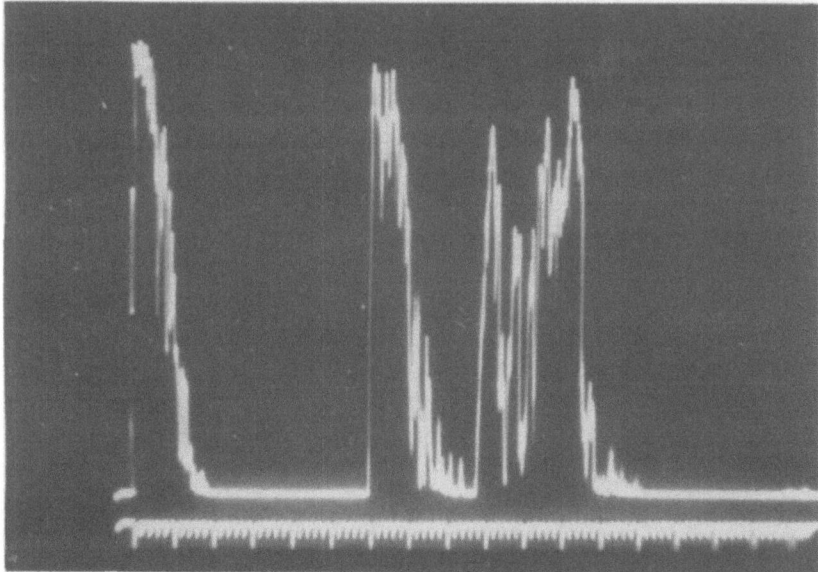

Figs. 6 and 7. Standardized A-scan echography: dermoid cysts.

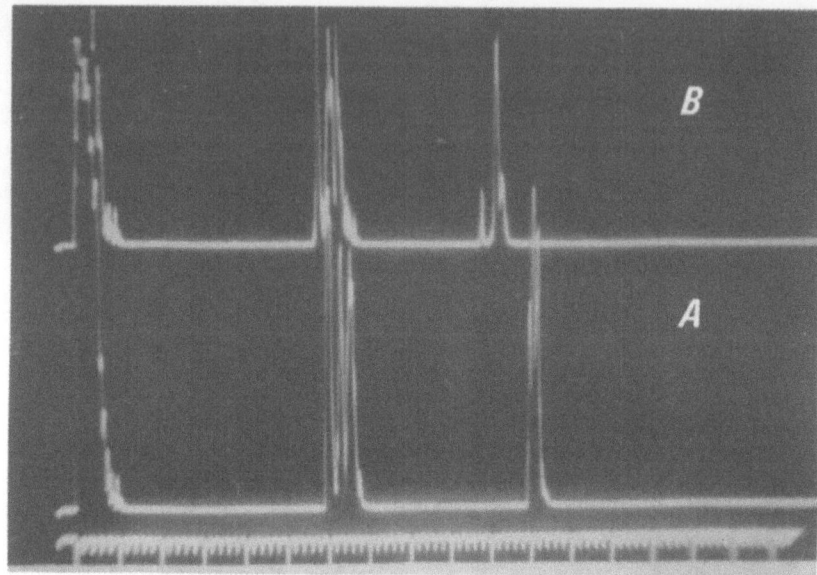

Fig. 8. The kinetic echography shows the presence of compressibility of the lesion:
  (A) Lesion before compression test;
  (B) Lesion during compression test.

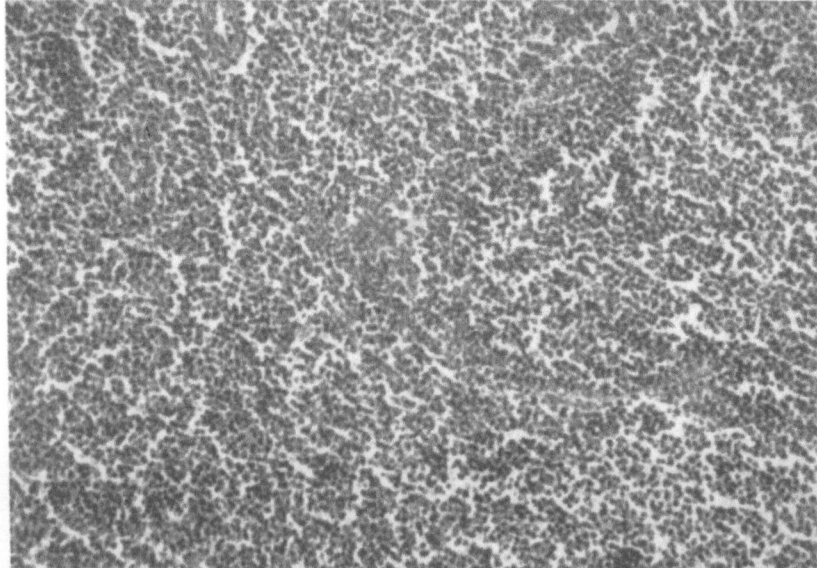

Fig. 9. Lymphoma of the lacrimal gland: poorly cohesive tumor cells are divided by fine collagenous trabeculae (H & E ×40).

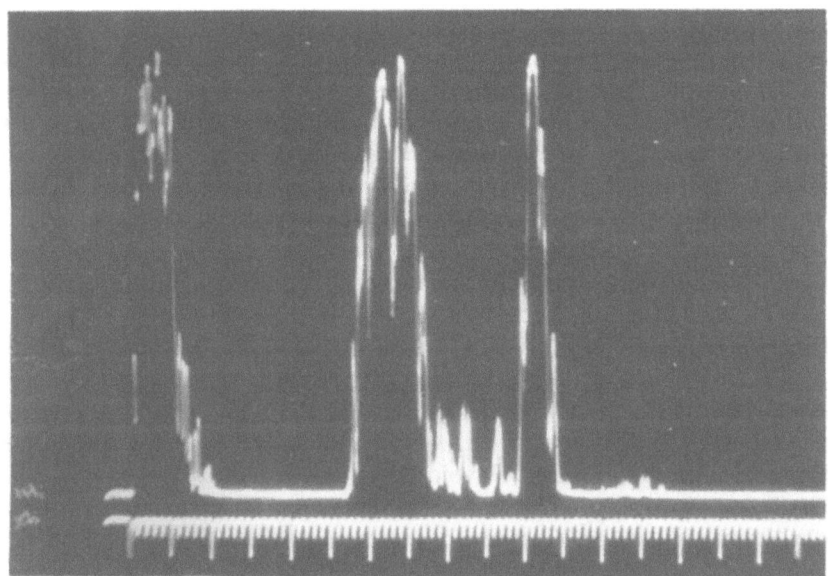

Fig. 10. Standardized A-scan echography: Lymphoma of the lacrimal gland.

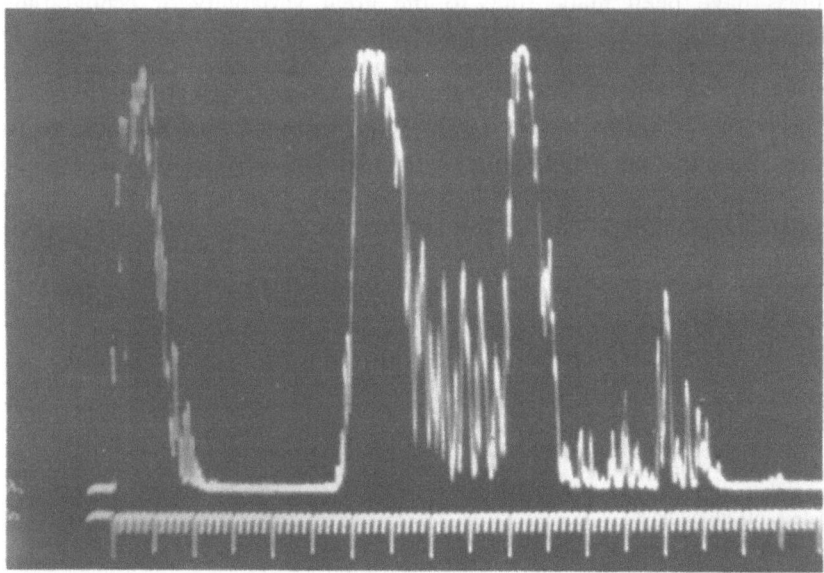

Fig. 11. Standardized A-scan echography at T—plus 6 dB shows weak sound attenuation.

The risk of making a wrong diagnosis is less important in these diseases as encapsulated tumors have to be removed in toto, even though different surgical approaches are performed as previously described. Thus an echographic precise tissue diagnosis is not important in these cases. On the other hand the schwannomas have low reflectivity, weak sound attenuation and opposite to the lymphomas the fellow lacrimal gland is not thickened (Table 5). In addition some diagnostic doubts can be present in a dacryoadenitis with a large cellular component, but in this case too, a diagnostic mistake can only lead to a wrong surgical approach and does not produce an irreversible damage to the patient.

The transconjunctival approach is used not only for dacryops in which both the clinical and echographic diagnosis is patognomonic but also for diseases requiring a biopsy for diagnosis. On the other hand an anterior transeptal orbitotomy is performed when the metastatic spread of the lesion through the periosteum must be avoided.

The lymphomas have a classical echographic pattern. Quantitative echography shows regular and homogeneous internal structure and low reflectivity ranging from 5 to 20% with an angle k of less than 30 degrees. The lesion is not compressible and moreover a thickening of the lacrimal gland in the fellow orbit can be detected. These data allow us to make a diagnosis of lymphoma with an accuracy of more than 99% (Table 6, Figs. 9, 10, 11) [8].

The dacryoadenitis is the lesion in which the greatest number of wrong diagnosis have been made, due to the great variability of echographic findings in these lesions. A careful evaluation of our data revealed diagnostic criteria based on the acoustic characteristics of quantitative echography. The reflectivity in the first 10 μsec can range from extremely high (80–95%) to extremely low (5–40%). These different acoustic findings however have in common a weak sound attenuation (angle k) which is always less than 30 degrees in both cases. Moreover, in contrast with the lymphomas, the lesion is moderately compressible due to the prevalence of the oedematous component over the cellular one (Table 7).

Table 7. Dacryoadenitis.

Quantitative echography
Regular homogeneous internal structure
High to low reflectivity (5–95%)
Weak sound attenuation (K < 30°)

Kinetic echography
No detectable blood flow
Immobile
Hard or partially soft

Topographic echography
Well outlined, encapsulated
Regular shape, often oval
Location in lacrimal fossa

On the basis of Pathology results high reflectivity is present in those cases of dacryoadenitis in which the oedematous component overcome the cellular one (Figs. 12, 13, 14), on the contrary low reflectivity is present in those lesions in which the lymphocitic component overcome the oedematous one (Figs. 15, 16). There is no difference between acute and chronic inflammation.

Finally the adenoid cystic carcinoma requires the most accurate diagnosis because a wrong surgical approach may worsen the prognosis for the patient. Echographically the lesion presents a regular and heterogenous

Table 8. Adenoid cystic carcinoma.

Quantitative echography
Regular heterogeneous internal structure
High reflectivity (80–95%)
Strong sound attenuation (K > 45° – about 60°)

Kinetic echography
No detectable blood flow
Immobile
Hard

Topographic echography
Well outlined, encapsulated or irregular with diffuse borders
Roundish — oval shape or irregular shape
Location in lacrimal fossa

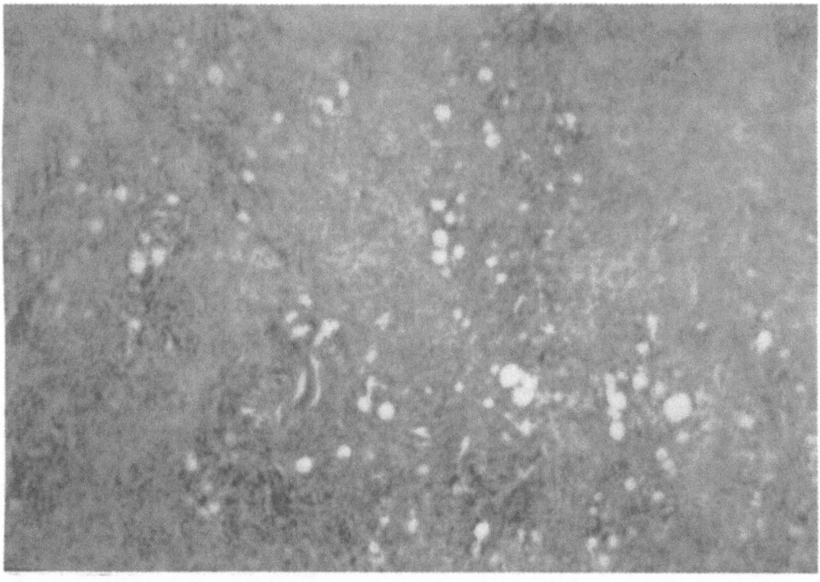

Fig. 12. Dacryoadenitis: parenchimal inflammation dominated by oedema and with poor lymphocytic infiltration.

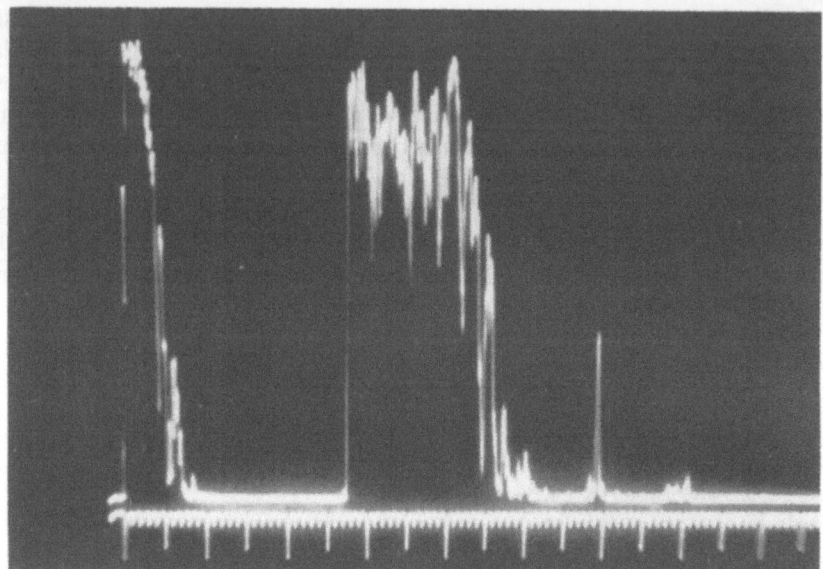

Fig. 13.

Fig. 14.

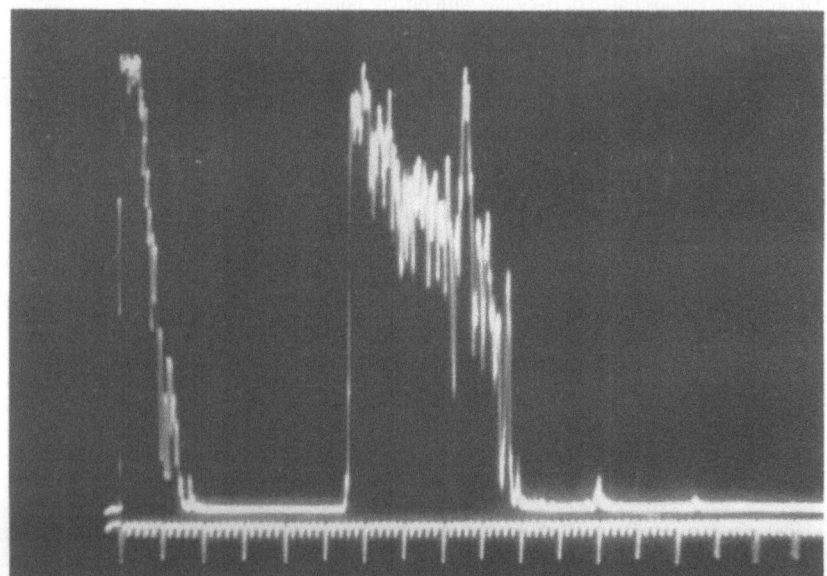

Figs. 13 and 14. Dacryoadenitis: standardized A-scan echography shows high reflectivity of the lesion.

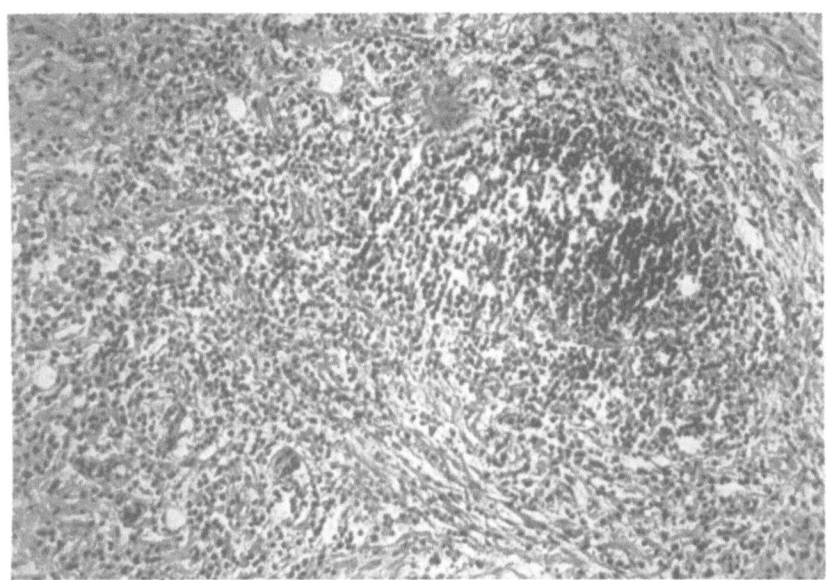

Fig. 15. Dacryoadenitis: parenchimal inflammation dominated by lymphocytic infiltration (H & E ×40).

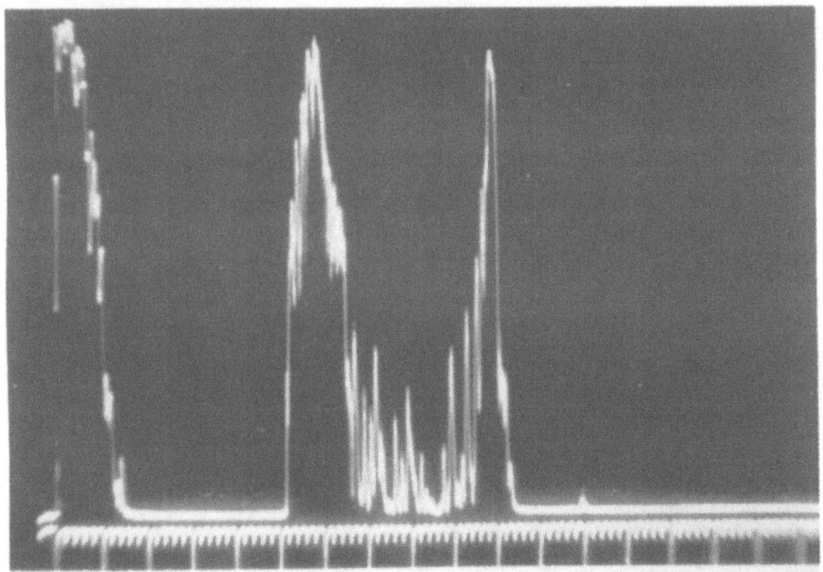

Fig. 16. Dacryoadenitis: standardized A-scan echography shows low reflectivity of the lesion.

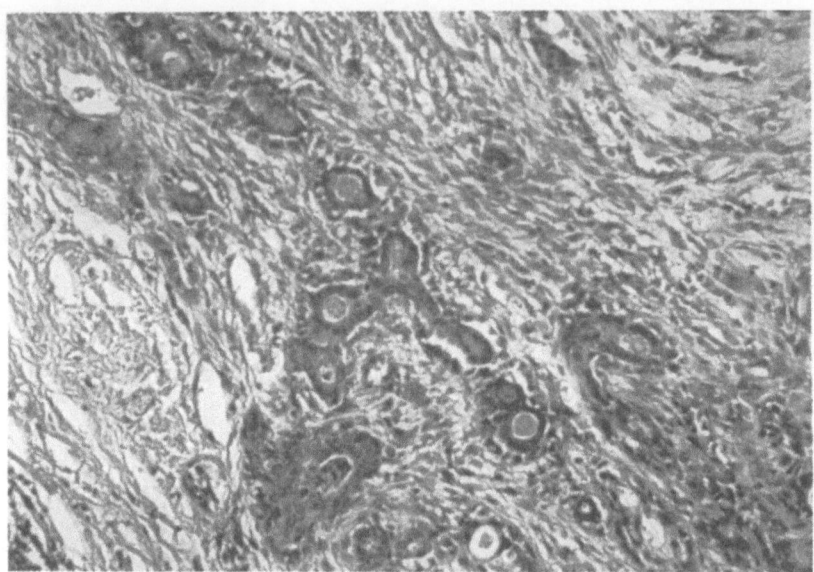

Fig. 17. Adenoid cystic carcinoma showing cribriform pattern (H & E ×100).

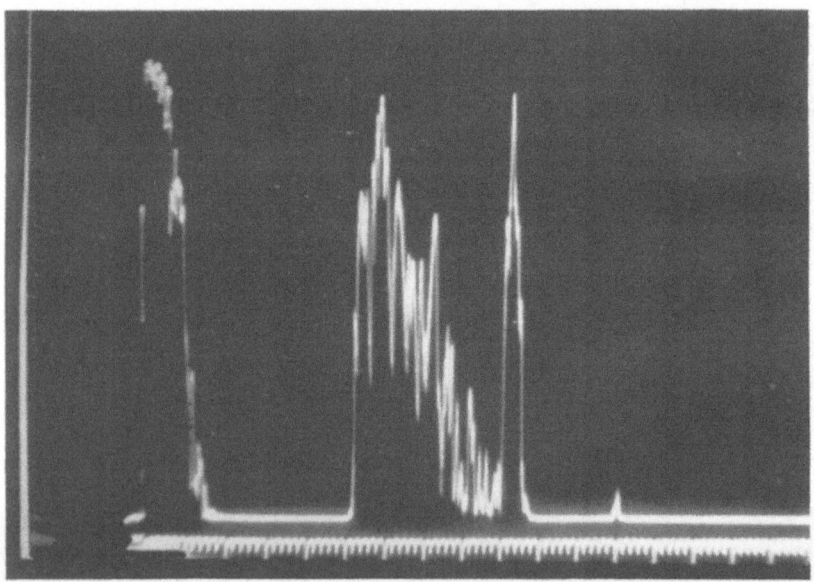

Fig. 18.

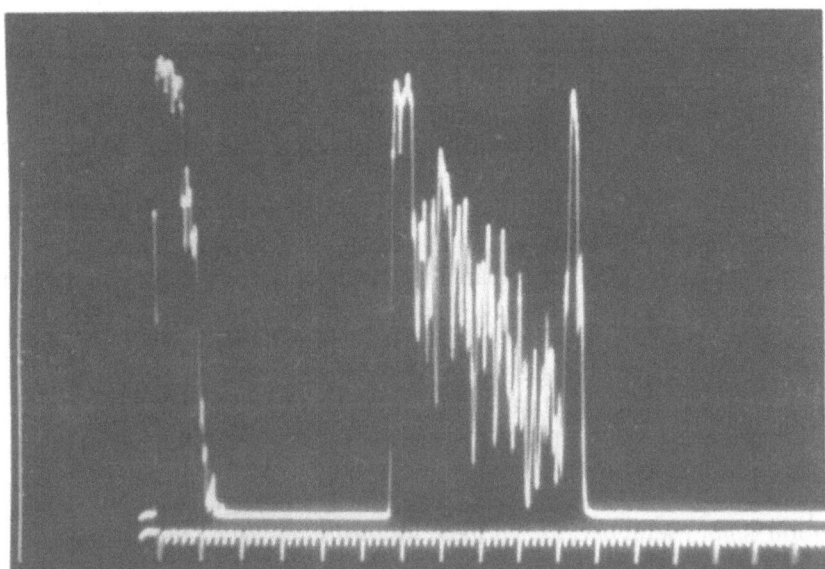

Fig. 19.

Fig. 20

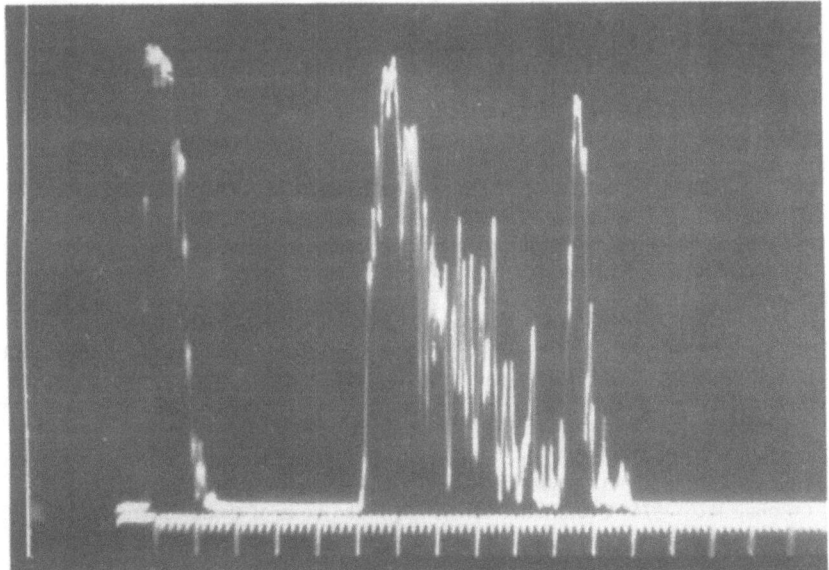

Figs. 18, 19, 20. Adenoid cystic carcinoma: Standardized A-scan echography.

internal structure and a high reflectivity. These findings are similar in benign mixed tumor. The only acoustic criterium which differs in these two kinds of tumors, the compression test being negative too, is sound attenuation which is great in adenoid cystic carcinoma with values equal or superior to 60 degrees in opposition to those observed in benign mixed tumor (Table 8, Figs. 17, 18, 19, 20) [3, 4].

On the basis of these data these lesions may be easily differentiated, even though a diagnostic doubt may still be present in schwannomas and in pseudolymphomas. The echographic pattern of the two cases of pseudo-lymphoma we observed showed high reflectivity, weak sound attenuation (angle k less than 30 degrees) and slight compressibility.

In conclusion we can state that:
– standardized echography can differentiate lesions of the lacrimal gland region in groups and sometimes is able to make a tissue diagnosis.
– when it is possible to make only a differential diagnosis in groups of lesions (e.g. cavernous hemangioma, mixed tumor), a further different-ation is not useful because all these lesions require the same surgical approach.
– In cases of malignant tumors and primarly in adenoid cystic carcinoma, it is useful to evaluate the sound attenuation inside the lesion which allows a correct diagnosis. This seems much more difficult with other diagnostic tests.

References

[1] Bellone G, Gallenga P E. 1973. Echography of mixed tumors of the lacrimal gland. Ophthalmologica 166: 156–160.
[2] Bonavolonta' G, Cennamo G. 1980. The role of ultrasonography in the choice of surgical to the orbit. Current concepts on ultrasound. Proceedings of the 2nd Italo–Jugoslavian US Meeting, Chieti, 1–3 Maggio.
[3] Cennamo G, Bonavolonta' G, Tranfa F. 1987. Le lesioni della fossa lacrimale. Studio ecografico retrospettivo. Clinica Oculistica e Patologia Oculare, VIII, 1, pp. 72–76.
[4] Dagher G, Andersen R L, Ossoinig K C, Baner J D. 1980. Adenoid cystic carcinoma of the lacrimal gland in a child. Arch Ophthalmol 98: 1098.
[5] Gallenga R, Bellone G, Gallenga P E, Pasquarelli A. 1971. Ultrasonografia clinica dell'occhio e dell'orbita. Atti LIII Congresso S.O.I., Malta.
[6] Ossoinig K C. 1981. Echographic differentiation of vascular tumors in the orbit. Proceed-ings of the 8th SIDUO Congress, September 16–19, 1980. Dr. W. Junk Publ.
[7] Ossoinig K C. 1974. Quantitative echography: The basis of tissue differentiation. J Clin Ultrasound 2: 33.
[8] Ossoinig K C. 1978. The role of clinical echography in modern diagnosis of periorbital and orbital lesions. Proceedings of the 3rd International Symposium on Orbital Disorders, Amsterdam, 1977. Dr. W. Junk Publ.

9. Ultrasound diagnosis of orbital schwannomas

O. BERGES* and R. GUTHOFF**

Summary

Macroscopic appearance of the schwannomas is often found by echography (5 on 11 cases: 45% of the patients). As a correlate, we can assume that confronted with an extraconal and/or dumb-bell lesion with cystic spaces, the first diagnosis to think of is that of orbital schwannoma. Differentiation with malignant peripheral nerve sheath tumor is impossible. Cystic spaces within the lesion are as well detected as by CT or MRI. New B-mode equipment with high energetic, high resolution good gray scale probes proved to be very helpful, giving as much information as Standardised A-mode.

Schwannomas represent 1% of the orbital tumors explored in the series of the Mayo Clinic.

They are slowly growing benign lesions, pre-operatively indistinguishable from localised (rare) neurofibromas. They are encapsulated by the peri-nevrum of the nerve which may be eccentrically present in the capsule macroscopically. There is an alternation within the same lesion of solid cellular areas: the so-called Antoni A pattern and areas of looser myxoïd tissue having stellae or ovoïd cells suspended in a mucinous background: the so called Antoni B pattern. The mucinous material may be very prominent and create pools.

Recurrence may occur if the lesion is not completely removed.

We have seen 11 cases of orbital schwannomas. 9 cases were benign and 2 cases were malignant. 3 cases were intraconal and 11 cases were extraconal. In 3 cases, CT and/or MRI demonstrated a dumb-bell lesion. The anterior portion of the lesion was well limited in 8 cases and bony erosion was detected by echography in 2 out of 4 cases. The reflectivity is usually low, but this low reflectivity as well as the strong attenuation may be due in some

* Foundation Rothschild, Paris, France
** Universitats Krankenhaus, Hamburg, FRG

R. Sampaolesi (ed.), Ultrasonography in Ophthalmology 12, 79–84.

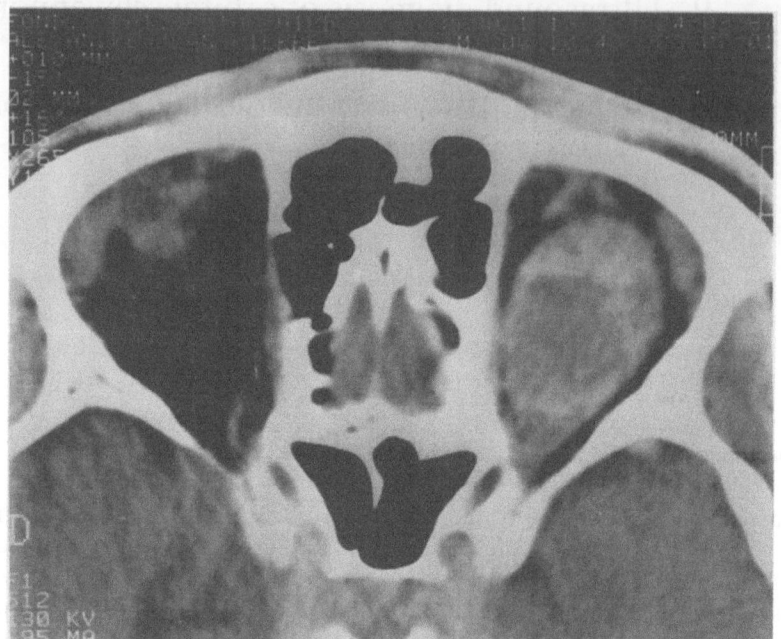

Fig. 1a.

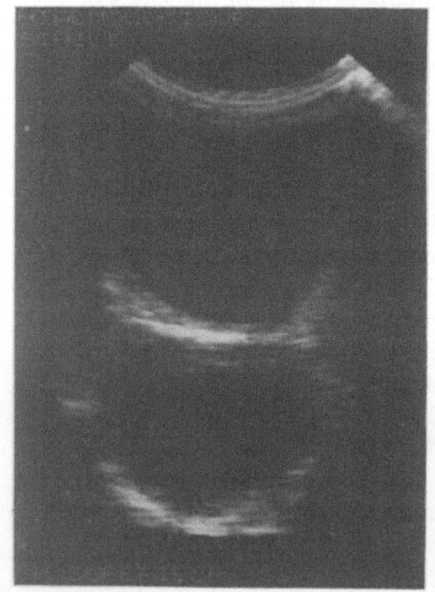

Fig. 1b.

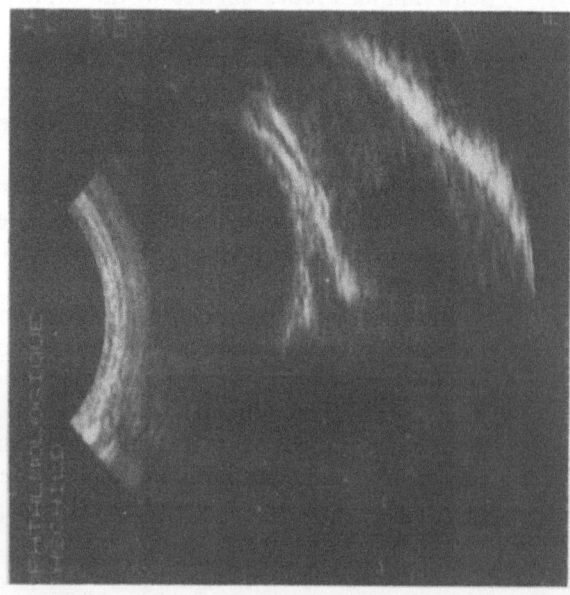

Fig. 1c.

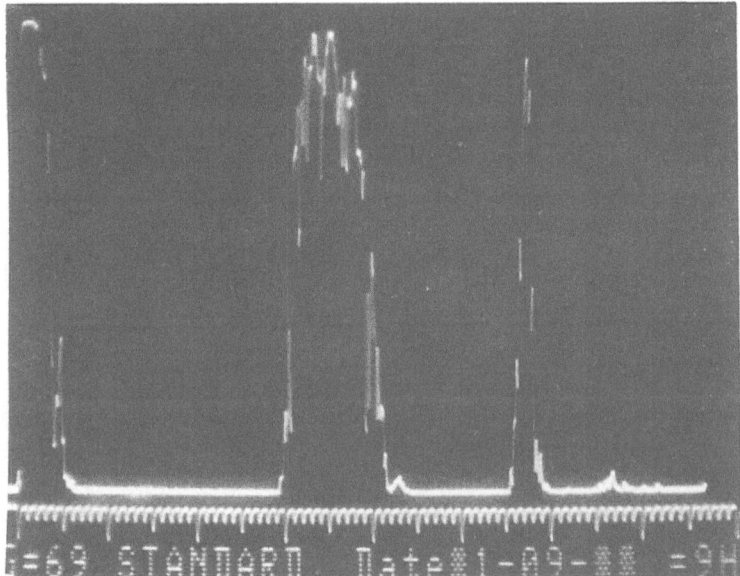

Fig. 1d.

Fig. 1e.

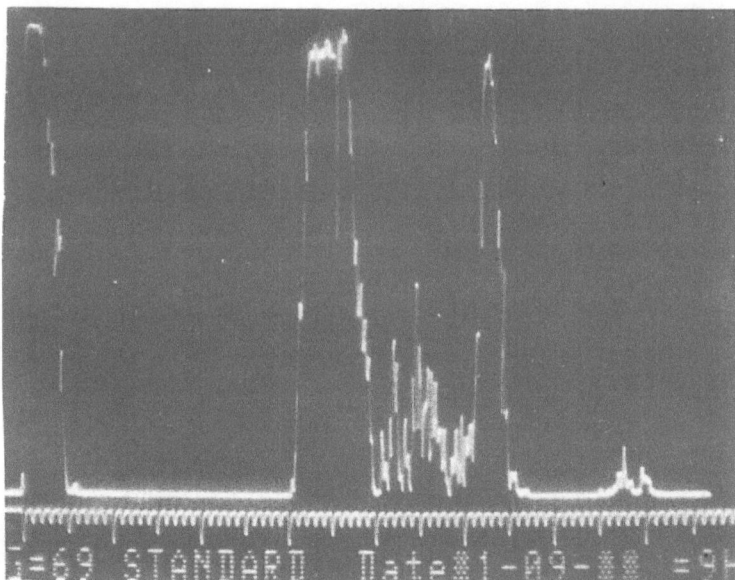

Fig. 1. Extraconal superior orbital schwanoma in a 45 year old caucasian male. (a) Contrast enhanced CT section parallel to the orbital roof: The cystic part of the lesion is evaluated with difficulty. (b) Trans ocular B-mode section of the cystic part of the lesion. (c) Sagittal B-mode section of the orbit demonstrating the anterior solid part and the posterior cystic part of the lesion. (d) A-scan of the cystic part of the lesion (Antoni A). (e) A-scan of the solid part of the lesion (Antoni B).

82

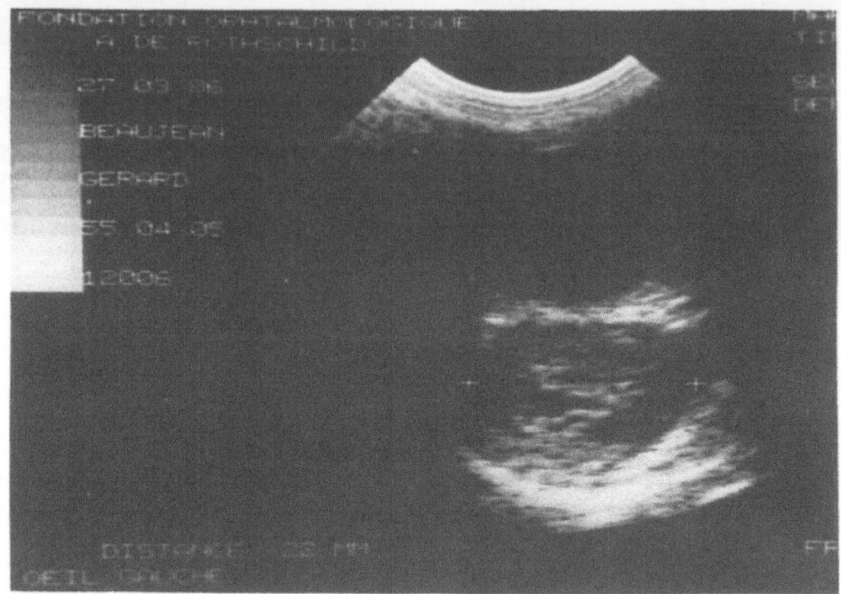

Fig. 2a.

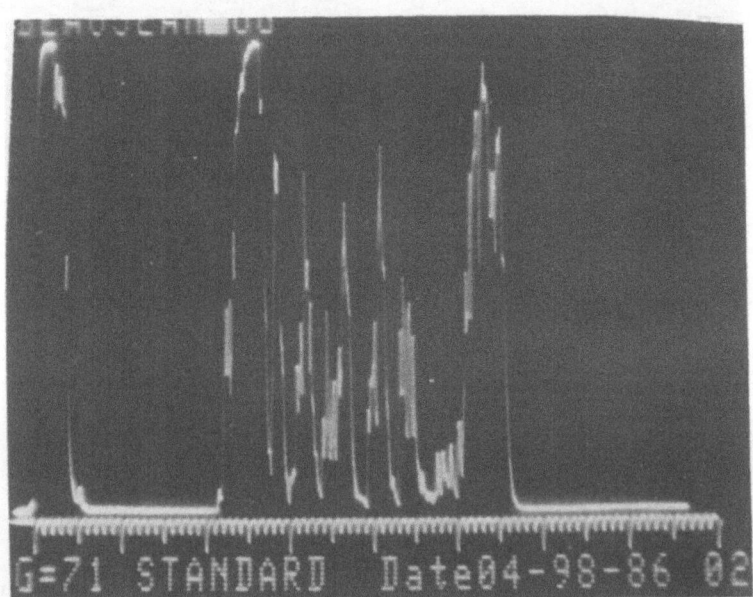

Fig. 2b.

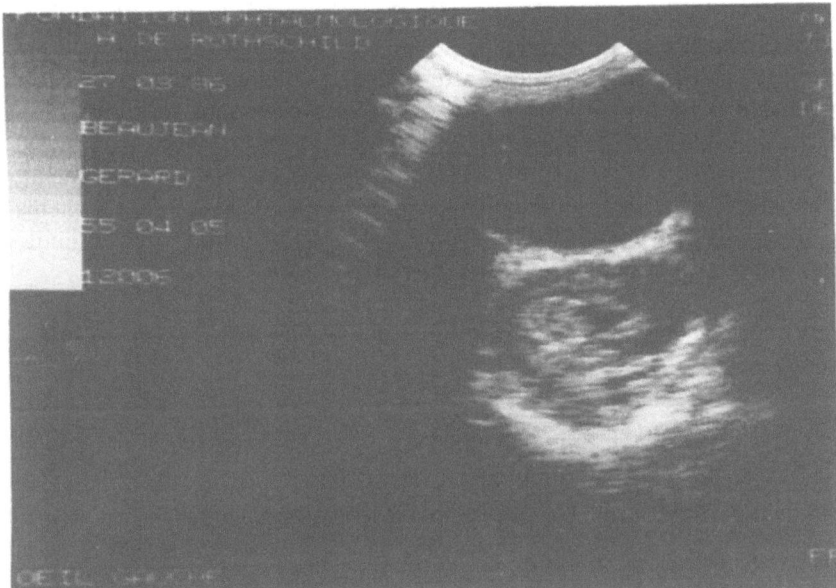

Fig. 2c.

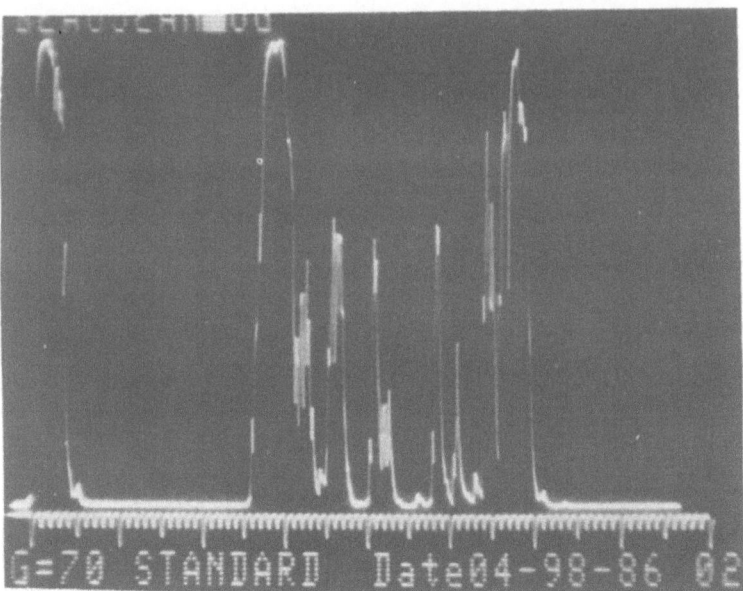

Fig. 2. Intraconal orbital schwannoma arising in a 55 year old caucasian male. (a) and (c): Trans ocular B-mode sections of the lesion at Tissue Sensitivity. (b) and (d): Trans ocular A-mode sections of the lesion at Tissue Sensitivity. Multiple small cystic spaces (Antoni B) are seen among the solid tumor which is very well limited.

cases to the obliquity of the beam to the lesion, especially when the lesion is posteriorly located at the orbital apex. In 2 cases, the part of the lesion, that corresponded to the Antoni A pattern, had a medium reflectivity with a regular internal echostructure. Cystic spaces, corresponding to the mucinous pools of the Antoni B pattern, were usually hypo- or anechoic.

Malignant peripheral nerve sheath tumors are extremely rare and it is usually difficult to differentiate between perineural fibrosarcomas, neuro-fibrosarcomas and malignant schwannomas. They also may be well limited by a capsule and may be cystic like the benign lesion.

References

Henderson J W., Orbital tumors. 2nd Ed. Brian C. Decken Division of Thieme Stratten, New York.
Jakobiec F A, Font R L. 1986. Peripheral nerve sheath tumors. In: Ophthalmic Pathology. An Atlas and Textbook. Vol 3. 3rd Ed. Spencer W H (ed) Orbit. Chap. 12: 2459–2860. W B Saunders Comp., Philadelphia, London, Toronto, Mexico City, Rio de Janeiro, Sidney, Tokyo, Hong Kong. pp. 2616–2631.
Kennedy R E. An evaluation of 820 cases. Trans Am Ophthalmol Soc 82: 134–157.
Offret G, Dhermy P, Brini A, Bec P. 1974. Anatomie pathologique de l'oeil et de ses annexes. Rapport de la Société Française d'Ophtalmologie. Masson et Cie Ed. Paris.

PART TWO

Biometry

10. Automatic measurement technique of the axial length using a new type of B-mode ultrasonography

KENJI YANASHIMA*, YASUNORI OKADA**, MISAKO ISHIDA*,
HIDEO SAKURAI**, MASAYA OHTA** and SEIJI KATO**

Summary

We developed a new type of B-mode echography equipment using the linear electronic scanning technique. This new equipment determines the axial length using a 2-dimensional B-mode tomogram and is far more comprehensive than the conventional one dimensional A-mode. The operator can easily judge the axis and can precisely estimate the axial length in a short period of time. Furthermore using this method we can achieve 95% reliability with but a single measurement and the measurement of the axial length is done more precisely and more quickly than with the conventional A-mode method.

Introduction

Recently, to correct visual acuity after extracting cataracts from the eye, intra-ocular lens (IOL) implantation has become common. To determine what power lens is needed, precise estimation of the axial length is required. The axial length is conventionally measured by A-mode echography. However, the A-mode method using only one-dimensional information is problematic because when using only the A-mode to calculate the axial length one cannot check whether the line used in measurement is the real axis or not. Furthermore the measurement takes a long time, lowering reliability. To solve this problem, we developed new equipment able to measure the axial length by conforming the optical axis on a B-mode tomogram [1, 4].

Method

This newly developed system utilizes a linear electronic scanning method to obtain a B-mode tomogram, after which the axial length is then determined

* National Rehabilitation Center for the Disabled, 4–1 Namiki Tokorozawa, Saitama, Japan
** NEC San-ei Instruments, Ltd., 1–57 Tenjin-cho Kodaira, Tokyo, Japan

R. Sampaolesi (ed.), Ultrasonography in Ophthalmology 12, 87–95.
© 1990. Kluwer Academic Publishers, Dordrecht

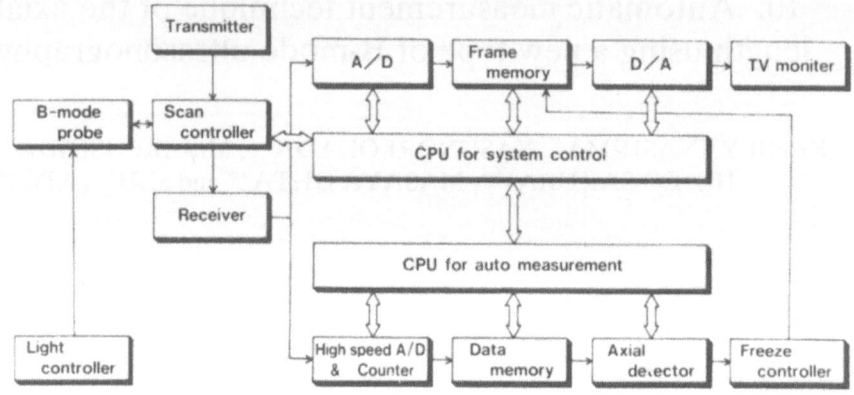

Fig. 1. System block diagram of the newly developed echography equipment.

by checking against the tomogram [5, 6]. The block diagram of the newly developed system is shown in the Fig. 1. The upper half of the Fig. 1 shows how the B-mode tomogram is generated. The lower part of the figure 1 shows how the axial length is automatically measured. The device consists of a high speed A/D converter of one echo line, different from the converter used for the tomogram, a data memory, a circuit to detect the axial length,

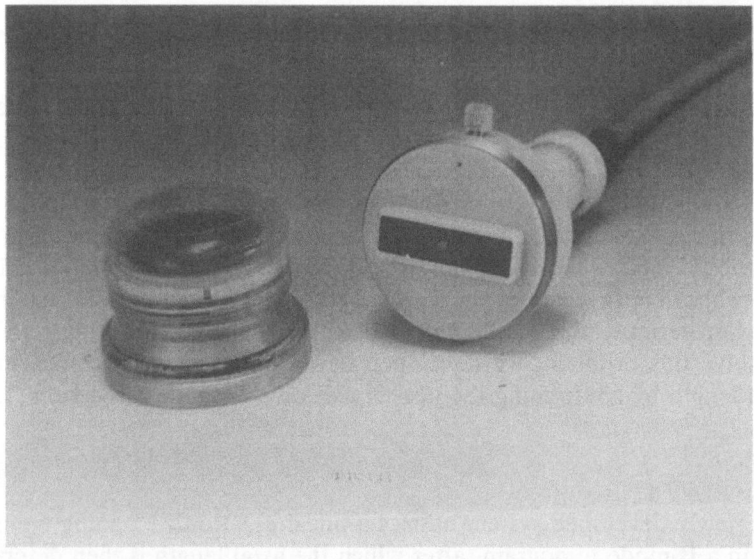

Fig. 2. The probe unit. The probe has a fixation lamp at the center of the scanner (right). The anterior surface of the probe is fitted with a water bag made of a transparent membrane (left).

an automatically controlled freezing circuit, and a CPU for measurement and calculation. Figure 2 shows the probe unit. The probe has a fixation lamp (Fig. 2, right) consisting of a single optical fiber at its center, thus reducing the acoustic influence of the echo beam to a negligible level [7].

The anterior surface of this probe is fitted with a water bag (Fig. 2, left) made of a transparent membrane. This membrane is very soft and keeps the pressure inside the water bag lower than that of the eye ball. The probe fits around the surface of the cornea touching not only one single point, as with conventional A-mode method, but covering the entire cornea, diminishing pressure on and distortion of the eye ball. The measurement of the axial length is done by processing a line on the cursor with window function in time and amplitude domain. Figure 3 shows the data from a normal subject. At first, the operator searches the tomogram for the optical axis, then the equipment automatically judges the axis. The length is statistically estimated by 128-serial data and if the results fall within the criteria, the display is automatically frozen. In Fig. 3, AL stands for the axial length, AD stands for the depth of anterior chamber, and LD stands for the thickness of the lens. The range, within which 99% of the data falls if the data follows a normal distribution, is also indicated and the operator can judge whether the results are acceptable or not. To ascertain the effectiveness of the equipment, the axial length of the eye ball was measured using the following three methods. Method 1 utilized the B-mode probe and method 2 utilized an A-mode probe using the same equipment and an algorithm to measure

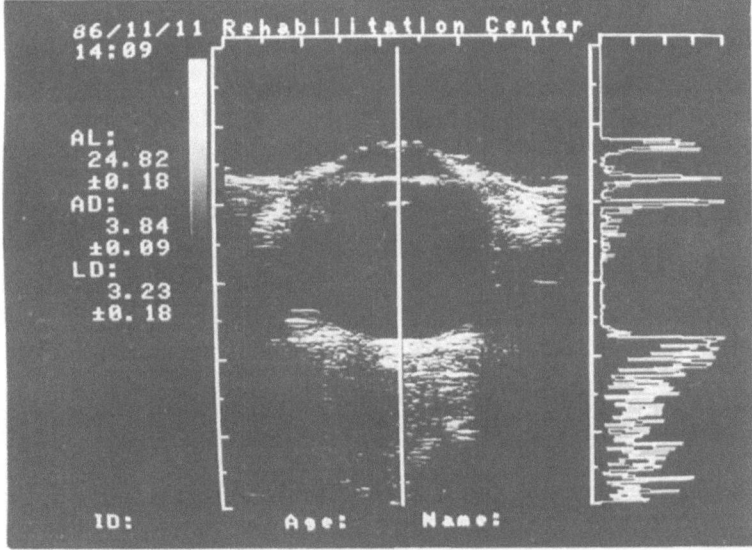

Fig. 3. The display of the data from a normal subject. Right: A-mode echogram coincided with the position of the cursor on the B-mode echogram (center). Left: AD: the depth of the anterior chamber AL: axial length LD: the thickness of the lens

90

whether the axial length is the same as when using the B-mode method. And finally method 3 used a STORZ ALPHA 20/20, which is widely used in Japan. To convert the value of the measurement into the real length of the eye ball for the ALPHA 20/20 a constant for the speed of sound of

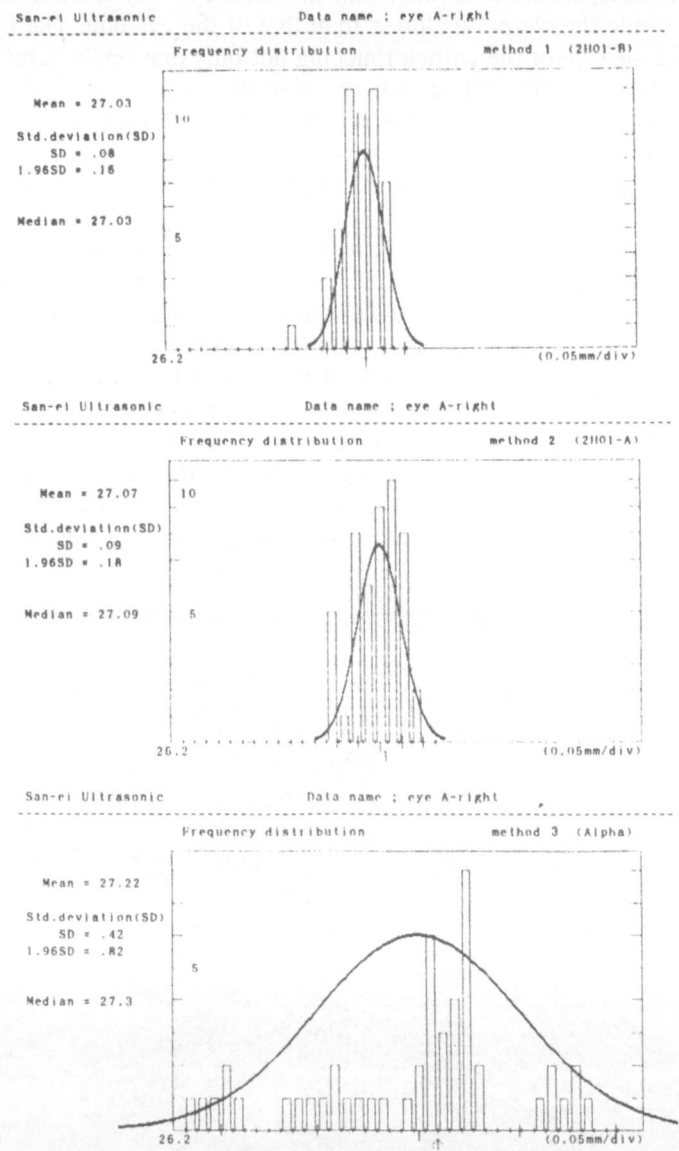

Fig. 4. The histogram to display the distribution of the axial length from a normal subject. Top: B-mode method Middle: A-mode method Bottom: A-mode method with ALPHA 20/20

1550 m/sec is used. For our machine a slightly different constant must be used, 1640 m/sec for the lens and 1540 m/sec for the rest. Each of these measurements of the open eye of a single patient resting in a supine position were taken 50 times. 50 times using method 1, 50 times using method 2, etc. All the data were included in the statistics without deleting any results.

Results

Figure 4 shows the data from the normal subject. Top of the Fig. 4 shows the results when using the B-mode method, and the middle of the Fig. 4 shows the results from the A-mode method. The bottom of the Fig. 4 presents the results when using the A-mode method with ALPHA 20/20. In the computer display the length was calculated in units of 0.01 mm. But in the histogram an interval of 0.05 mm is used to display the distribution of the axial length. In the Fig. 4, the mean value, the standard deviation and the median for the each method are shown on the left. Moreover, the normal distribution was drawn around the mean value and the standard deviation. In the Fig. 5, the Kolmogorov–Smirnov method was used to check how well the distribution of the results from these three methods fit normal distribution curves. The area between the two lines indicates the statistically significant range within 95%. From this we can see that the data derived using the B-mode method utilizing our equipment (Fig. 5, top) does indeed fit a normal distribution curve. The deviation of the data derived using the ALPHA 20/20 cannot be regarded as fitting the normal distri-bution. These results were pretty much the same for both eyes in all subjects. Therefore one cannot compare results obtained using our equip-ment with those obtained using a ALPHA 20/20 using nonparametric technique assuming a normal distribution. Only comparisons using the difference between the median and the mean value will be considered. Table 1 shows the value of the median and the difference between the

Table 1. The value of the median and the difference between the median and the mean value derived using three methods.

	Method 1		Method 2		Method 3	
	m (mm)	d (mm)	m (mm)	d (mm)	m (mm)	d (mm)
A	27.03	0	27.10	+0.03	27.31	+0.09
B	26.97	0	27.11	+0.02	27.11	+0.14
C	25.80	+0.01	25.53	+0.02	25.94	+0.19
D	25.17	−0.01	25.45	−0.04	25.59	0
E	21.11	0	20.78	−0.02	21.14	0
F	21.01	−0.01	20.97	+0.02	21.07	+0.03

m = median.
d = (median) − (mean).

median and the mean value derived using these three methods. Method 1 and method 2 reveal a high degree of invariability for the values of the median and also very little difference between the median and the mean value for each method. However, with method 3 ising the ALPHA 20/20

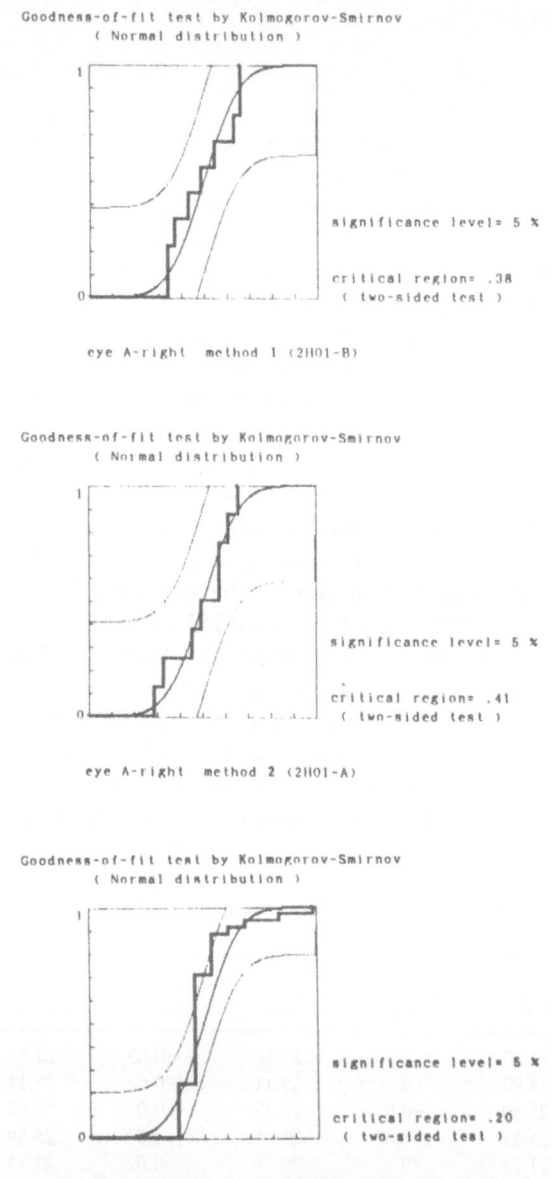

Fig. 5. Goodness-of-fit test using the Kolmogorov-Smirnov from the data of Fig. 4. Top: B-mode method Middle: A-mode method Bottom: A-mode method with ALPHA 20/20.

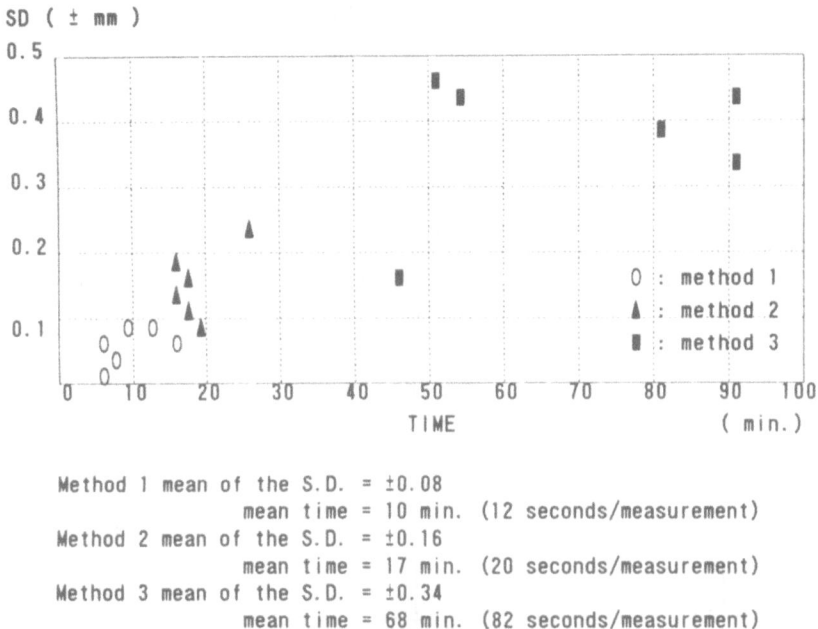

Fig. 6. The relationship between the standard deviation of the data and time required to take 50 measurements from 3 normal subjects (6 eyes).

there is a small difference between the mean value and the median. Figure 6 shows the relationship between the deviation of the data and the time taken for each method. The vertical axis indicates the standard deviation of the data and the horizontal axis indicates the time required to take 50 measurements. With method 1, the mean of the standard deviation is +/− 0.08 mm, the smallest of the three methods. The mean time is 10 minutes, 12 seconds for each measurement, also the shortest of the three.

Discussion

As we have seen there are some problems in measuring the axial length using the A-mode method. Even utilizing the automatic or manual method to measure the axial length, it is very difficult to judge the direction of the echo beam with the A-mode method. Conventional methods using the A-mode increase measurement error. Figure 7 shows how the echo beam diverges in three different methods, the direct method on the left, the eye cup method in the center, and the linear scanning method on the right. In the A-mode method, the measurement error can be as much as approximately 0.5 mm. However, using our method as shown on the right, the measurement error is quite small, because the echo beam does not diverge

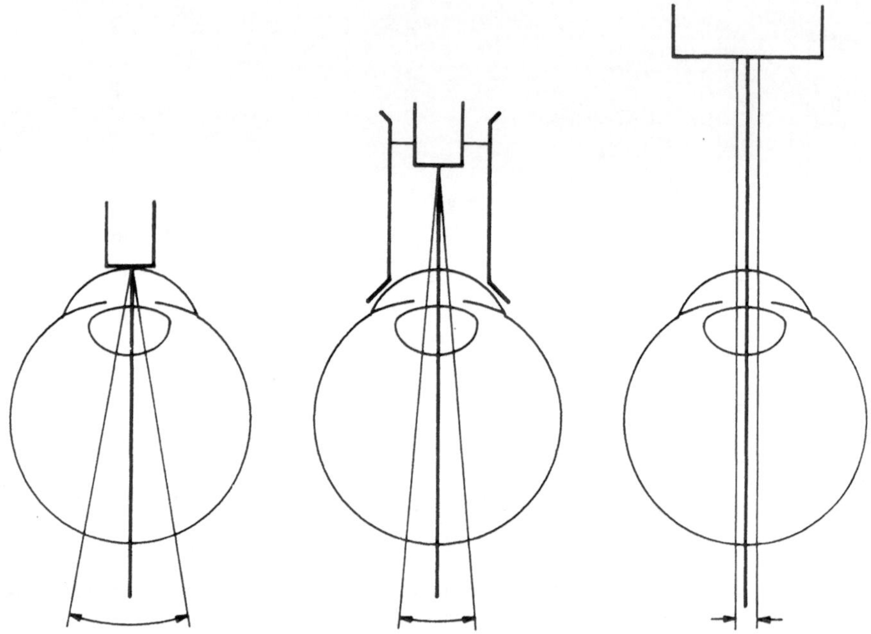

1) **Single probe**
   direct contact

2) **Single probe**
   with eye cup

3) **Linear array probe**
   with water bag

Fig. 7 How the echo beam diverges in three different methods. Right: Water bag with linear
scanning method Left: The direct method with a single probe Center: Eye cup method
with a single probe

and is parallel to the direction of the visual axis. Figure 8 shows the width of
the echo beam in the single focusing method and the dynamic focusing
method with linear scanning. The upper section of the Fig. 8 shows a case of
the mechanical scanning. The beam from the probe is focused at a certain
depth and the beam diverges out of the focal point. Thus the width of the
beam causes a measurement error. The lower section shows a case where
the electronic dynamic focusing method was used. The new equipment
utilizes a narrow beam focused along all points on the line within the eye
ball. This diminishes measurement error. The reason why the new technique
adopted the electronic linear scanning method is as follows;
1) the equipment can obtain high resolution using the high-tech electronic
   dynamic focusing method.
2) the equipment can greatly increase the frame rate and, therefore, the
   movement of the eye can be instantaneously determined.
3) No part of the probe has to be mechanically moved, and thus, there is no
   vibration when the operator grasps it.

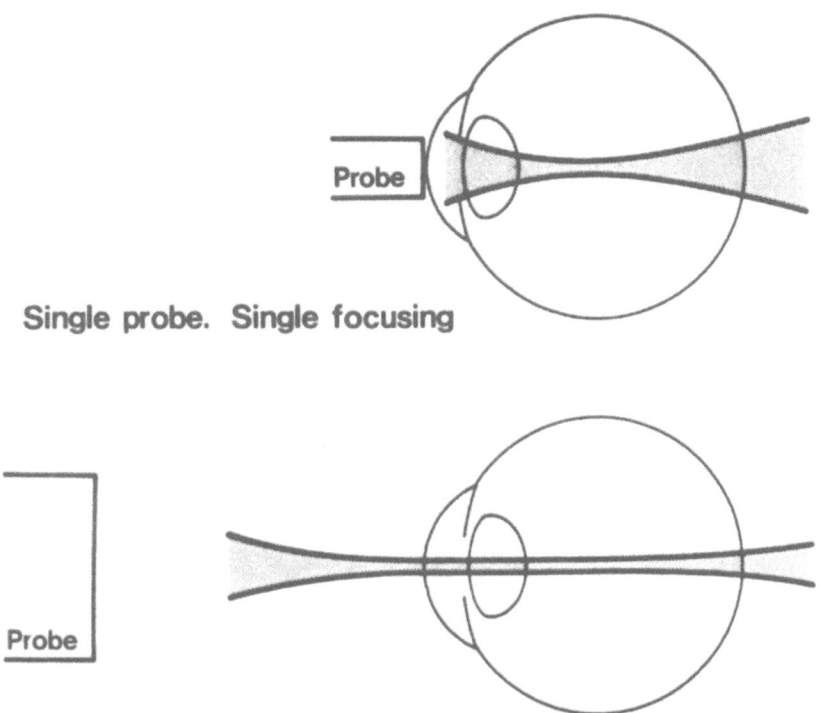

Single probe. Single focusing

Phased array probe. Dynamic focusing

Fig. 8. The width of the echo beam in single focusing method and dynamic focusing method. Upper: Single focusing method with a single probe Lower: Dynamic focusing method with a linear scanning method

References

[1] Poujol J. 1985. Echography in Ophthalmology. Masson Publishing USA. Inc.
[2] Bronson N R, Fischer Y L, Pickering N S et al. 1976. Ophthalmic contact B-scan Ultrasonography for the clinician. Westport International Publications.
[3] Coleman J D, Carlin B. 1967. A new system for visual axis measurements in the human eye using ultrasound. Arch Ophthalmol 77: 124.
[4] Fraceschetti A, Gernet H. 1965. Importance of ultrasonic echography for measurement of the optical components of the eye. Trans Amer Acad Ophthalmol Otolaryngol 69: 465.
[5] Okada Y, Yanashima K, Akeo Y. 1987. Automatic measurement of axial length using the ultrasonic B-mode method. Folia Ophthalmol Jpn 38: 384.
[6] Okada Y, Sakurai H, Ohota M et al. 1987. An automatic technique for measuring the axial length using B-mode. JSUM Proceedings (November) 569, Japan.
[7] Fushimi H, Nakabayashi Y, Ohota M et al. 1987. Development of probe with soft water bag for diagnosis of superficial organs. JSUM Proceedings (November) 309, Japan.

11. Transducer performance parameters and their influence on biometric results

W. HAIGIS and W. BUSCHMANN

Summary

Eleven transducers with working frequencies ranging from 5.1–11.9 MHz
and bandwidths from 1.5 to 6.2 MHz were used on 3 commercial ultrasonic
instruments with different operational principles to measure the length of a
well defined phantom. In all cases, the true length could be reproduced with
no dependency on frequency. The accuracy of biometric length determination
was best in the instrument using high frequency counters and worse, when
results were derived from the digitized video echogram. The dominant
influence on biometric results is given by system sensitivity rather than
transducer working frequency. From clinical measurements, a minimum
transducer tone-burst sensitivity of ≈ -25 dB or ≈ 50 dB pulsemode
sensitivity respectively has to be postulated in order to obtain acceptable
biometric results.

Introduction

Modern biometry devices are High-Tech products with impressive features.
Equipped with 'digital intelligence', they do not only measure ocular distances, but also process biometric data to end up e.g. with a recommendation
for an intraocular implant lens. However, it must be remembered that the
quality of biometric data is determined by the performance of all subcom-
ponents of the ultrasound apparatus with the transducer playing a key role.
Without proper sensitivity and frequency performance of this system component, insufficient results may be obtained.

It has been shown earlier (Haigis, 1985; Haigis and Buschmann, 1986,
1988) that often significant deviations between nominal and acoustical
working frequencies of transducers may be found. Also, considerable differences in individual sensitivities were measured when comparing different

University Eye Hospital, Wuerzburg, FRG

R. Sampaolesi (ed.), Ultrasonography in Ophthalmology 12, 97–105.

transducers. In diagnostic ultrasound, especially in quantitative echography performing tissue characterization, frequency plays an important role, since e.g. frequency-dependent attenuation in itself is a tissue characterization parameter. Also, overall sensitivity (to which transducer sensitivity is contributing) must clearly be high enough to detect all structures of interest.

In biometry, the frequency spectrum of a transducer and the pulse length are in close dependance and hence the axial resolution. It was, therefore, the aim of this study to examine the influences of transducer frequency and sensitivity on biometric results with special allowance made for biometry devices with different functional operating principles.

Materials and methods

Within the last years, experimental data on 67 single-element transducers of different make and kind were collected. The nominal frequencies of these transducers—most of which were designed for ophthalmic biometry —ranged from 5 to 20 MHz. Based on recommendations by the International Electrotechnical Commission (IEC, 1986) and the American Institute of Ultrasound in Medicine (AIUM, 1982), the following parameters were measured for each transducer:

– working frequency (IEC, 1986)
– spectral center frequency (AIUM, 1982).
– (−6 dB)-bandwidth (AIUM, 1982)
– sensitivity at center frequency (AIUM, 1982)

In addition to the sensitivity at center frequency (termed 'AIUM-sensitivity' in the following) a second sensitivity parameter was determined, named UTA3-sensitivity. By this, the attenuation setting on the UTA3-instrument (Ultrasonic Transducer Analyzer UTA3 of KB Aerotech) necessary to produce a 100 mV_{pp}-echo from a plane saline/W38-reflector (Haigis and Buschmann, 1985) is understood, with a transducer-reflector distance equivalent to 30 μsec. The 'AIUM-sensitivity' essentially expresses the relation of received echo amplitudes to transmitter pulse amplitudes when the transducer is driven with a tone-burst of at least 15 cycles at center frequency. The 'standard plane echo interface' (IEC, 1986) in this case was given by a highly reflecting glass plate, 30 μsec apart from the transducer.

Measurement set-up and methods together with first results on a limited number of transducers were described in detail at the SIDUO XI Symposium (Haigis and Buschmann, 1988).

As an important result from these measurements it follows that the IEC recommendation to use the working frequency in order to characterize the acoustical frequency behaviour of a single-element pulse-echo transducer is experimentally supported. A detailed description and discussion of the data for all 67 transducers will be published elsewhere (Haigis, 1988).

Out of these 67 transducers, 11 specimen were selected for biometrical measurements on a test phantom with 3 different ultrasonic machines. The transducers were choosen to cover a wide range of frequency and bandwidth. They were operated on the units they were designed for and, if possible, on the other biometry devices, too. A schematic representation of their frequency spectra is given in Fig. 1. Numerical performance parameters for all transducers are compiled in Table 1. Working frequencies ranged from 5.1 to 11.9 MHz with bandwidths from 1.5 MHz (transducer #1, bandwidth/center frequency = 30%) to 6.2 MHz (transducer #4, bandwidth/center frequency = 67%).

From Fig. 1 it can be seen that although most transducers were characterized by symmetric spectra, some of them showed asymmetric and even scalloped spectra with non-neglectable low frequency components (transducer #10).

As a test phantom, an acrylic cylinder (referred to as 'calibration block') supplied with one of the instruments was used. Its dimensions were $\varnothing$ 25 × 15.55 ± 0.05 mm. The sound velocity of this calibration block was determined to be 2347 ± 14 m/sec (Haigis and Buschmann 1985). It follows from this (dimensional and velocity) data that on a biometry instrument with a preset velocity of 1532 m/sec the length of the calibration block should come out to be 10.15 ± 0.07 mm.

The length of this test phantom was determined with
- a GBS (Grieshaber Biometric System)
- an Ocuscan 400 (Sonometrics)
- an Ophthascan S (Biophysic Medical).

Of these the GBS and the Ophthascan S process biometric data digitally, whereas the Ocuscan 400 is a true analogue machine. In the GBS being a dedicated biometry-only device, the analogue ultrasound signals of interest

Table 1. Performance parameters of transducers used for biometrical measurements on calibration block. (f_{nom} = nominal frequency, f_{work} = working frequency, f_{cent} = center frequency, bandw. = (−6 dB)-bandwidth, A_{UTA} = UTA3-sensitivity, A_{AIUM} = AIUM-sensitivity).

Nr transducer	f_{nom} (MHz)	f_{work} (MHz)	f_{cent} (MHz)	bandw. (MHz)	A_{UTA} (dB)	A_{AIUM} (dB)
1 OCU 5 MHz	5	5.1	5.0	1.5	44	−29
2 NM 6–5F #152	6	6.2	6.2	1.6	56	−23
3 NM 8–K #81	8	7.6	7.5	2.0	55	−20
4 NM 6–5K #39	6	9.1	9.3	6.2	60	−23
5 OCU 10 MHz	10	10.0	9.8	2.8	50	−28
6 Ophtha Bio XDR	10	10.0	10.1	5.4	51	−20
7 12 MHz 3.5 #1	12	10.5	10.4	2.3	52	−25
8 TQM #104	10	10.6	11.2	3.2	50	−21
9 TQM X	10	10.9	10.8	3.2	45	−27
10 TQM #103	10	11.6	10.8	4.8	53	−26
11 TQM #15	10	11.9	11.7	4.6	53	−22

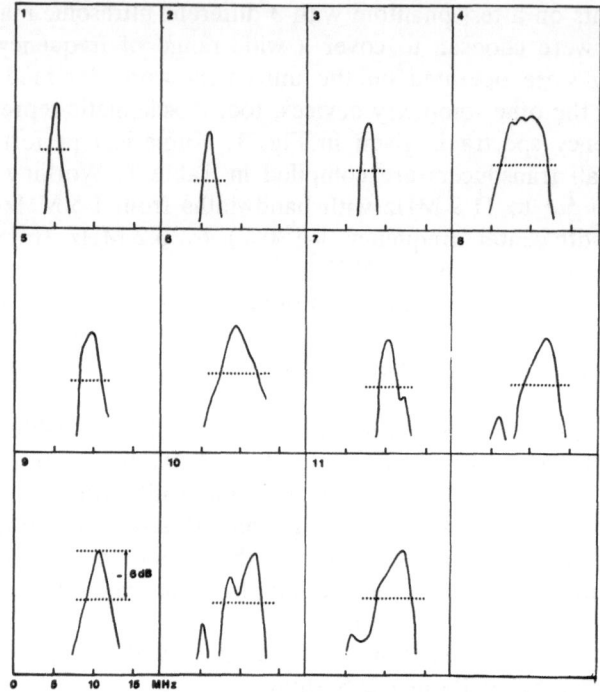

Fig. 1. Schematic representation of frequency spectra of transducers used for length measurements on calibration block. Numbers in the upper left corners of each spectral plot denote transducer numbers as used in Tables 1 and 2. For each spectrum, a dotted line indicates the −6dB bandwidth. Abscissae represent frequency, scaled as depicted for transducer #9 (lower left corner).

trigger four 40 MHz-counters, thus measuring tissue distances in units of 25 nsec. The Ophthascan S is a digitizing ultrasonic system, designed primarily for diagnostics but also offering biometry as an option. In this case biometric distances are derived from the stored digitized echogram.

The latter unit was operated in the biometry mode with the distance derived from the echo rising edges (and not from their peak positions). The Ocuscan 400 was run in the 'normal' A-mode with a number of photographs taken, which were subsequently digitized with a Hewlett Packard Digitizer hp 9874A (Haigis, 1987) and fed into the computer for distance-calculations.

Influence of transducer parameters on biometric results

For all measurements a water stand-off was used. Typical echograms, from which the length of the calibration block was derived, are shown in Fig. 2 for the 3 instruments. Numeric results are compiled in Table 2 and graphi-

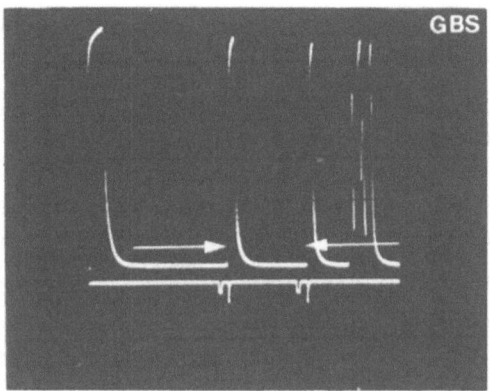

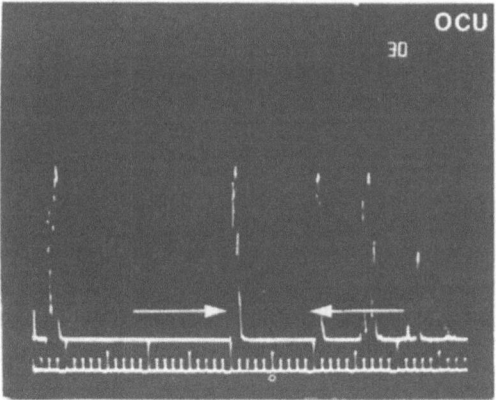

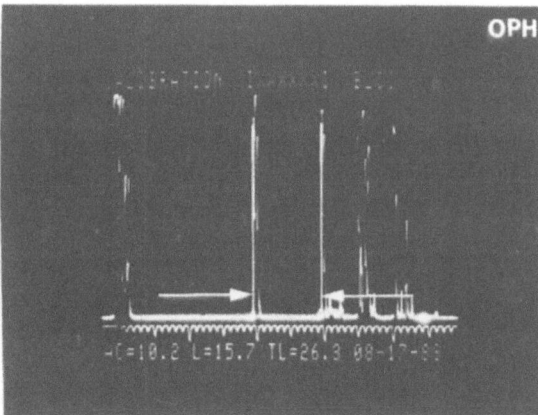

Fig. 2. Measuring length of calibration block: Typical echograms on GBS (top), OCUSCAN 400 (middle) and Ophthascan S (bottom). Rising edges of top and bottom surface echoes of calibration block are indicated by arrows.

Table 2. Results of measuring the length of the calibration block with different transducers and different biometry devices. (GBS = Grieshaber Biometric System, OCU = Ocuscan 400, OPH = Ophthascan S, mean = arithmetic mean of at least 11 single independent measurements, stdev = standard deviation). The bottom line denoted 'syserr' indicates system inaccuracy (cf. text).

Nr f_{work} (MHz)	GBS		OCU		OPH	
	mean (mm)	stdev	mean (mm)	stdev	mean (mm)	stdev
1 5.1	10.230	± 0	10.146	± 0.041	—	
2 6.2	10.206	± 0.008	10.142	± 0.067	10.109	± 0.108
3 7.6	—		10.180	± 0.053	10.183	± 0.055
4 9.1	10.190	± 0	10.175	± 0.050	10.127	± 0.096
5 10.0	10.190	± 0	10.204	± 0.053	—	
6 10.0	—		—		10.182	± 0.057
7 10.5	—		10.174	± 0.004	10.100	± 0.147
8 10.6	10.190	± 0	—		—	
9 10.9	10.217	± 0.011	—		—	
10 11.6	10.190	± 0.005	—		—	
11 11.9	10.193	± 0.007	—		—	
syserr		± 0.020		± 0.034		± 0.200

cally displayed in Figs. 3–5. In each one of these diagrams, the mean and standard deviation of the calibration block length as measured with each individual transducer is plotted. The horizontal lines correspond to the 'true' length of 10.15 ± 0.07 mm. On the right side of each figure, the inherent system inaccuracy is symbolized by an error bar originating from the 'true' length value.

In the GBS, the system inaccuracy is given by 1 counter digit ≡ 25 nsec equivalent to ≈ 0.02 mm. For the Ocuscan this figure equals the reproducibility (± 0.034 mm) of the resulting length value, when one and the same photograph is repeatedly evaluated. The Ophthascan error bar is given by the change in the instrument's distance readout induced by incrementing or decrementing the lighted gates on the display by 1 step.

As a surprising result no evident frequency dependance of the measured length can be found for either instrument. On the whole, every ultrasonic unit with every transducer reproduces the 'true' length within the error margins, these being significantly smallest in the case of the GBS. The different functional principles of the 3 devices are reflected in the standard deviations of the individual means, which are essentially influenced by the inherent system inaccuracies although these may be averaged down through repeated measurements.

During all measurements the transducers were hand-held as in a clinical situation and care was taken to adjust them thus that echo rising edges as steep as possible were obtained, because in all 3 ultrasonic systems the

GBS

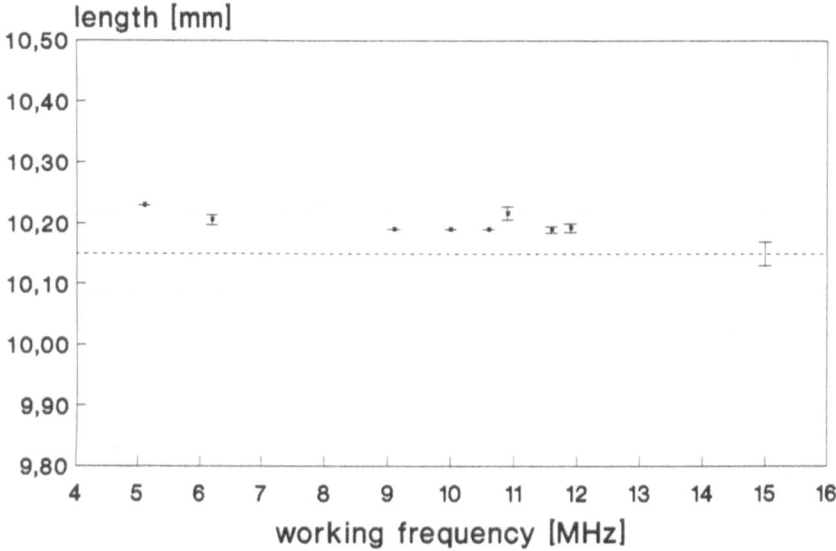

Fig. 3. Length of calibration block measured with GBS and transducers of different working frequencies.

OCU

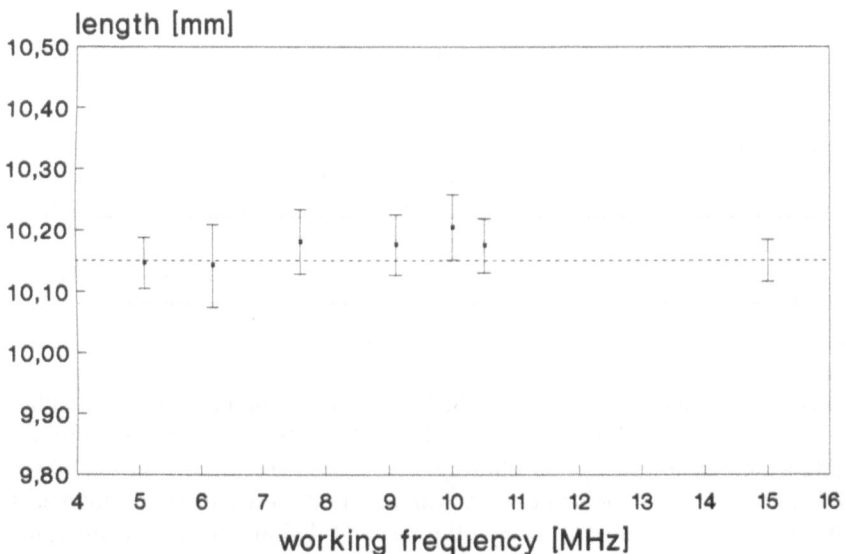

Fig. 4. Length of calibration block measured with OCUSCAN 400 and transducers of different working frequencies.

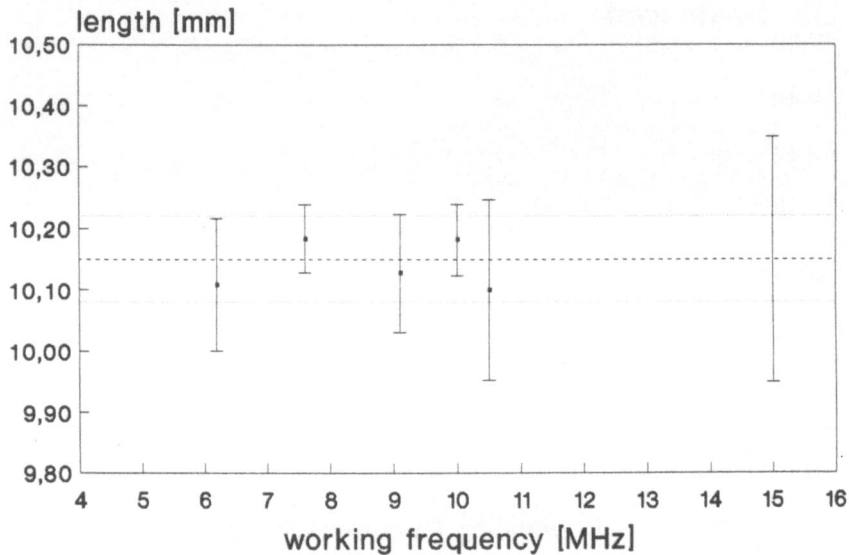

Fig. 5. Length of calibration block measured with OPHTHASCAN S and transducers of different working frequencies.

distance evaluation is determined by the position of the rising edges. To achieve a small echo rise time, overall system sensitivity (including transducer sensitivity) had to be high enough. With the strongly reflecting surface echoes of the calibration block under controlled experimental conditions this was easily achieved. However, measuring axial lengths clinically we found that measurement accuracy is significantly influenced by transducer sensitivity. Under clinical conditions, i.e. performing biometry on patients, it was often not possible to adjust for steep rising edges, when transducers with AIUM-sensitivities below ≈ -25 dB (corresponding to UTA3-sensitivities smaller ≈ 50 dB) were used.

We conclude that frequency effects which would influence the echo envelope and thus the echo rise time were neglectable in the measurements described. Overall system sensitivity was in all cases high enough to provide steeply rising echoes. Also, different forms of the frequency spectra (symmetric, asymmetric or scalloped) had no obvious influence on the results.

It has to be noted, too, that the 'classical' method of evaluating biometric data by means of echogram photographs (as in the case of our OCUSCAN 400 measurements) yields no worse (in fact: better) results than sophisticated ultrasonic equipment working on the basis of digitally 'frozen' echograms.

References

AIUM, American Institute of Ultrasound in Medicine, 1982. Standard methods for testing single-element pulse-echo ultrasonic transducers, Interim Standard, J. Ultrasound Med. 7, (Suppl. 1).

Haigis W, Buschmann W. 1985. Echo reference standards in ophthalmic ultrasonography, Ultrasound Med Biol 11: 149.

Haigis W. 1985, Performance measurements in ophthalmic ultrasonography with respect to IEC-recommendations. In: R W Gill M J Dadd (eds) WFUMB '85, Proc. of the 4th Meet. of the World Fed. for Ultras. in Med. & Biol., Pergamon Press, Sidney, New York, p. 433.

Haigis W, Buschmann W. 1986. Frequenzmessungen an Schallköpfen zur Qualitätssicherung in der ophthalmologischen Ultraschalldia-gnostik. In: Ultraschalldiagnostik 85, O Schnaars (eds) G. Thieme Verlag, Stuttgart, p. 776.

Haigis W. 1987. Computer-assisted clinical A-mode analysis in ophthalmic ultrasonography. In: Ophthalmic echography, K C Ossoinig (ed) Doc. Ophth. Proc. Ser. 48, Martinus Nijhoff/Dr. W. Junk Publ., Dordrecht, p. 187.

Haigis W, Buschmann W. 1988. Clinical performance measurements on ultrasonic transducers. In: Ultrasonography in Ophthalmology, Proc. of the SIDUO XI Symp., Capri, Italy, April 27—May 1, 1986, J M Thijssen et al. (eds) Kluwer Academic Publ., Dordrecht, The Netherlands, in press.

Haigis W. 1988 (to be published). IEC, International Electrotechnical Commission, IEC Report, 1986. Methods of measuring the performance of ultrasonic pulse-echo diagnostic equipment, Publication 854, Bureau Central de la Commission Electrotechnique Internationale; 3, rue de Varembe, Geneve, Suisse.

References

12. Clinical usefulness of linking biometry systems to personal computers

W. HAIGIS

Summary

It was described how biometry, although readily associated with IOL calculation, is also an important constituent of other applications in ophthalmology. The benefits of using a commercial biometry unit as an acquisition device with a separate computer to process biometric data according to specific applications were pointed out. Based on this approach a clinical biometry system with the GBS as ultrasonic component was introduced. By linking the biometry unit to the world of IB-PC/XT/AT Personal Computers and their compatibles, an open system had been set up, which is easily adaptable to future requirements. Standard database software could be applied, which is widely in use and easy to handle. Some of the system's performance features were illustrated with clinical examples.

Introduction

With the increasing number of intraocular lens (IOL) implantations in the last years, ultrasonic biometry has become more and more important. The growing interest in IOL implantation, also among private practitioners, is reflected in the appearance of new ultrasonic biometry equipment on the market. Whereas 'traditional' diagnostic ultrasound instruments mostly are multi-purpose devices, which may also be used for measuring tissue dimensions, this does not hold in reverse for modern biometry equipment. These instruments are very often designed to serve as stand-alone units, eventually giving a recommendation for an intraocular lens to be implanted. Biometry is provided as a necessary prerequisite for this purpose; mostly no diagnostic features are offered by the instrument. To calculate e.g. IOL powers it is necessary for the instrument's own microprocessor to have the ultrasonic data converted to digital form. Once digital, these data may well be handed

University Eye Hospital, Wuerzburg, FRG

R. Sampaolesi (ed.), Ultrasonography in Ophthalmology 12, 107–115.
© *1990. Kluwer Academic Publishers, Dordrecht*

over to Personal Computers for further processing. The benefits of this approach will be described in the following.

Biometrical applications in ophthalmology

Intraocular lens calculation is but one field, where biometry is needed. Data on the axial length of the eye and/or other intraocular distances are necessary e.g. for computing the power of corneal contact lenses in cases of aphakia, for exophthalmometry (together with Hertel's parameters), or for measuring the dimensions of various other healthy or pathologic structures in the eye (e.g. membranes, tumours etc). Also, all sorts of growth monitoring applications (e.g. regular/pathologic increase of axial length with age, tumour growth in response to treatment, follow-ups to therapeutic measures, etc.) base on data obtained by ultrasonic biometry.

In these applications, the normal or pathologic tissue dimension may be important with respect to its
- absolute value
- relative value, as compared to another structure (e.g. fellow eye)
- change with time.

Also, in all applications, additional information has to be added to the data obtained in a single biometric session, e.g. optical data (IOL-, contact lens calculation), biometric data from former sessions (growth monitoring), topographic information (volume measurements), etc.

Processing of all this information consists of performing the necessary calculations and producing an output in an appropriate form, e.g. as-plot or printout.

A commercial biometry unit with IOL power calculation option may well be suited to fulfil the purpose it is designed for. It is, however, a 'dedicated' instrument and can therefore not cover the total scope of biometric applications in ophthalmology. Usually, no sufficient long term data storage facilities are provided. Also, computations with algorithms other than the 'built-in' ones are not possible. The user is left to 'manually' perform the job. Patient files get filled up with numeric data e.g. from subsequent axial length measurements, and to present these data in an appropriate from (e.g. of a growth curve) is a time-consuming job, not suitable for clinical routine and subject to errors.

Advantages of a PC-based biometry system

The above described shortcomings may be overcome, if the typical biometrical application is split into its two functional stages:

- acquisition of primary ultrasonic data
- data processing according to the applicational needs.

Acquisition of biometric data may be performed with any suitable ultrasound system, whereas processing should be done by a user-programmable computer. To remove error sources originating in manual data transfer, it must be possible for the ultrasound device to be connected to the computer, i.e. it has to be equipped with an appropriate interface.

Such a system configuration allows not only to meet most biometry application requirements, but also offers additional features like data storage, all kinds of statistical evaluations etc.

As soon as 1981, when small powerful computers had become available, our working group started processing biometric data digitally (Prahs, 1981a, b). When the GBS (Grieshaber Biometric System), developed by the Bonn working group (Lepper and Trier, 1981), appeared on the market, it was (and still is) the only one instrument with a user-programmable computer. Since, up to now, the commercially supplied GBS software only covers IOL calculations, we developed additional IOL programs (Haigis, 1988) as well as routines to handle, store away and present biometric data in the management of congenital glaucoma (Haigis and Buschmann, 1987). The GBS' computer (Commodore VC64), although well suited to act as a controller for the biometry part of the instrument and to perform specific tasks like IOL power calculations, is in fact today considered a 'home computer' and—with its peripheral storage devices—is not able to handle data masses which are too big.

In addition, since the early 1980s, another computer type has established itself as an industrial standard: the IBM PC/XT/AT and the world of compatibles with their MS/DOS (PC/DOS) operating systems. Thus, we decided to configure a clinical biometry system with an IBM-compatible PC for data processing and with the GBS as primary biometric data source.

Configuration of clinical biometry system

The system configuration is depicted in Fig. 1. The GBS controlling VC64 is equipped with a modified RS232C/V.24 interface to allow 3-wire communication with an IBM-AT compatible PC COMMODORE 40/40. Handshake is software-induced. Programs are loaded from the GBS system's 5¼" floppy drive or optionally from an EPROM-bank connected to the VC64. On the PC side, we tried to keep the system open and easy-to-handle by using well-known standard MS/DOS-software. Thus, patient database management is written in dBase III+ code, whereas most of the calculation routines are programmed in Turbo-Pascal 4.0. With this concept, future requirements may easily be met by adding or replacing the respective software modules.

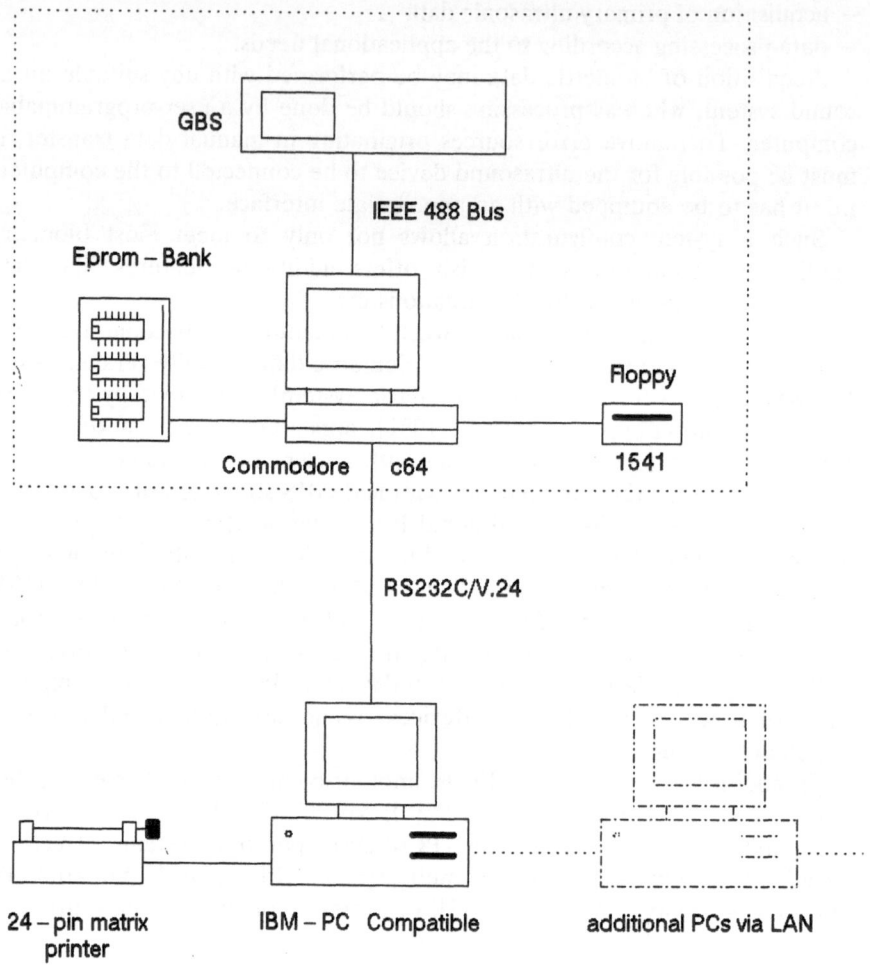

Fig.-1. System configuration: GBS (Grieshaber biometry system) linked to Personal Computer (compatible with IBM PC/XT/AT) via RS232C/V.24 interface using 3-wire software handshake. The PC may be part of a Local Area Net (LAN), e.g. a hospital information system.

System features

At present, the following processing features are implemented:
– receive data from GBS
– store data in patient file

– patient database management (edit, append, delete)
– calculate IOL power
– calculate corneal contact lens power
– present individual growth curves for axial length increase with age
– statistic utilities.

Data transfer from the GBS to the PC is achieved through a keystroke on the GBS' vc64 console. After successful reception of the GBS transmission, the data is automatically appended to the database, together with a system-defined patient id.

IOL calculation — making allowance for aniseiconia — is based on the GERNET formula (Gernet et al., 1970, 1978; Haigis, 1988). Fig. 2 shows an

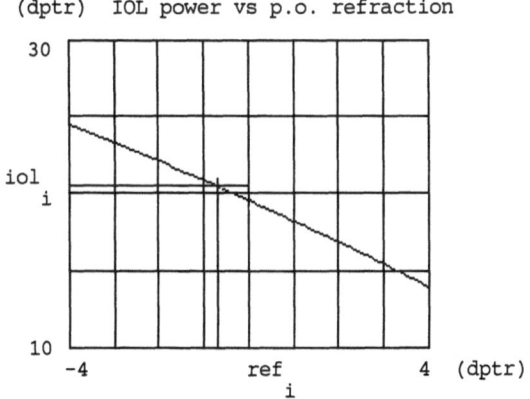

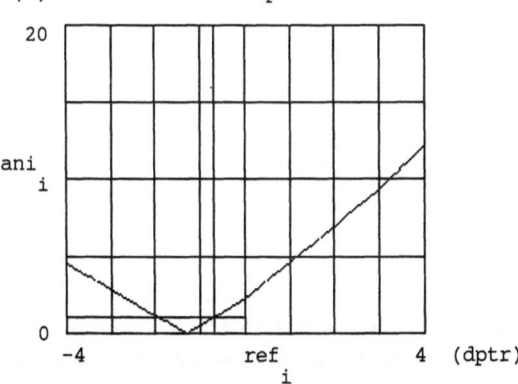

Fig. 2. Graphic screen output for IOL calculation: (Top) Calculated IOL (PPCL) power for different predicted post-operative refractions; (Bottom) Aniseiconia for different predicted post-operative refractions. Solid lines in top and bottom diagram connect respective data for IOL recommendation: with selected IOL-power (20.5 dptr) in top diagram a post-operative refraction (–0.7 dptr) is obtained, yielding an expected aniseiconia (1.1%) in bottom diagram.

112

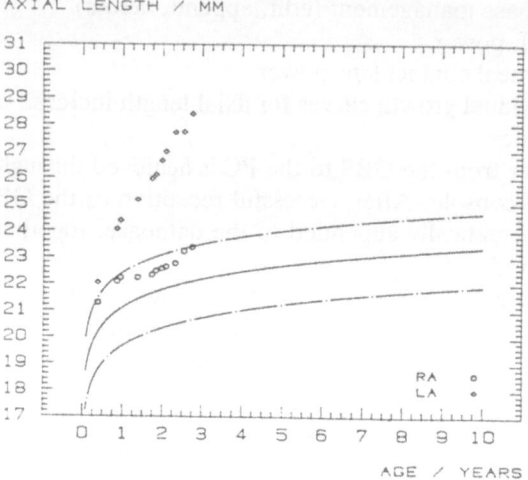

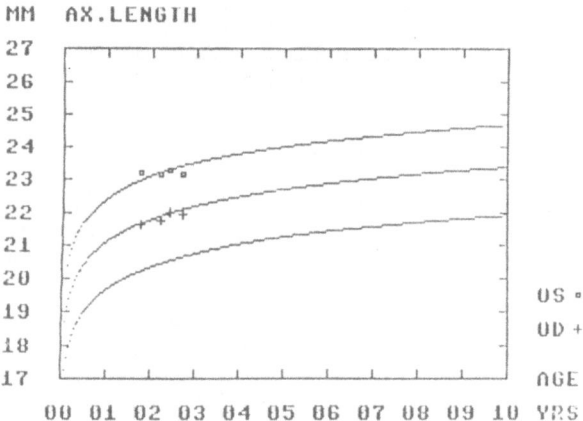

Fig. 3. Growth of axial length: (Top) Plot of axial length increase in congenital glaucoma. (Bottom) Printout (9-pin matrix printer) of axial length growth with age.

example for a graphic output from the calculation routine. IOL power as a function of predicted refraction is plotted in the upper part, the respective aniseiconia for different post-operative refraction values in the lower part of Fig. 2. A hardcopy of this screen may be obtained on the system printer.

An example for generating growth curves out of stored axial length data is depicted in Fig. 3. The plot at the top (Haigis and Buschmann, 1987) was obtained with a Hewlett Packard Plotter hp 7225A, connected to the GBS-system via a IEEE488-interface, the lower part presents a screen hardcopy with a 9-pin matrix printer (which is now replaced by a 24-pin printer).

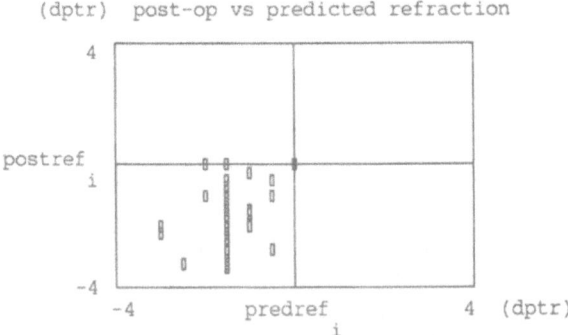

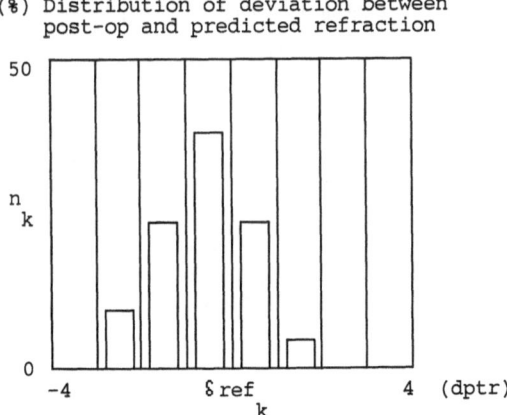

Fig. 4. (Top) Post-operative vs predicted refraction. (Bottom) Distribution of deviation between post-operative and predicted refraction (cf. text).

The standard growth curves and confidence intervals shown in Fig. 3 are based on data of Sampaolesi (1981) and from our own laboratory (Prahs, 1981b), yielding identical results.

Statistical evaluations may be performed with a variety of stored data. A comparison between predicted and actually achieved post-operative refraction is shown in Fig. 4. A graphic output like this may be obtained directly on keystroke. The plots in this figure stem from a different database of myopic patients, which was used to test the statistical evaluation routines. With the described software package installed in late April 1988, there is at present not enough verified data in the main database to allow proper comparison between predicted and actual post-operative refraction. A detailed interpretation of the distribution of refraction deviations will be published as soon as enough data is available.

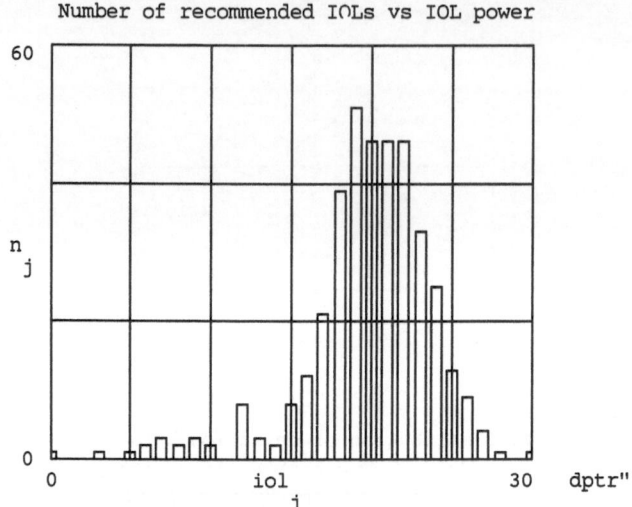

Total number of recommended IOLs : 384

Fig. 5. Example of statistical evaluations: screen output of IOL statistics (distribution of re-commended IOL powers).

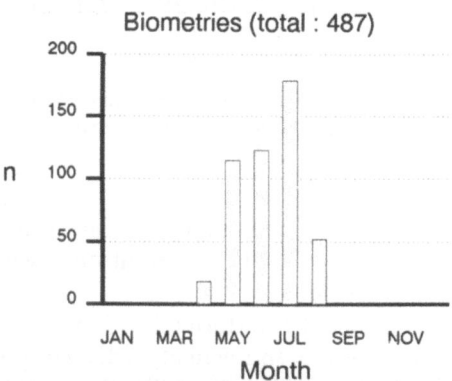

Fig. 6. Example of statistical evaluations: examination statistics data (number of ultrasound biometries per month) handed over to GEM Graph Software for graphical presen-tation. (Biometry evaluation software package was installed in late April; data for August comprise Aug. 1–5).

It is evident that a statistical evaluation like the one shown in Fig. 4 is mandatory for quality control purposes.

Another example of statistical evaluation of IOL-data is depicted in Fig. 5. It shows the distribution of powers of IOLs as they were recommended for implantation. Again, this graph may readily be output to the screen or hardcopied to the printer or given to the operation room technicians in order to have them update their IOL storage.

With all data saved in dBase files, it is easy to export them to e.g. presentation software or other commercial software packages. Fig. 6 is an example of handing statistical data over to a graphic presentation software package (GEM Graph). Here, the number of biometries performed per month is shown, starting with late April, when the software was installed, and ending with the first week of August, 1988.

References

Gernet H, Ostholt H, Werner H. 1970. In: Ostholt H., H. Gernet, H. Werner (eds.) Ein neues Haftschalen-Nomogramm für Aphakie. 122. Vers. d. Ver. Rhein.-Westfäl. Augenärzte. Balve, Verlag Zimmermann. p. 54.

Gernet H, Ostholt H, Werner H. 1978. Intraokulare Optik in Klinik und Praxis. Rothacker, Berlin.

Haigis W, Buschmann W. 1987. Computer-assisted recording of eye growth in congenital glaucoma. In: Euroson 1987, Proc. of the 6th Congr. of the Europ. Fed. of Soc. f. Ultras. in Med., Helsinki, Finland, June 14–18, 1987. S. Bondestam, A. Alanen, D. Jouppila (eds) publ. by the Finn. Soc. for Ultras. in Med & Biol., p. 272.

Haigis W. 1988. (to be published).

Lepper R D, Trier H G. 1981. A new device for ocular biometry. In: Doc. Ophthal. Proc. Ser. 29, Thijssen J M, A M Verbeek (eds) Dr. W. Junk Publ., The Hague, p. 473.

Prahs B. 1981a. A computerized method to analyse echograms for the calculation of intraocular lenses. In: Doc. Ophthal. Proc. Ser. 29, Thijssen J M, A M Verbeek (eds) Dr. W. Junk Publ., The Hague, p. 245.

Prahs B. 1981b. Des mesures biometriques dans les glaucomes congenitaux primaires. Bull. Soc. Ophthalmol. Fr. 93, p. 405.

Sampaolesi R. 1981a. Ocular echometry in the diagnosis of congenital glaucoma. In: Doc. Ophthal. Proc. Ser. 29, Thijssen J M, A M Verbeek (eds) Dr. W. Junk Publ., The Hague, p. 177.

13. Continuous biometry of the crystalline lens during accommodation

JOHN K. STOREY, CINDY TROMANS and EZRA RABIE

Summary

Apparatus consisting of a DIAS Biometer, a 100 MHz oscilloscope, a BBC SE 460 chart recorder and a Kretz 10 MHz plane wave transducer was used to plot rapid changes in AC depth, lens thickness and vitreous length over a period of time. Responses were recorded for several random accommodative stimuli presented to emmetropic and myopic eyes which were matched for age and sex. The speed and nature of dimensional change for positive and negative accommodation was measured. Comparisons between the refractive groups were made. This ultrasound method for examining dynamic aspects of accommodation is compared to work previously carried out ultrasonically and optically.

Introduction

Previous investigations of dynamic aspects of accommodation have largely been performed using optical methods to measure changes in refractive power of the eye. However, ultrasound can be used to measure continuous dimensional changes which occur within the three ocular segments (anterior chamber, crystalline lens and vitreous) during accommodation.

Coleman and Weininger (1969) developed an M-mode system which recorded movement of ocular surfaces and showed how this demonstrated movement of the lens surfaces during accommodation. Manabe (1974 and 1976) developed an A-mode biometer which could measure changes that occurred in one surface of the eye e.g. the anterior surface of the crystalline lens. Lepper and Trier (1981) described a method to measure the dimensions of the three ocular layers simultaneously and in 1987 presented a system with greater resolution in order to examine dynamic aspects of accommodation. These changes were displayed using a pseudo M-mode technique.

Manchester Royal Eye Hospital, Oxford Road, Manchester M13 9WH, England

R. Sampaolesi (ed.), Ultrasonography in Ophthalmology 12, 117–123.

Van de Heijde and de Vries Knoppert (1987) used continuous biometry during consensual accommodation to detect small displacements of the healthy lens and of intra-ocular lenses in pseudophakic eyes.

The purpose of our study was to monitor consensual dimensional changes that occurred on axis within the eye during accommodation, whilst assessing response time and the magnitude of change for various accommodative stimuli in emmetropes and myopes. This was achieved with a purpose built biometer, a high frequency oscilloscope and a chart-recorder as described by Rabie (1986).

Apparatus

The biometer used in this study was an A-scan instrument built to our specifications by the Department of Instrumentation and Analytical Science (DIAS), UMIST. A pulser drove the 10 MHz Kretz plane wave transducer at a pulse repetition frequency rate of 1 KHz so that the returning echoes for each ocular interface were converted for display and direct measurement. The trace was amplified linearly with full wave rectification and it appeared on the screen of the 100 MHz oscilloscope (Iwatsu SS5711). The time periods between successive echoes were converted into analogue voltages and displayed digitally to 0.01 mm on three panel meters representing anterior chamber depth, lens thickness and vitreous length. Each panel meter was fitted with a calibration screw to permit adjustment for the appropriate ultrasound velocity that is 1532 m/sec for aqueous and vitreous and 1641 m/sec for the lens.

The 3 Hz chart recorder used by Rabie (1986) was replaced by a British Brown-Boveri Co. (BBC) SE 460 instrument which had a faster recording rate. The analogue voltages from the panel meters of the biometer were fed into three channels of the chart-recorder. With direct recording only changes every 1/3 sec (3 Hz) could be monitored, so to improve this to 1/36 sec the instrument was fitted with a 4 K storage plug-in unit which digitised and stored the incoming analogue voltage. In practice, 40 sec of memory could be stored, and when printed out over a period of 8 min, discernible changes to 1/36 sec (36 Hz) were obvious on the trace.

Method

Twenty-four subjects, 11 males and 13 females, aged 18–30 years were chosen. Twelve were classed as emmetropic with a refective range of +1.00 to −0.50D and twelve were classed as myopic ranging from −2.50 to −9.00D. All subjects had less than 1D of anisometropia and 1D of astigmatism. An immersion technique was used to monitor one eye whilst the consensual eye fixated a distance target at 4 metres. The refractive error of the consensual eye was corrected with an ultra-thin contact lens to avoid problems that might be created by vertex distance.

Once a good trace had been established on the oscilloscope, the chart-recorder was activated and minus lenses of 2D, 4D and 6D were placed before the consensual eye to stimulate accommodation. It was essential to maintain steady alignment of the eye under inspection, so it was decided to place the full burden of convergence upon the consensual eye. This was established with a horizontal line of targets at 4 metres which were viewed through a mirror supported at 45° above the head. As the stimulus was changed the subject's fixation was directed to an appropriate target to achieve this. If over any part of the 40 second recording period, the trace failed to be satisfactory, then the experiment was repeated until a steady trace was obtained. The stored trace was then printed out.

Results

Figure 1 shows an example of a print-out from the chart-recorder. It can be seen that when the stimulus was presented, there was an initial increase in

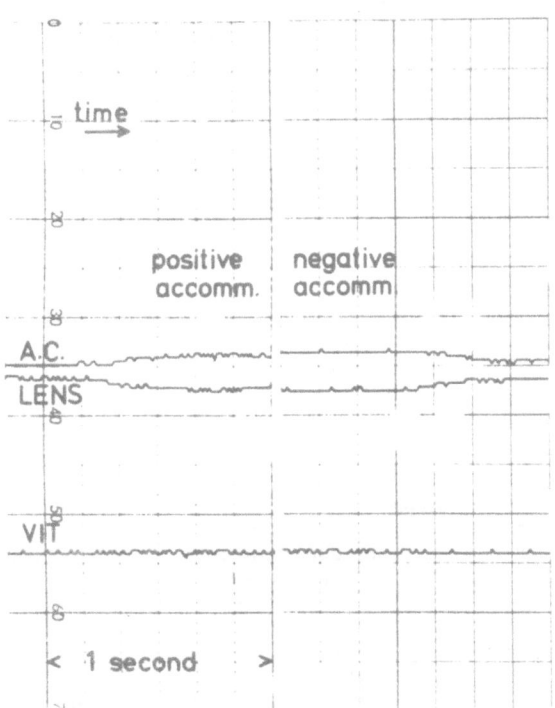

Fig. 1. shows an annotated example of a print out from the chart-recorder showing positive and negative accommodation responses to a 2D stimulus in an emmetropic eye.

the thickness of the crystalline lens and a corresponding decrease in the depth of the anterior chamber (Positive Accommodation) which was then followed by a period of at least three seconds of steady state accommodation (break in record). When the stimulus was removed, the thickness of the lens decreased and the anterior chamber deepened (Negative Accommodation). The criterion for judging the beginning of the response was that there should be an alteration from the steady state and for the end of the response that a steady state had been reached. With the present set-up we were unable to measure the transient period between the introduction of the stimulus and the beginning of the response. Response times were measured to 1/36 sec for the anterior chamber and crystalline lens. Response times were not measured for the vitreous length as it was often difficult to distinguish between the beginning and end of the period due to the small changes involved.

The myopic anterior chamber depth was significantly deeper than the emmetropic group ($p < 0.05$), there was no significant difference between lens thickness in the two groups and there was a highly significant difference in vitreous length and axial length ($p < 0.001$) between the two groups. The rate of change of the anterior chamber and crystalline lens with increasing stimulus was very similar for the myopes and emmetropes, but vitreous length decreased more with increasing stimulus in the myopes than with the emmetropes. There was no significant change in axial length on accommodation within either group.

Table 1. Mean response time for positive and negative accommodation for the anterior chamber of emmetropes and myopes.

Accommodative stimulus	Response time emmetropes		Response time myopes	
(D)	(sec)		(sec)	
	+	−	+	−
2	0.37	0.34	0.33	0.31
4	0.50	0.48	0.42	0.38
6	0.60	0.46	0.77	0.46

Table 2. Mean response time for positive and negative accommodation for the crystalline lens of emmetropes and myopes.

Accommodative stimulus	Response time emmetropes		Response time myopes	
(D)	(sec)		(sec)	
	+	−	+	−
2	0.39	0.35	0.33	0.31
4	0.55	0.47	0.49	0.39
6	0.63	0.46	0.87	0.55

Tables 1 and 2 show the mean response times for changes in anterior chamber depth and lens thickness for the two groups. It appears that the response time for negative accommodation is faster than the positive response time in both groups and for both the anterior chamber and crystalline lens. However, this does not appear to be statistically significant due perhaps to the variability of results within the two groups. The response times of the myopic group appear to be faster than the emmetropic group for 2D and 4D of stimulus, but slower than the 6D stimulus.

Discussion

Storey and Rabie (1983) compared changes in anterior chamber depth, lens thickness and axial length at fixed points of accommodation in 9 emmetropes and 5 myopes and found that myopes showed more reduction in vitreous length than the emmetropes. The results here on a larger number of subjects (12 emmetropes and 12 myopes) supported this general finding. However, Storey and Rabie noted a greater change in lens thickness per dioptre of accommodation in the myopic group which was not noted in this present study. As far as we can tell this was not due to the higher myopia in the 1983 experiments and maybe because less subjects were used in that study.

The speed of response to the accommodative stimulus was found to be similar to the results from studies using infra-red optometers. Campbell and Westheimer (1960) found that for 6 subjects the mean positive and negative accommodation were 0.64 and 0.56 sec respectively. Heron (1972) found response times of 0.60 sec for positive accommodation and 0.61 sec for negative accommodation. Tucker and Charman (1979) found positive accommodation response times of 0.74 and 0.75 sec and negative response times of 1.56 and 0.82 sec for 2 subjects. Manabe (1976) and Tucker and Charman (1979) found that negative accommodative responses take more time than positive ones.

In this study it was found that the speed of the response of both the lens thickness and the anterior chamber depth was dependent upon the magnitude of the accommodative stimulus. For both groups and for lens and anterior chamber it appeared that the response time for negative accommodation was faster than the response time for positive accommodation although this did not prove to be statistically significant. Weale (1963) showed that the lens substance is elastic with differences in elasticity between the nucleus and cortex. Fisher (1969) examined capsular energy changes during accommodation. It is possible that this difference may be due to an interplay of these forces within the lens. Perhaps, an analogy may be drawn between the lens and its capsule and a coiled spring in that energy is stored within the accommodated lens which is then released at a quicker rate during negative accommodation.

For accommodative stimuli of 2 and 4 dioptres, the myopic groups appeared to have slightly faster response times than the emmetropic group. Fledelius (1981) proposed that myopes were superior accommodators by examining nearwork scores and amplitudes of accommodation. He also stated that this fact appeared to be paradoxical because one might expect 'lazy' accommodation once myopia had developed since little accommodation is required for close work if a correction is not worn.

The myopes, however, appeared to take longer to accommodate to the higher 6 dioptre stimulus. At this level of stimulation more backward movement of the lens was noted in the myopic group than in the emmetropic group. Also at this level the response time of the crystalline lens appeared slower than that of the anterior chamber. Therefore, it may be that the vitreous offers some resistance to the backward movement of the lens or as Coleman (1970) has suggested in his unified model of accommodation that the vitreous has a positive supportive role during accommodation. However, Fisher (1982) stated that from his series of mechanical experiments on the crystalline lens that the differences between the anterior and posterior polar movement of the lens were solely inherent in the zonule lenticular complex. This was because there was no vitreous present in the apparatus when the lenticular polar movements were measured in vitro. It is still interesting to speculate on why the vitreous shortens during accommodation in some eyes and not in others and whether accommodation may play a role in the development of myopia.

References

Campbell FW, Westheimer G. 1960. Dynamics of the accommodation response of the human eye. J Physiol 151: 285–295.

Coleman DJ. 1970. Unified model for accommodative mechanism. Am J Ophthalmol 69: 1063–79.

Coleman DJ, Weininger R. 1969. Ultrasonic M-Mode technique in ophthalmology. Arch Ophthal 82: 475–479.

Fisher RF. 1969. The significance of the shape of the lens and capsular energy changes during accommodation. J Physiol 201: 21–47.

Fisher, RF. 1982. The vitreous and lens in accommodation. Trans Ophthalmol Soc UK 102: 318–322.

Fledelius HC. 1981. Accommodation and juvenile myopia. Doc Ophthal Proc Series 28: 103–8.

Heron G. 1972. A study of accommodation using an infra-red optometer. MSc. Thesis, University of Manchester.

Lepper RD, Trier HG. 1981. A new device for ocular biometry. Doc Ophthal Proc Series 29: 473–477.

Lepper RD, Trier HG. 1987. Measurement of accommodative changes in the human eye by means of a high-resolution ultrasonic system. In: KC Ossoinig (ed) Ophthalmic Echography, Dr W Junk Publishers, Dordrecht, pp. 157–162.

Manabe T. 1974. Studies in the dynamic changes in the lens due to accommodation. Acta Soc Ophthal Jap 28: 1213–17.

Manabe T. 1976. Studies on dynamic changes in the lens due to accommodation. Acta Soc Ophthal Jap 30: 979–83.

Rabie E P. 1986. PhD. Thesis, University of Manchester.

Storey J K, Rabie E P. 1983. Ultrasound — A research tool in the study of accommodation. Ophthal Physiol Opt 3: 315–320.

Tucker J, Charman W N. 1979. Reaction and response times of accommodation. Am J Optom 56: 490–502.

Van de Heijde G L, Van de Vries-Knoppert, W A E J. 1987. Ultrasonic measurement of accommodation in phakic and pseudophakic eyes. In: K C Ossoinig (ed) Ophthalmic Echography, Dr W Junk Publishers, Dordrecht, pp. 171–176.

Weale R A. 1963. New light on old eyes. Nature 198: 994.

14. Biometric investigation of the effect of gravity on the crystalline lens during accommodation

C. TROMANS and J. K. STOREY

Summary

The reliability of the Storz Alpha Biometric Ruler was found to compare very favourably with the Kretz 7200MA A-scan instrument.

The Storz Alpha II Biometric Ruler was used to measure the position of the crystalline lens with the subject upright, prone and supine.   Initial measurements were recorded under cycloplegia. On another visit a random seies of accommodative stimuli were presented and the ocular dimensions recorded from the contralateral eye. Age, sex, refraction and amplitudes of accommodation were noted. This study aims to provide a guide to the possible effects of head posture on ocular dimensions and to determine whether any assistance to accommodation is provided by gravity.

Introduction

The aim of this experiment was to investigate accommodation in various head positions, upright, prone and supine in order to determine whether gravity has any effect on the dimensions or position of the crystalline lens.

The mobility of the crystalline lens was investigated by Storey and Phillips (1971) using an A-scan ultrasound system. However, in this experiment, as a water-jacket with a hard contact surface was used, only lens thickness and vitreous length measurements were obtained accurately. The results were expressed as differences in the length of the vitreous with different head positions and so it was concluded that the position of the crystalline lens was affected by gravity.

As A-scan biometry for the calculation of intra-ocular lens implant power is now a routine clinical proceedure prior to cataract extraction, many commercial biometers for this purpose are available. One such instrument is the Storz Alpha II Biometric Ruler which was designed for axial lens

Manchester Royal Eye Hospital, Oxford Road, Manchester, M13 9WH, England

R. Sampaolesi (ed.), Ultrasonography in Ophthalmology 12, 125–129.

measurement and IOL calculation but has other important features which were utilised in this experiment.

The Alpha II transducer is fitted with a 'Soft Probe' which incorporates a water column sealed with a thin silicone rubber membrane to allow coupling with the eye without indentation of the cornea. The design of the probe lends itself to use in various positions and with minimal effect on the measurement of anterior chamber depth.

A-scan measurements are displayed on a digital histogram derived from 480 single measurements and anterior chamber depth, lens thickness, vitreous length and axial length can be printed out as numerical values. The Alpha II takes 60 consecutive readings in less than 50 milliseconds and repeats this process 8 times to give 480 readings in approximately 1/2 second. The result is given as an axial length and its components with a standard deviation to indicate the reliability of the measurements taken during this period. Up to 32 measurements may be stored and subsequently averaged to give a final measurement with standard deviation. So, this instrument can provide statistical evidence of accuracy of is measurements.

Prior to this study, Rabie and Storey (1984) compared the Storz Alpha 20/20 biometer which, like the Alpha II, is fitted with a 12.5 MHz focussed transducer and the Kretz 7200 MA S-scan ultrasonoscope equipped with a 10 MHz plane wave transducer. Measurements with the Kretz instrument were made using the immersion method and for the best accuracy all measurements were take from film negatives of the oscilloscope traces using a travelling microscope. The results from the two instruments correlated very well and as a double check, aphakics were used as models where the axial length could be calculated optically from refraction and keratometry. The Storz instrument measured on average 0.09 mm longer than the Kretz which was reasonable in view of the differences in beam widths of the two transducers.

Method

The Alpha II was used to measure anterior chamber depth, lens thickness, vitreous and axial length in three positions (upright, prone and supine) in 10 subjects (5 male, 5 female). The age range of the subjects was 20 to 25 years and the refraction ranged from +0.75D to −4.00D (mean −1.40D). Refractive error in the consensual eye was corrected using an ultra thin soft contact lens.

The subject was left in the desired position for a minimum of 5 minutes prior to measurement. One drop of Benoxinate 0.4% local anaesthetic was then instilled into the eye under measurement and the subject instructed to look with the other eye at a target at a distance of 4 metres. Ten readings showing a good histogram trace and a standard deviation of less than 0.05 mm were accepted and subsequently averaged to give the ocular dimensions.

This proceedure was carried out initially under cycloplegia and then two days later was repeated for an nearly unaccommodated eye at 4 metres (in tables as OD). Changes in stimulus were made by the use of minus power soft contact lens on the consensual eye.

Results and discussion

For cycloplegia and with and without accommodation, no significant change in lens thickness was found between the three positions, also no significant changes in axial length were noted. Significant changes were found, however, in the anterior chamber depth (Table 1) and vitreous length (Table 2). The graphs in Figs. 1 and 2 show anterior chamber depth dimensions and vitreous length dimensions for the prone and supine positions along the abscissa against the upright position on the ordinate axis. Two 45° lines are marked on each graph. Points falling below the 45° line show an increase in the dimension when in the prone or supine position and points falling above that line indicate a decrease in the dimension when prone or supine.

Figure 1 shows that the anterior chamber deepens in the supine position for all conditions. In the prone position there is a significant shallowing of the anterior chamber for the 6 dioptre stimulus, the other points lying close to the 45° line. Figure 2 shows that the vitreous length decreases in all cases in the supine position and increases in all except the 4D stimulus in the prone position.

These findings are in general agreement with those of Storey and Phillips

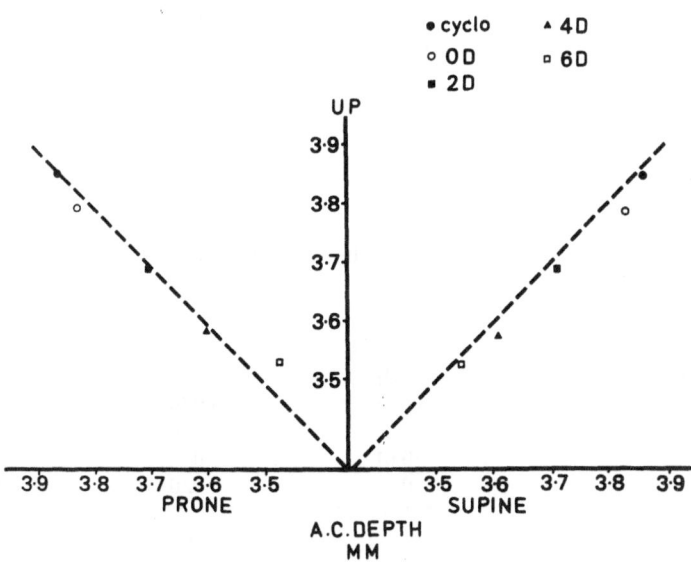

Fig. 1. Graph to show how the depth of the anterior chamber alters in the prone and supine positions when compared to upright.

128

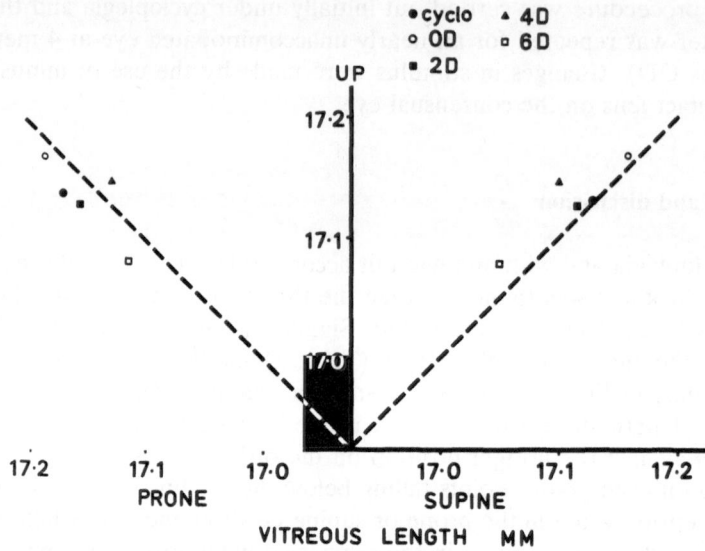

Fig. 2. Graph to show how vitreous length alters in the prone and supine positions when compared to upright.

Table 1. Mean difference in the anterior chamber depth between different positions (mm).

Accommodative stimulus	Prone-up	Prone-sup	Sup-up
Cyclopentolate	+0.04	+0.04	0
0D	+0.02	+0.03	−0.01
2D	+0.03	+0.04	−0.01
4D	−0.03	+0.02	−0.05[a]
6D	+0.04[a]	+0.07[b]	−0.03

[a] p<0.05.
[b] p<0.01.

Table 2. Mean difference in vitreous length between different positions (mm).

Accommodative stimulus	Prone-up	Prone-sup	Sup-up
Cyclopentolate	+0.01	0	+0.01
0D	+0.03[a]	+0.01	+0.02
2D	+0.01	+0.02	−0.01
4D	−0.01	0	−0.01
6D	0	+0.01	−0.01

[a] p<0.05.
[b] p<0.01.

(1971). The crystalline lens, although not showing any significant change in thickness itself, is falling forward into the anterior chamber in the prone position and falling backwards into the vitreous in the supine position. This effect is less with cyclopentolate than with a 6 dioptre accommodative change. This is to be expected since under cycloplegia the ciliary ring is dilated and so the crystalline lens is held tightly in place by the zonular fibres. However, during accommodation the ciliary ring contracts, loosening the zonular tension to allow the capsule to mould the lens contents into an accommodated state. This would also allow the crystalline lens to become more mobile.

As the lens gravitates forward in the prone position it may be supposed that optically this would assist the accommodation by increasing the effective power of the crystalline lens. As we noted no change in axial length or lens thickness for each step of accommodation, this indicated no actual change in lens power, assuming the lens radii remained constant. So it was decided to simply measure the total apparent amplitude of accommodation. Ten subjects, aged 20 to 25 years had their accommodation measured with a near point rule in all three positions under constant illumination. In all subjects the monocular apparent amplitude of accommodation was increased in the prone position as compared to the upright position and nine out of ten subjects showed a slightly decreased amplitude of accommodation in the supine position as compared with the upright position. This would agree with a change in effective lens power, i.e. the eye would become more myopic if the lens falls forward and would become more hypermetropic if the lens fell backwards and so alter the apparent amplitudes of accommodation accordingly. Clearly, an accurate assessment of refraction is required in all three positions to ascertain these findings.

Acknowledgement

We would like to thank Cyanamid UK for their most generous support.

References

Storey J K, Phillips C I. 1971. Ultrasonic investigations on mobility of the crystalline lens. In: M Massin, J Poujol (eds) Transactions of SIDUO IV. Centre de National D'Ophthalmologie des Quinze-Vingts, Paris 1973, pp. 261–264.

Rabie E P, Storey J K. 1984. The reliability of ultrasonic axial length measurement. In: W N Charman (ed) Trans. 1st International Congress on Frontiers of Optometry. British college of Optometrists, London, pp. 51–57.

15. In vivo determination of the speed of ultrasound in cataracted lenses

M. MASSIN and I. LAMBRINAKIS

Summary

A primary measurement in microseconds of the length of the different parts of the eye is made before the operation of cataract.

A secondary measurement is made after the cataract extraction, with or without an IOL, always in microseconds, and immediately converted into mm with the speed of 1532 m/sec for the aqueous and the vitreous and of 2730 m/sec for the PMMA of the IOL.

So it becomes easy to calculate the length of the cataracted lens and the speed of the ultrasound through it.

The total number of our patients is 63. We have found values between 1582 and 1708 m/sec with a mean of 1644,45 m/sec and a standard deviation of 30, m/sec.

The interest of these results is discussed.

Introduction

Nowadays the ultrasonic biometry is in daily use for many purposes: diagnosis of closed angle glaucoma, preoperative calculation of an aphakic refraction, pre-operative calculation of an IOL. The most important measurement concerns the total axial length.

Our to-day machines give us the time, expressed in microseconds, that the ultrasound needs for going from the probe to the interface and back to the probe. And we change this time into mm, by using the speed of the ultrasound through the ocular media. If it is well known for the aqueous and the vitreous, 1532 m/sec at 37° Celsius, and for the clear lens, 1641 m/sec at the same temperature, it is not the same for the cataractous lens. As our machines give a direct result in mm, calculated after the average speed through a normal eye, the result is obviously wrong when they are used on eyes with cataracts.

Hôp. des Quinze-Vingts, Paris, France

R. Sampaolesi (ed.), Ultrasonography in Ophthalmology 12, 131–134.
© *1990. Kluwer Academic Publishers, Dordrecht*

Material and methods

Our investigation was conducted on a group of 63 eyes belonging to 63 patients, all operated on for cataract extraction. 48 eyes received an IOL and 15, which were myopic, did not. The youngest patient was 42 years old and the oldest 82.

All our measures were made with an EO2 of Biophysic Medical fitted out with a probe of 8 MHz. This probe was directly applied to the cornea, according to the method of contact. We did not think that the interposition of a water zone was useful, since we have shown in a previous work that the accuracy was the same for the appreciation of the total length: 0.25 mm.

For each eye we took 2 measurements, both expressed in microseconds.

In the preoperative one we put apart the time for the anterior segment (AS) and the vitreous where the speed of the ultrasound is known: 1532 m/sec and the time for the lens where it is not.

The postoperative measurement was taken at least 1 month after the surgery. For the aphakic eyes it was easy to know the real length. For the pseudophakic eyes we had to take into account the time of the IOL and the particular speed of the ultrasound through the PMMA: 2730 m/sec.

Having such determined the real value of the total length of the eye, and thinking it was the same before the operation, it became easy to calculate the preoperative length of the cataractous lens, and according to it the speed of the ultrasound through this lens.

Results

Our 63 measurements of the speed of the ultrasound through the cataracted lenses were distributed following a Gauss binomial curve whose the main values were:

Mean: 1644.54 m/sec
Standard deviation: 30.05 m/sec
Extreme values: 1582.6 m/sec–1708 m/sec

Analysis and discussion

Before obtaining these results, and to be quite sure of their value, we had to avoid several causes of errors.

We have already discussed the accuracy of the contact method. Delmarcelle thinks, as we ourselves do, that this precision is between 0.1 and 0.3 mm for a 8 MHz probe.

The measurement itself needs a special training of the operator since he must, at the same time, check the position of the probe, the fixation of the patient, and above all the features of the echoes. We know indeed that the measurement is right when the ascending part of the echo is straight with no hook.

All our measurements were made on well dilated pupils to avoid iris echoes and we had some trouble with the strong echoes of repetition generated by the IOL. We generally had to reduce the gain to get easier to read echoes.

Several attempts have been done in the past to measure the speed of the ultrasound through cataracted lenses, but they always were in vitro experiments, on lenses removed from the eye. Our presentation concerns in vivo measurements, with the lens in its normal position within the eyeball.

The following authors have published their results:
Jansson and Kock in 1962 have found an average speed of 1640.5 m/sec on 12 lenses.

Coleman, in 1975, has found 1629 m/sec on 50 lenses.

Pallikaris, in 1981, on 37 lenses has found a mean of 1641.35 m/sec with a st. dev. of 28 m/sec and extreme values of 1588 and 1692 m/sec.

It seems that the differences of speed can be explained by the water contents of the different types of cataracts. Capsular and intumescent cataracts contain more water and the speed of ultrasound becomes lower. On the contrary, in nuclear cataracts, the water content decreases and the sound goes faster.

Conclusions

We have found a mean value for the speed of ultrasound in vivo through cataracted lenses of 1644.45 m/sec, not far from the speed through a normal lens. As our machines are programmated with a speed of 1641, the total length they indicate is not so wrong, finally.

Errors may only happen with intumescent cataracts for whom the length is overevaluated and with nuclear cataracts where it is underevaluated. These errors may not be negligible. As the st. dev. is 30 m/sec, 2 st. dev. are 60 m/sec. Translated into mm it becomes 0.32 mm for a lens thickness between 4 to 5 mm, and into diopters, for the calculation of an IOL following the SRK formula, 0.8 diopters.

So it seems advisable to adjust slightly, of 0.5 diopters, the rough values given by the computer for the IOL power, when the cataract is intumescent or when it is nuclear.

References

Massin M, Poujol J, Hieronymus. 1971. Etude statistique de différents facteurs influant sur la précision des mesures biométriques. Ultrasonographia Medica (SIDUO III), Verlag der Wiener Med. Akad., II, pp. 467–472.

134

Delmarcelle Y, Francois J, Goes F, Collignon-Brach J, Luyckx-Bacus J, Verbraeken H. 1976. Biométrie oculaire clinique, oculométrie. Rapport Bull Soc belge Opht 172: 117.

Jansson F, Kock E. 1962. Determination of the velocity of ultrasound in the human lens and vitreous. Acta Ophthal (Kbh) 40: 420–433.

Coleman D J, Lizzi F L, Franzen L A, Abramson D A. 1975. Ultrasonography Ophthalmology, Bibl Ophthalm Karger (Basel) 83: 246–251.

Pallikaris I, Gruber H. 1981. Determination of sound velocity in different forms of cataracts, In: Ultrasonography in Ophthalmology, Proceedings of the 8th SIDUO Congress. Doc Ophth Proc Series 29: 165–169.

16. Biometry and characterization of the lens‡

G. CENNAMO*, N. ROSA*, P. DAPONTE**, and G. IACCARINO*

Summary

We measured the lens thickness in a group of patients with normal lenses compared to a group of patients with different age and with various types of lens opacities.

We obtained these measurements with standardized A-scan using the immersion technique and on the basis of R.F. signals obtained by A-mode ultrasonic measurement. The measurements in microseconds were obtained along the optical axis of the lens, utilizing Ossoinig's immersion shell and using a 15 MHz probe.

Introduction

Several authors studying cataractous lenses obtained from intracapsular extraction have shown that there is an increased or decreased sound speed in these lenses according to the different types of opacities [6–8].

There is an increased sound speed in lenses with nuclear opacities while there is a decreased sound speed in lenses with cortical opacities. The different behaviour can be related to a different pathogenethic mechanism: in cortical cataracts there is an increase in water percentage and a decrease in protein, while in nuclear cataract there is an increase of density. On the basis of these data we decided to evaluate the thickness of the lens in patients with normal and cataractous lenses.

In a previous study [4] we evaluated 61 eyes with normal lenses and 64 eyes with mild-moderate opacities, and visual acuity better than 20/70 and age ranging from 30 to 80 years utilizing standardized A-scan echography with immersion scleral shells [5–7], because this technique between the classical echographic techniques is the most precise, and the only one which allows an accuracy of +/−0.005 mm (Fig. 1).

* University of Naples, Italy
** University of Calabria, Italy
‡ This paper has been awarded in 1988 by the Italian Society of Ophthalmology.

R. Sampaolesi (ed.), Ultrasonography in Ophthalmology 12, 135–140.

136

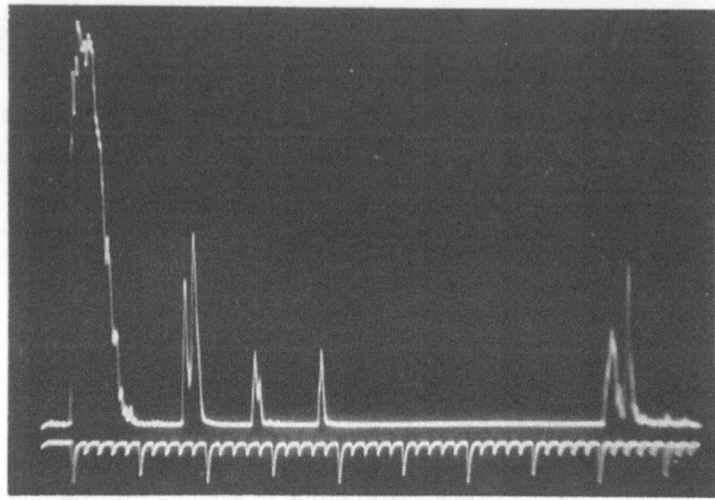

Fig. 1. Axial eye length obtained with standardized A-scan echography utilizing immersion scleral shells.

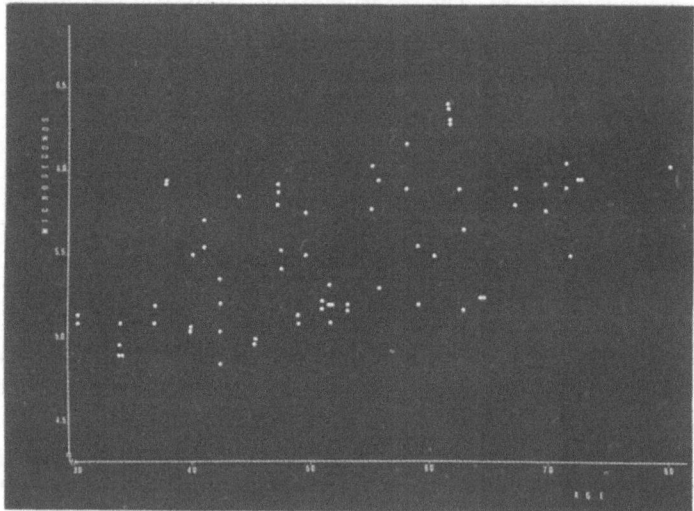

Fig. 2. Thickness of normal lenses in μsec, related to the age, obtained with standardized A-scan echography.

Five measurements for each eye were taken, and all the measurements had never a difference greater than 0.1 μsec. As we know the thickness of the lens is age related [3], we reported our results on a graph; from these data we could see that in normal lenses (Fig. 2) there is a more homogeneous distribution, while in cataractous ones (Fig. 3) it is more randomized; this is

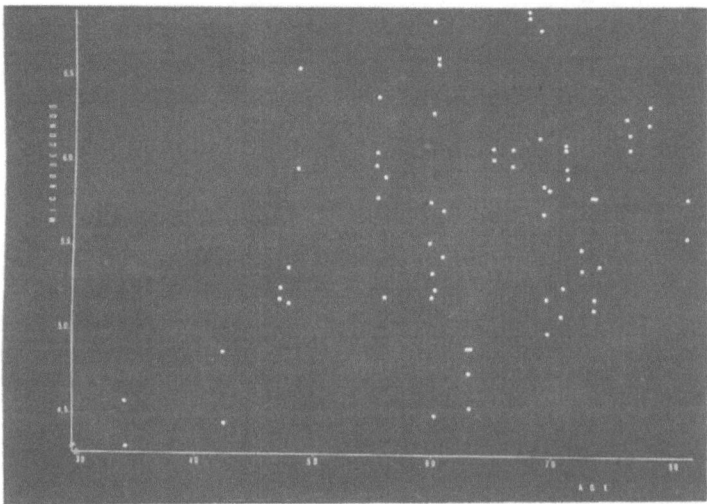

Fig. 3. Thickness of cataractous lenses in microseconds, related to the age, obtained with standardized A-scan echography.

due to the different sound speed in the lens with opacities. For this reason we proposed the ecographic biometry as an objective method to evaluate the progression of the lens opacities [1].

Material and methods

On the basis of our results, we decided to try to check if the difference in sound speed was already present in an early stage of the cataractous process.

For this purpose we used R.F. signals with a more sophisticated method, utilizing:
1) Sonometrics Ophthalnoscan 200 with a 15 MHz probe
2) Data precision D 1000 pre amplifer
3) Data 6000 analog-digital converter
4) IBM At personal computer 30 Mbyt hard disk

To measure the thickness of the lens along the optical axis, we used the same technique previously described, but with a 15 MHz probe, we increased the resolution from 0.2 to 0.1 mm.

The measurements were obtained electronically with an accuracy of +/−0.001 μsec.

With this technique 37 normal lenses and 98 lenses with mild opacities were examined; the visual acuity was never worse than 20/30.

Eyes of patients with glaucoma, diabetes or abnormal axial eye length were excluded from this study [2].

All the patients were examined after dilation with cyclopentolate eye

138

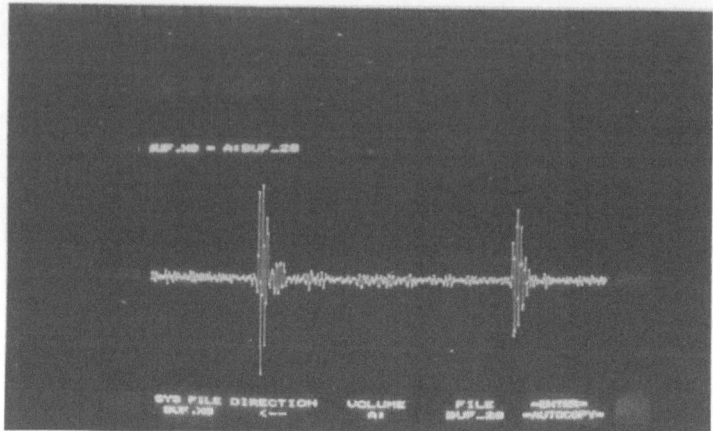

Fig. 4. Echogram obtained from a normal lens along the axial eye length utilizing R.F. signal.

drops, 2 drops every 10 minutes for 1/2 hour, to avoid mistakes due to the accomodation.

For each eye 10 measurements were obtained, and never was found a difference greater than 0.01 μsec (Fig. 4).

Results

The thickness of the lens in normal eyes was similar to that of the group studied with standardized A-scan echography, and the distribution was even less wide (Fig. 5).

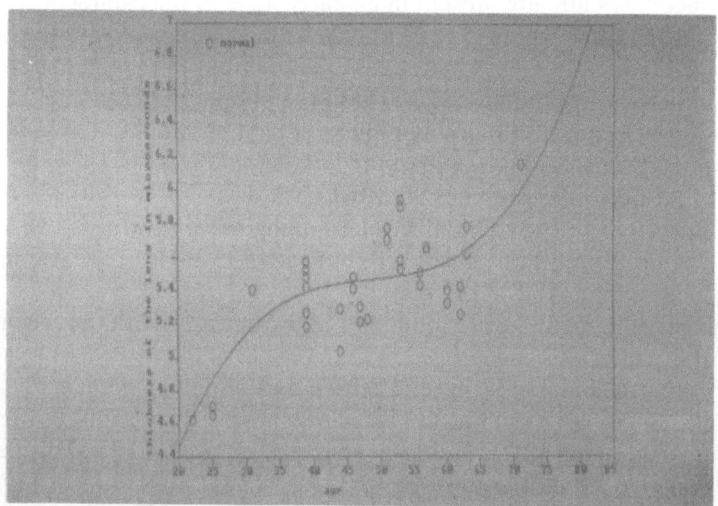

Fig. 5. Thickness of normal lenses in μsec, related to the age, obtained with R.F. signal.

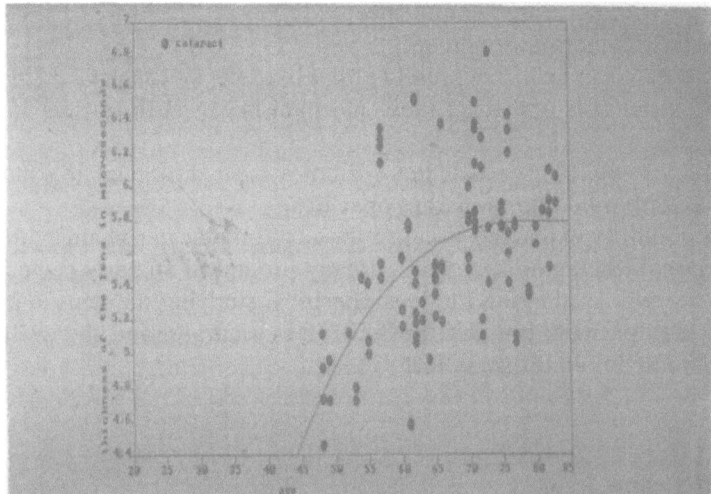

Fig. 6. Thickness of cataractous lenses in μsec, related to the age, obtained with R.F. signal.

In lenses with mild opacities the distribution is much more randomized, and is similiar to that found in patients with more advanced opacities (Fig. 6).

Conclusions

Opaque lenses can be divided in 3 groups:
1) Lenses with increased sound speed

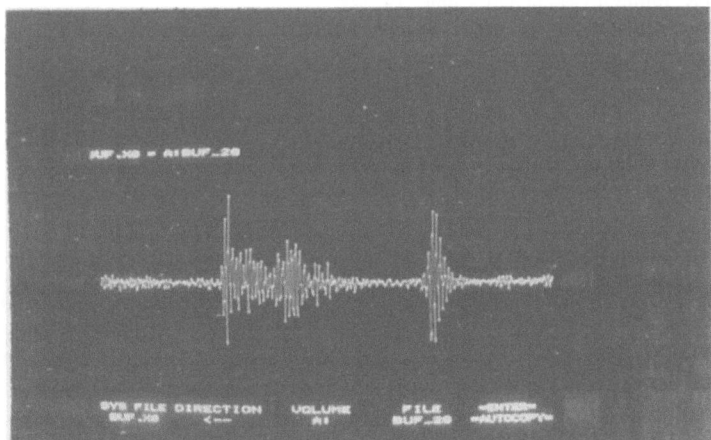

Fig. 7. Echogram from a patient with cataractous lens and visual acuity of 20/70 obtained along the axial eye length with R.F. signal.

140

2) Lenses with decreased sound speed
3) Lenses with normal sound speed

These data confirm the presence of a double mechanism in the pathogenesis of the lens opacities; these mechanism are both present in the 3rd group.

Moreover, we can see that there is not a great difference in sound speed in lenses with mild and moderate opacities.

This could be explained because the macromolecular changes that cause the difference in sound speed are already present in an early stage.

We are also evaluating the lens opacities, studying the acustic interfaces due to the opacities, but this method is less accurate, and the evaluation is possible only in a later stage (Fig. 7).

References

[1] Bonavolonta' A, Cennamo G, Rosa N, Arienzo G, Corvino C. 1986. Controlled Clinical Evaluation of Bendazac Lysine in Senile Cataract: Comparison of Different Tests. Proceedings XXV International Congress of Ophthalmology, Roma.
[2] Cennamo G, Rosa N, Gabai R. 1984. Biometric Evaluation of the Lens in Glaucoma. Proceedings VII S.O.E. Congress, Helsinki.
[3] Cennamo G, Rosa N. 1985. Ecografia e Glaucoma. Proceedings XIX S.O.M. Congress, Capri.
[4] Cennamo G, Rosa N, Daponte P. 1986. Studio Ecografico del Cristallino Catarattoso. Proceedings 2nd IACRR Int. Congress, Cefalù.
[5] Gallenga P E, Cennamo G. Indicazioni dell'esame ecografico nella pseudofachia. In: Manuale di Lenti Intraoculari (ed) Medicina Internazionale.
[6] Loffredo A, de Lellis A, Cennamo G. 1983. Ultrasound Velocity in Different Types of Lens Opacities. Hillman J S, Le May M M (eds) Ophthalmic Ultrasonography. Dr. W. Junk Publishers, The Hauge/Boston/Lancaster.
[7] Ossoinig K C. 1979. Standardized echography: basic principles, clinical applications and results. Internat Ophthalmol Clinics 19: 127.
[8] Pallikaris I, Grüber H. 1981. Determination of sound velocity in different forms of cataracts. Docum Ophthal Proc Series vol. 29 ed. by Thijssen J M, Verbeek A M, Dr. Junk Publishers. The Hauge pp. 165–169.

17. Formulas and results of intraocular lens implantation

H. GERNET

The optical eye length cannot be measured by ultrasound because the macular cones do not respond to ultrasound. Given an apopropriate equipment the only measurable distance by ultrasound is the distance to the inner retinal surface, i.e. the inner eye length. To add 0.2 mm to the inner eye length gives us the optical eye length.

In our measuring technique this addition has nothing to do with a fudge factor, it is necessary. For clinicians it would be very helpful if all available ultrasound equipments would work this way even in long eyes.

The theoretical formula

$$D_L = \frac{n - L \times D_C}{(L - d) \times (1 - \frac{d \times D_C}{n})}$$

(Gernet, Ostholt, Werner, 1970)
equal to

$$P = \frac{N}{L - C} - \frac{NK}{N - KC}$$

(Sanders, Retzlaff, Kraff, 1982)

Fig. 1.

In Fig. 1 the by Retzlaff, Sanders and Kraff (1982) so called and nowadays 18 years old theoretical (geometrical optical) formula is written above in its original form [1] and below in the 6 years old form published by Sanders, Retzlaff and Kraff [2].

Dunantstr.6, 44 Muenster, FRG

R. Sampaolesi (ed.), Ultrasonography in Ophthalmology 12, 141–143.

The prototype of the second formula type is the well known and widely applied original SRK formula against which I've made objections for 6 years because in short eyes with SRK undesired hyperopias occurs. This was demonstrated in my letter to the editor of the Journal of the American Implant Society in 1983 [3].

After IOL implantation following SRK in certainly some millions of cases Sanders, Retzlaff and Kraff [4] have changed opinion in creating the SRK II formula, recently in 1988. I personally find it a little curious that these autors speak of 'formula generations'. One can see in their figures that Sanders, Retzlaff and Kraff are more than half way back to our so called theoretical formula. Considering our results which would have resulted from SRK I, I have no doubt that they too — in some years and after some other undesired postoperative refractive errors in short and in long eyes — will come back to our geometrical optical formula of 1970 [1].

Preoperative planning and postoperative results (n = 335)			
Deviations			
up to ± 1 D	up to ± 2 D	up to ± 3 D	up to ± 4 D
79,4%	19,1%	1,5%	0%
(266)	(64)	(5)	(0)
98,5%			

Fig. 2.

Figure 2 shows the results of our first 335 early IOL plannings following our geometrical optical formula. The results prove the quality of our results, 98.5% within ± 2 D. Up to now our experiences include more than 2000 IOL plannings following this formula for clinicians and practitioneers.

Further results of our first 197 refractive balances show that our geometrical optical formula in short and in long eyes is superior to the regression formulas including SRK. The same is valid for all in between eye lengths even if the differences are smaller and are therefore more difficult to demonstrate.

Other disadvantages of the regression formulas are the impossibility to make refractive balances and to evaluate preoperatively and therefore to avoid undesired aniseikonias postoperatively. The mathematician S. Zörkendörfer and I developed sophicated computer programs to make the IOL planning easy for eye clinicians and practitioners.

References

[1] Gernet H, Ostholt H, Werner H in Ostholt H, Gernet H, Werner H. 1970. Ein neues Haftschalen-Nomogramm für Aphakie. Sitzungsbericht 122. Versammlung des Vereins Rheinisch-Westfälischer Augenärzte 122: 54–55.

[2] Retzlaff J, Sanders D, Kraff M: 1982. A manual of implant power calculation. 3rd printing, 7: 1982.

[3] Gernet H: 1983. Intraocular lens calculations. Am Intra-Ocular Implant Soc J 9: 195–196.

[4] Sanders D R, Retzlaff J, Kraff MC: 1988. Comparison of the SRK II formula and other second generation formulas. J Cataract Refract Surg: 14: 136–141.

18. Axial length measurements and IOL power calculations in microphthalmic eyes

H. JOHN SHAMMAS

Summary

The two eyes of 58 year old man with microphthalmia measured 16.4 mm, requiring a 41.5 diopter lens for emmetropia. The right eye was pseudophakic with a 21.5 diopter posterior chamber lens in place, that has resulted in a 20.00 diopter error. This was due to an erroneous measurement of the axial length and the use of a regression formula.

Introduction

Measurement of the axial length is an integral part of intraocular lens (IOL) power calculations prior to cataract surgery. In large series the axial length was rarely found to be shorter than 19.5 mm [1–3]. We report, herein, a case of bilateral microphthalmia with very short axial lengths, necessitating high power intraocular lenses for emmetropia

Case report

This 58 year old man has been aware of his eye problems since early childhood. Through the years, he has been extensively evaluated at major university centers and was diagnosed to have bilateral microphthalmia, high hyperopia and a delineated form of retinitis pigmentosa.

Six weeks earlier, he had undergone a phacoemulsification cataract extraction with primary implantation of a 21.5 diopter posterior chamber lens that has resulted in a post-operative refraction of +10.75 +0.50 × 180° improving his vision to 20/50. His visual acuity was 20/100 in the left eye with +10.50 +0.75 × 15°. The corneal diameter was 9.5 mm vertically and

Department of Ophthalmology University of Southern California, Los Angeles, California, USA

R. Sampaolesi (ed.), Ultrasonography in Ophthalmology 12, 145–148.
© *1990. Kluwer Academic Publishers, Dordrecht·*

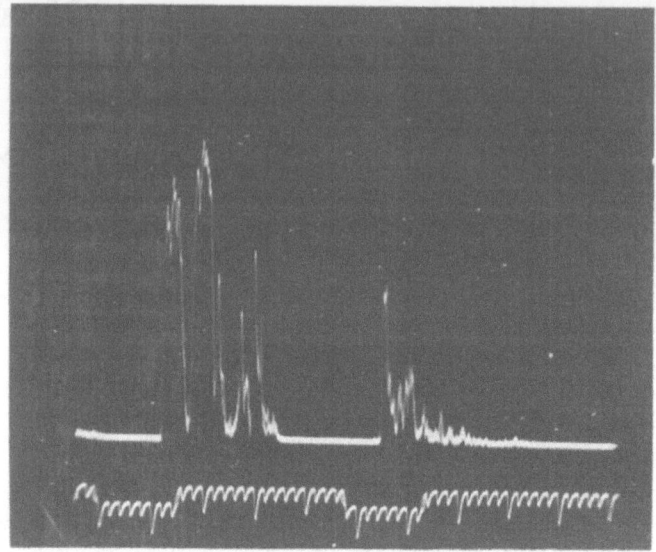

Fig. 1. (Shammas): A-scan measurement of Axial length.

horizontally in both eyes. He was referred to our office for IOL power calculations.

Bilateral axial length measurements were performed with the Kretz 7200 MA ultrasound unit using an immersion technique [4]. Both eyes measured 16.4 mm (Fig. 1) with keratometric readings of 51 diopters. The anterior chamber depth measured 2.9 mm, the lens thickness 4.0 mm and the vitreous cavity 9.5 mm. We used the Shammas modification of Colenbrander's formula. Both eyes were found the need 44 diopter lenses for emmetropia. Due to the microphthalmia and the unusual high hyperopia, we recommended a conservative use of 38 diopter lenses.

The referring ophthalmologist operated first on the left eye, removing the cataract and inserting a 38 diopter posterior chamber lens. Two months later, he removed the wrong implant from the right eye and replaced it, also, with at 38 diopter lens. The final refraction was +1.50 sphere in both eyes.

Discussion

High hypermetropia exceeding +11 diopters is extremely rare and is usually associated with microphthalmic deformities [5]. In our patient, the diagnosis of microphthalmia was based clinically on the small corneal diameter and the deep-set eye appearance. The hyperopia in our patient was not as high as in other reported cases [5]; this was due to the partial emmetropizing influence of the associated steep corneas.

Table 1. Measurement of the different ocular compartments in mm.

	Microphthalmia	Average eye
AC depth	2.9	3.5
Lens thickness	4.0	4.4
Vitr. cavity	9.5	15.6
Axial length	16.4	23.5

Echography confirmed the diagnosis of microphthalmia by measuring short axial length in both eyes (Fig. 1). The small anterior chamber depth, short vitreous length and small corneal diameters are characteristic of a harmoniòus nanophthalmos; it presumably results from arrested development of the globe, sometime after the seventh week of gestation [6]. Table 1 shows a comparison between the different ocular compartments in our patient and an average 23.5 mm eye [1]. Although the anterior segment is slightly shallower in the microphthalmic eye, the major decrease in size is in the posterior segment. Nanophthalmos contrasts with a newly described category of posterior microphthalmia where only the vitreous cavity is shortened while the corneal diameter and anterior chamber depth are normal [7,8]. In extreme cases, microoophthalmic globes are markedly reduced in size and are associated with other structural anomalies.

Intraocular lens power calculations in microphthalmic eyes present special problems due to the extreme shortening of the axial length and the lack of data in such cases. In our patient, a 38 diopter lens was used, yielding a refraction of +1.50 diopters. The exact IOL power needed for emmetropia was recalculated using the available postoperative data and was found to be 41.5 diopters. Table 2 shows the calculated power for emmetropia for our patient using the different available formulas. Theoretical formulas predict stronger power lenses; second generation formulas (Shammas) [9] are more accurate than the first generation formulas (Binkhorst) [10]. On the other hand, the S.R.K. [11] and the S.R.K. II [12] linear equations predict much weaker lenses.

Table 2. IOL power calculations using different formulas.

Formulas	Calculated IOL for emmetropia	Actual IOL for emmetropia	Difference
Binkhorst	50.00	41.50	+8.50
Shammas	44.00	41.50	+2.50
SRK	30.00	41.50	−11.50
SRK II	33.00	41.50	−8.50

The IOL power calculations performed in the referring ophthalmologist's office resulted in an 11 diopter postoperative refraction surpise after the first operation. A 21.5 diopter lens was used instead of a 41.5 diopter. The 20

148

diopter lens power error is due to a wrong axial length measurement and the use of the SRK formula:

1. The eye measured 20 mm instead of 16.4 mm. The technician used a contact technique and had problems identifying the echospikes. Since no representative pictures were taken, one can only postulate that the measurement was taken between the corneal and some scleral or orbital spike instead of the retinal spike. The longer axial length measurement is responsible for approximately 8.5 diopters lens power error.

2. The use of the SRK formula is responsible for approximately 11.5 diopter lens power error (Table 2) for a total error of 20 diopters.

Although microphthalmia and high hyperopia are relatively rare, it is inevitable that some of these eyes will develop cataracts and will undergo implant surgery. Surgeons should be aware of the extremely short axial length associated with microphthalmia and the need of high power intraocular lenses for emmetropia.

References

[1] Shammas H J. 1987. A-Scan Biometry of 1000 cataractous eyes. Documenta Ophthalmologica 48: 57–63.

[2] Goes F. 1987. Biometry of lens implantation in the capsular bag. Documenta Ophthalmologica 48: 51–55.

[3] Hoffer J J. 1980. Biometry of 7500 cataractous eyes. Am J Ophthalmol 90: 360–368.

[4] Shammas H J. 1984. *Atlas of Ophthalmic Ultrasonography and Biometry*. The C. V. Mosby Co., St. Louis. pp. 276–285.

[5] Fledelius H C, Rosenberg T. 1987. Extreme hyperopia and posterior microphthalmos in three siblings. An oculometric study. Documenta Ophthalmologica 48: 87–91.

[6] Cross H E, Yoder F. 1976. Familial nonophthalmos. Am J Ophthalmol 81: 300–306.

[7] Boynton J R, Purnell E W. 1975. Bilateral microphthalmos without microcornea associated with unusual papillomacular retinal folds and high hyperopia. Am J Ophthalmol 79: 820–826.

[8] Spitznas M, Gerke E, Bateman J R. 1983. Hereditary posterior microphthalmos with papillomacular fold and high hyperopia. Arch Ophthalmol 101: 413–417.

[9] Shammas H J F. 1982. The fudged formula for intraocular lens power calculations Am Intraocular Impl Soc J 8: 350–352.

[10] Binkhorst R D. 1975. The optical design of intraocular lens implants. Ophthalmic Surgery 6: 17–31.

[11] Sanders D R, Kraff M C. 1980. Improvement of intraocular lens power calculation using empirical data. Am Intraocular Implant Soc J 6: 263–267.

[12] Sanders D R, Retzlaff J, Kraff M C. 1988. Comparison of the SRK II formula and other second generation formulas. J Cat Refr Surg 14: 136–141.

19. Ultrasound diagnosis of unilateral axial myopia

H. JOHN SHAMMAS

Summary

Seven patients presenting for cataract surgery were diagnosed by ultrasonography to have Unilateral Axial Myopia in the cataractous eye. Bilateral axial length measurements revealed a difference of 4.5 to 6.7 mm between the two eyes. All patients were amblyopic in the cataractous eye and ultrasonography established the correct diagnosis, preoperatively.

Introduction

Axial length measurements and intraocular lens power calculations have become an integrated part of cataract preoperative workup. They have enabled ophthalmic surgeons to avoid large postoperative refractive errors due to an erroneous choice of the implant power [1]. We herein present seven patients with unilateral mature cataracts that have been diagnosed by ultrasonography to have Unilateral Axial Myopia in the cataractous eye.

Material and methods

We reviewed seven cases of Unilateral Axial Myopia examined in the past five years. All patients were examined because of a decreased vision in one eye and were found to have a mature cataract in that eye. We compiled the following information:
– Patient's age and sex;
– Eye involved;
– Bilateral axial length measurements;
– Implant needed for emmetropia;
– Pre- and post-operative vision.

Department of Ophthalmology, University of Southern California, Los Angeles, California, USA

R. Sampaolesi (ed.), Ultrasonography in Ophthalmology 12, 149–154.

150

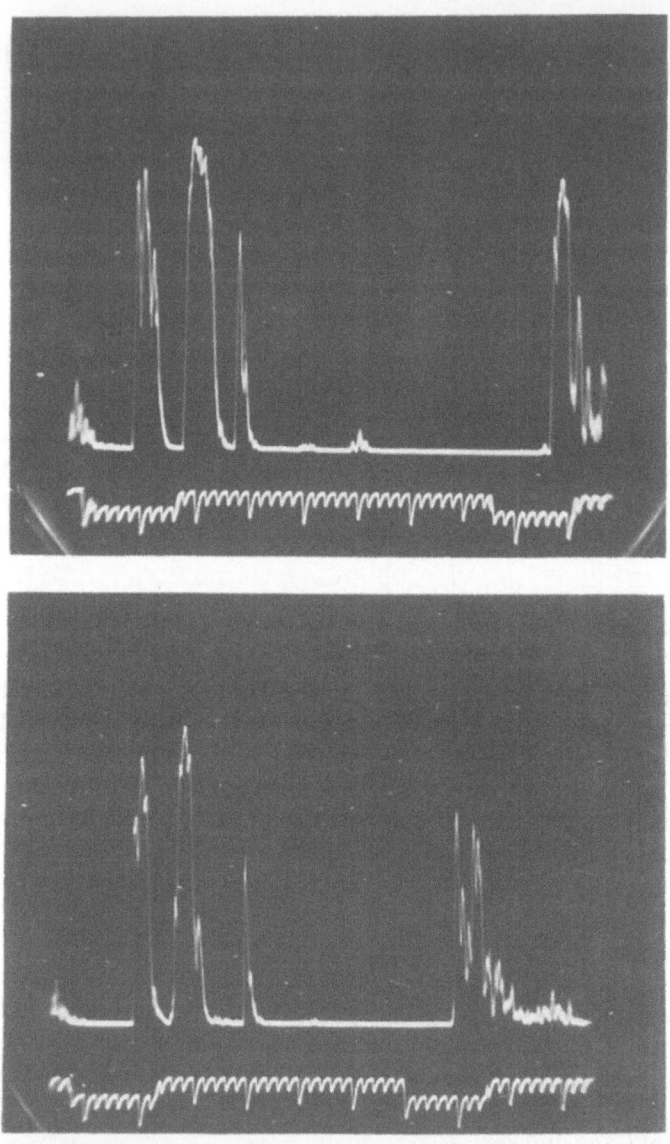

Fig. 1. A-scan echograms in a case of Unilateral Axial Myopia showing the increased length of the cataractous eye (1a) compared to the fellow eye (1b).

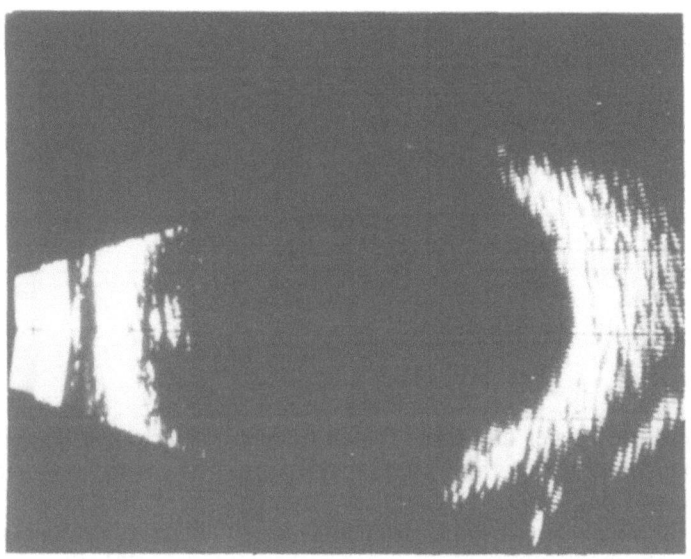

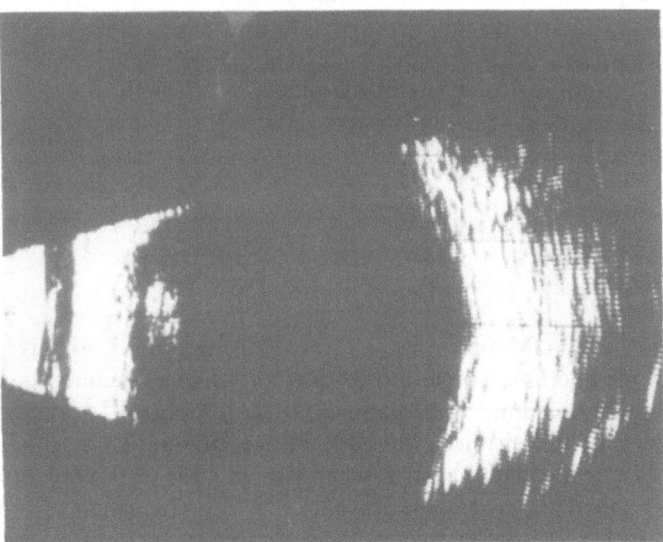

Fig. 2. B-scan ultrasound in a case of Unilateral Axial Myopia showing the increased curvature of the posterior pole in the cataractous eye (2a) compared to the fellow eye (2b).

Table 1. Cataracts in eyes with unilateral axial myopia.

	Cataractous eye		Fellow eye	
	Average	Range	Average	Range
Axial length	28.07 mm	26.0 to 30.2	22.98 mm	21.5 to 24.2
Implant for EMM	6.2 D	−3.9 to 11.0	19.7 D	17.5 to 21.4
Preop vision	HM	LP to CF	20/25	20/20 to 20/30
Postop vision	20/100	20/200 to 20/70	—	—

Results

There were four males and three females. Vision deteriorated rapidly at an average age of 47 with a range of 40 to 55 years. The right eye was involved in 4 cases and the left eye in three.

Bilateral axial length measurements were obtained with the Kretz 7200 MA ultrasound unit using an immersion technique [2]. Figure 1 shows the typical ultrasound pictures of Unilateral Axial Myopia. The difference in axial length (Table 1) between the cataractous and fellow eyes ranged from 4.5 mm to 6.3 mm with an average difference of 5.8 mm. The average implant power needed for emmetropia was 6.2 diopters in the cataractous eyes compared to 19.7 diopters in the fellow eyes. Table 1 shows the range of values. The preoperative vision was light perception in all five cases that underwent surgery. Postoperatively the visual acuity ranged from 20/200 to 20/70.

Discussion

Unilateral Axial Myopia is a rare congenital anomaly, causing anisometropia and amblyopia in the affected eye. It remained undetected in our patients throughout their childhood; they were all presented to our office when they lost vision in the affected eye, due to the progression of the cataract. When the patients were examined for the first time, the myopia was not detected for two main reasons: (1) the patients were not wearing the myopic correction due to the associated anisometropia and amblyopia and (2) The preoperative refraction was unreliable due to the opaque media.

The loss of vision in our patients occurred between the ages of 40 and 55 years. The development of a unilateral cataract in young non-diabetic patients is hard to explain and may be the result of degenerative changes in these highly myopic eyes [3]. Surgery is recommended in spite of the associated amblyopia when the cataract becomes mature and vision drops to light perception. In our patients, it restored isometropia and partial vision;

furthermore, each patient reported an increase in the field of vision by over 20° on the temporal side of the operated eye.

The diagnosis of Unilateral Axial Myopia in eyes with a mature cataract should be made *preoperatively* and the patient informed of the associated amblyopia and possible retinal anomalies. Such a diagnosis necessitates bilateral axial length measurement [4]; in each of our cases, the difference between the two eyes exceeded 4.5 mm. Such a difference can be unsuspected at the time of examination and an uniformed technician will disregard the results, blame it on a difficulty with the A-Scan echograms and record a reading similar to the normal eye. In one case, it resulted in a post-implant refraction of $-18.75 -2.00 \times 180°$ and possible litigation [4]. A B-Scan examination (Fig. 2) and repeated measurements of both eyes will establish the correct diagnosis.

References

[1] Shammas H J. 1984 *Atlas of Ophthalmic Ultrasonography and Biometry*. The C.V. Mosby Co., Publishers, St. Louis.
[2] Shammas H J. 1984. A comparison of immersion versus contact technique for axial length measurement.
Am Intra-Ocular Implant Soc J 10: 444–447.
[3] Perkins, E S. 1979. Morbidity from myopia. The Sightsaving Review 49: 11–19.
[4] Salz J J, Reader A L. 1988. Lens implant exchanges for incorrect power: Result of an informal survey. J Cataract Refract Surg 14: 221–224.

20. Biometry of retina choroid layer

F. CENNAMO*, G. CENNAMO* and P. DAPONTE**

Summary

The authors describe signal analysis techniques in order to detect the echoes in signals with noise. Then a measuring station is illustrated. By means of a polynomial synthesizer, arbitrary echographic signals are simulated, varying the superimposed noise. The improvements obtained with the proposed techniques are shown and compared with the traditional ones.

Introduction

In recent years, the use of RF signal analysis has been increasingly widespread in the ophthalmic field since new electronic equipment has become available [4, 5]. This equipment presents (i) a high sampling rate (100–200 MHz) (ii) digital processing in short time even in complex operations and (iii) wide internal memory.

In the RF signal analysis it is very important to define and to value the noise sources which can occur in the echographic signals [3, 8]. Such noise is due to (i) the eye-probe-echograph complex, (ii) the conditioning and acquisition system, (iii) non-homogeneous tissues and (iv) the presence in the eye of thin membranes (100 μm).

In the present paper the authors show echographic signal analysis techniques in the presence of noise. Such techniques allow:
– the detection in the echographic pattern of single echo sources also with low signal to noise ratio;
– the increase of frequency resolution by using an opportune algorithm.

The measuring station is based on the use of a polynomial synthesizer which allows the simulation of echographic waveforms with superimposed noise. Finally the simulation results are compared with the ones obtained by

* University of Naples, Italy
** University of Calabria, Italy

R. Sampaolesi (ed.), Ultrasonography in Ophthalmology 12, 155–164.
© *1990. Kluwer Academic Publishers, Dordrecht*

working on echographic signals available at the data bank of the Institute of Ophthalmology, II School of Medicine, University of Naples.

Echographic signal analysis techniques

The thin layer measurement can be obtained in the echographic field, either in time domain or in frequency domain. In the first case the time interval between pulses reflected from the anterior and posterior surfaces of the tissue under examination gives immediately the thickness measurement if the sound velocity is known. In the second case, by considering that the power spectrum can be interpreted as a plot of tissue reflectivity vs frequency, the above-mentioned time interval is obtained as the inverse of the difference between two successive frequencies of the power spectrum [6]. So it is very important to set up some algorithms to detect the echoes in the echographic pattern and to compute the power spectrum with great accuracy. With this aim the authors have set up two techniques: Cepstrum and Chirp Z-transform.

Cepstrum

Cepstrum analysis is a technique suitable for the investigation of different arrival times of continuous signals received in a multipath environment.

The Cepstrum of a signal is defined as the power spectrum of the logarithm of the power spectrum of that signal:

$$C(\tau) = \mid F\left[\log \mid F[f(t)] \mid^2\right] \mid^2.$$

The presence of a delayed echo will manifest itself as a ripple in the log spectrum. The 'frequency' of this ripple is easily determined by calculating the spectrum of the log spectrum wherein this 'frequency' will appear as a peak. However, the units of 'frequency' of this ripple in the log spectrum are in units of time; thus, the independent variable (abscissa) in the spectrum of the log spectrum is time [7, 10].

Chirp Z-transform

By using the Fast Fourier Transform (FFT) to obtain a frequency resolution $\leqslant \Delta F$, with a sampling rate equal to $1/T$, $N = (1/T\Delta F)$ points are necessary. So if we want ΔF to be very small a high value of N is required; in addition, such high frequency resolution is required only for a narrow frequency range, while outside this range a lower resolution is acceptable.

With Chirp Z-Transform (CZT), it is possible to define the center frequency and the width of the spectrum to be examined [11]. So CZT permits evaluation of a region of interest of the frequency spectrum and discrimination of details not revealed by lower resolution time to frequency domain processing. In addition, conventional FFT processing imposes a severe limitation on the size of input data: input data length (number of input data points) must equal a value that is a power of two. This limitation causes loss of information and degrades the frequency-domain output, on the coutrary, CZT is not restricted to 'powers of two' processing. The CZT implemented in the proposed measurement station can process any size input data up to 32 000 input points; in addition, it allows a resolution which is 65 times greater, half the processing time in comparison with power spectrum analysis. Moreover CZT has been used with TSENG window, which allows us, by means of four design parameters, to control the pattern falloff rate, the overall sidelobe level, the near-sidelobe level and the depth of a steerable wide dip [9, 13, 14].

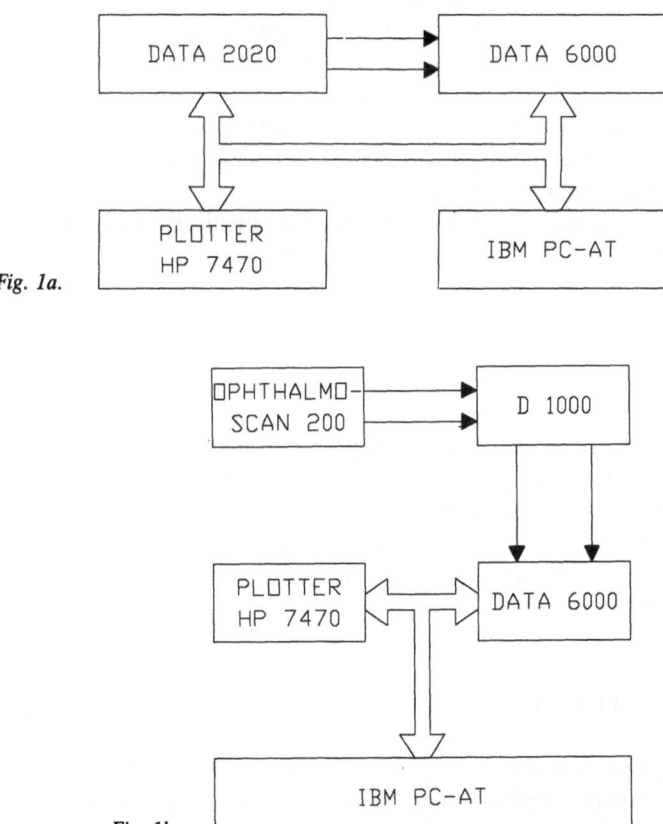

Fig. 1a.

Fig. 1b.

Fig. 1. Block diagram of the measuring station for the acquisition of simulated (a) and real (b) echographic signals.

Measuring station

The proposed measuring station for acquisition and processing of the simulated and real signals is shown in Fig. 1a and b. In the simulation phase (fig.
1a) the station consists of (i)a DATA 2020 polynomial synthesizer [2]
(ii)a DATA 6000 waveform analyzer with 1 MHz—16 bit sampling rate
(iii)a personal computer and (iv)a plotter.

By means of the polynomial waveform synthesizer it is possible to
generate waveforms defined through mathematical formulae [Y(t) = f(t)],
to receive acquired signals from DATA 6000, and to add noise to the
waveform.

So it is possible to simulate the echographic signals to generate the
echographic signals acquired by DATA 6000 adding a noise signal or other
waveforms. In this way we are able to optimize the successive processing
operations. Both DATA 2020 and DATA 6000 are linked, via a standard
interface IEEE-488 to a personal computer.

For acquisition of real echographic signals the measuring station is
configured as shown in Fig. 1b. The echographic signal from an echograph
OPHTHALMOSCAN mod.200 provides the input of an amplifier D1000,
connected to a DATA 6000 waveform analyzer with a plug-in mod 620
(100 MHz—8 bit sampling rate). The DATA 6000 is linked, via standard
interface, to personal computer.

With the proposed measuring station the substitution of the echographic
system is possible, resulting in a considerable improvement in performance
especially with regard to its flexibility. In fact the Data Precision 2020
enables us to easily generate a waveform with specific corrections for transducer and amplifier gains and/or attenuation. Since the Data 2020 uses a
mathematical expression to create a corresponding waveform, it only needs
to know what the transfer function is for system configuration. This information may then be used to amplify and modulate the desired signal (in
water) and correct it to obtain the optimum result.

The technique is also applicable to an ultrasonic transducer and may be
used to optimize signals for specific reasons. This optimization may be the
enhancement of signal penetration by increasing low frequency amplitudes or
improving resolution by increasing high frequency content and amplitude.

Results on simulated signals

Signals representing the echo sequence backscattered from human tissues,
are modulated in amplitude and in phase because of sound interfaces. We
have simulated the echographic signals coming from the eye with the
following formula [12]:

$$s(t) = A(t) *\cos[\varphi(t)],$$

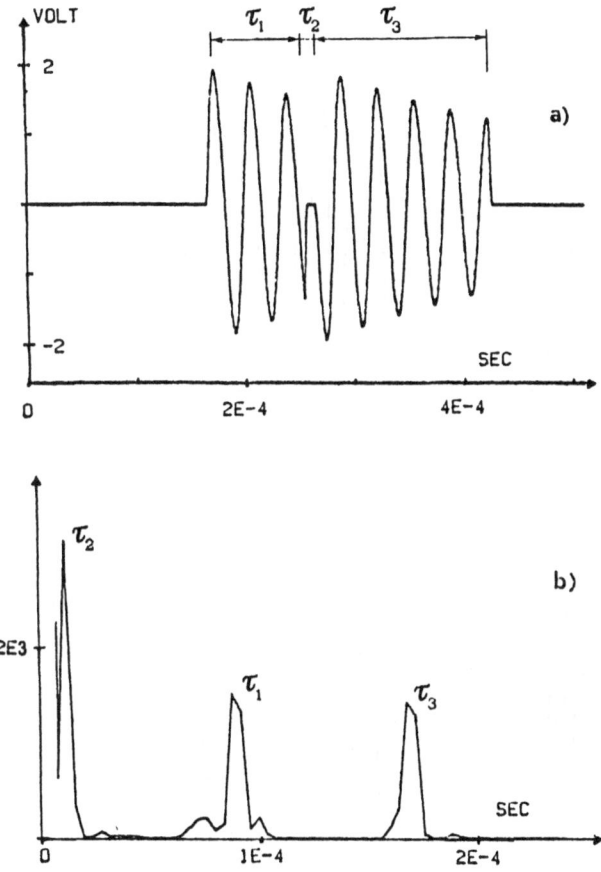

Fig. 2. (a) Simulated signal and (b) its Cepstrum.

where A(t) is the amplitude and φ(t) the phase-angle of the signal. These simulated signals were generated with the DATA 2020 polynomial synthesizer.

Figure 2a shows a simulated signal coming from a human tissue, considering that its thickness is large enough to allow the detection of separation surfaces. In fact, the time interval τ_1 represents the echo coming from the anterior surface, the τ_3 time interval the echo coming from the posterior surface, while τ_2 is the time interval between the two echoes. The second echo has been dephased with regard to the first one to simulate an acoustic impedance variation.

With the analysis of the simulated signal carried out with the use of the Cepstrum (shown in Fig. 2b), we can see clearly the correspondence between

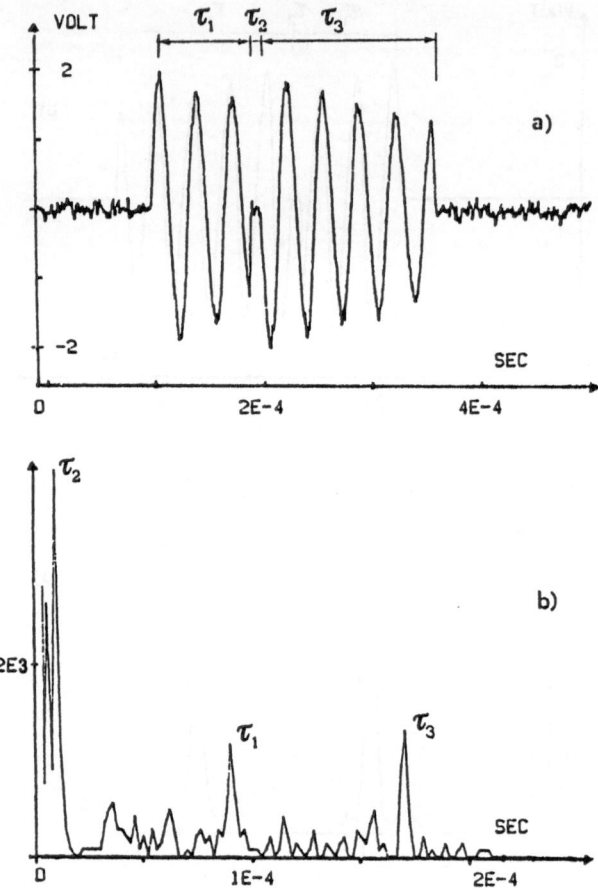

Fig. 3. (a) Simulated signal with noise and (b) its Cepstrum.

the duration of the echoes (τ_1, τ_2, τ_3) and the time intervals obtained with the Cepstrum technique. Several tests have been carried out, varying the signal to noise ratio and the ratio between their bands. Figure 3a and b show the results obtained with the Cepstrum technique on a signal with S/N = 20dB and Bnoise = 2MHz. In addition to this limit, the Cepstrum technique does not allow us to detect with accuracy the duration of the echoes [1].

In Figures 4a and d the results of CZT with Tseng window are reported, which were obtained from the simulated signal with and without noise. These results are compared with the ones obtained with the logarithmic power spectrum (Fig. 4a and c). It is evident that by reducing the signal to noise ratio it is not possible to measure the frequency interval with the logarithmic power spectrum (Fig. 4c, S/N < 5 dB). On the other hand, by using the CZT with Tseng window, it becomes possible to measure the frequency interval (with or without noise).

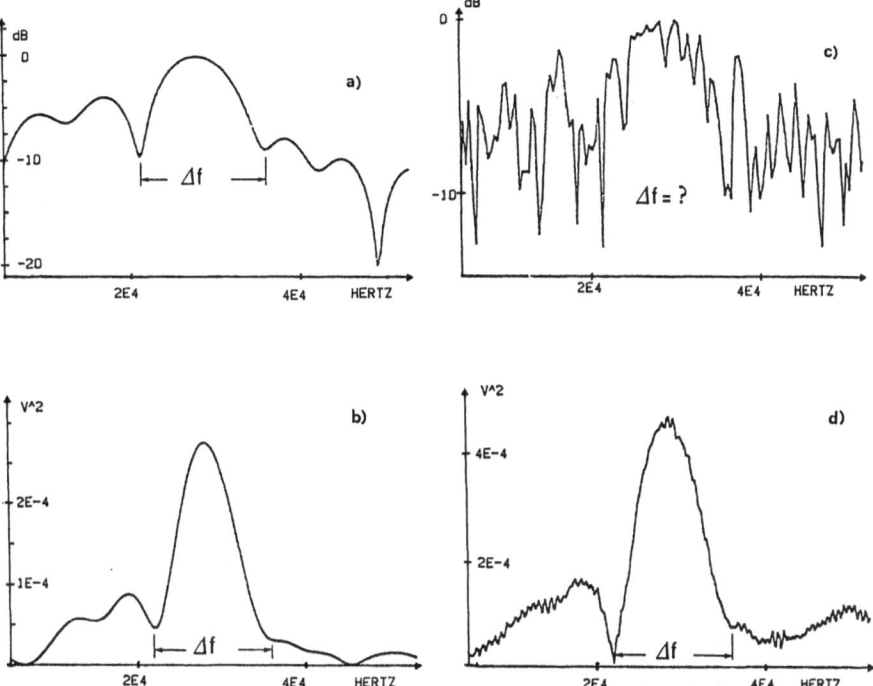

Fig. 4. (a), (c) Logarithmic power spectrum of the simulated signal without and with noise; (b), (d) CZT and Tseng windows applied on the same signal.

Results on real signals

By using the echographic signals of the data bank of the Institute of Ophthalmology — University of Naples, it has been possible to apply the proposed techniques on real signals. In Fig. 5a an RF signal is shown coming from the retina-choroid area, with τ showing the retina time thickness. Figure 5b shows the Cepstrum of the RF signal, related to retina-choroid area. This layout is characterized by a pulse at τ time, from which it is possible to evaluate the retina thickness.

The CZT algorithm has also been applied to the real signals and we have compared the spectra obtained by means of CZT with Tseng (Fig. 6a) and Hamming (Fig. 6b) windows. This comparison shows up as the Tseng window allows an accurate measurement of frequency interval, while the Hamming window, because of noise, does not allow an accurate measurement of the upper limit.

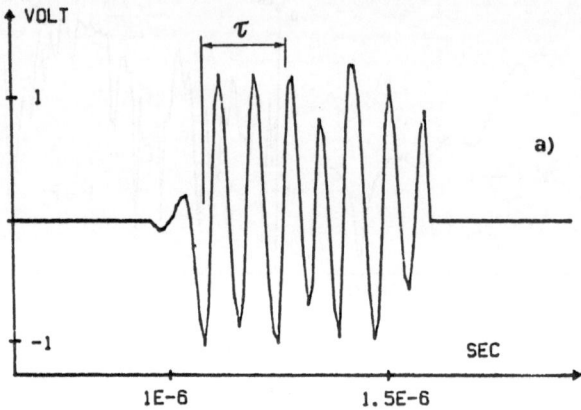

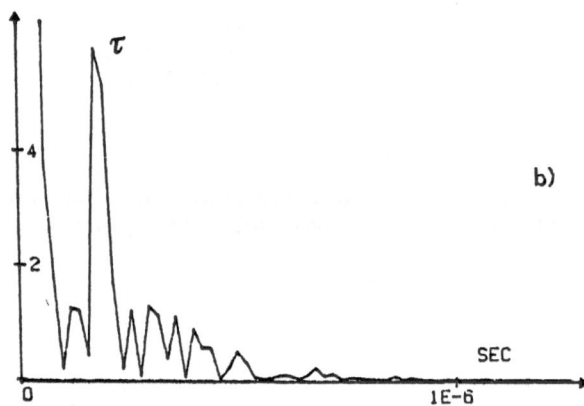

Fig. 5. (a) RF signal coming from the retina-choroid area; (b) Cepstrum of the RF signal, with τ showing the retina time thickness.

Conclusions

The Authors have illustrated some techniques to process the echographic signals in the presence of noise. The Cepstrum technique allows the detection of echoes in the echographic pattern. Moreover by means of Chirp Z-transform and the Tseng window it has been possible to increase the frequency resolution. The use of a polynomial synthesizer has been shown to simulate echographic signals.

The Authors think they can improve these techniques by means of new equipment with a 200–250 MHz sampling rate and with the possibility of

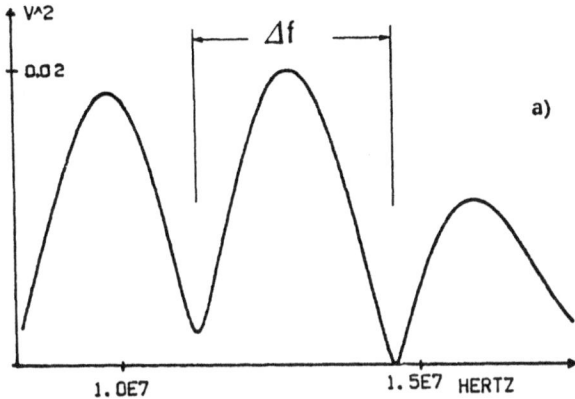

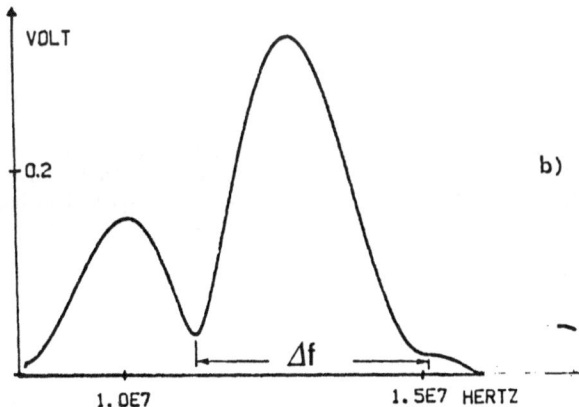

Fig. 6. CZT with Tseng (a) and Hamming (b) windows of the RF signal.

defining memory partitions with low commutation time among such partitions. Initial tests on the techniques and equipment are in progress to obtain further improvements, particularly in the study of successive echogram acquisitions, useful for the classification and analysis of tissue movements and their characteristics, such as ocular muscles and neoplastic masses.

References

[1] Betta G, Daponte P. 1988. Elaborazione ottimale di segnali ecografici in presenza di rumore. Atti della LXXXIX Riunione Annuale Associazione Elettrotecnica Italiana, Capri, (Italy) mem. 1 & 3.

[2] Brodeur L. 1985. Waveform synthesizer relies on equations to define complex signals. Electronic Design, May 16.

[3] Bushmann W, Haigis W, Linnert D. 1981. Influence of equipment parameters on results in ophthalmic ultrasonography. Proc. of 8th SIDUO Congress, W. Junke Publishers, pp. 487–497.

[4] Cennamo F, Cennamo G, Daponte P. 1986. Ocular tissue characterization in vivo by RF signals analysis. Proc of XXV Int. Congress of Ophthalmology, Roma, Kugler Publications, pp. 231–237.

[5] Cennamo F, Luciano A M, Savastano M. 1985. Real time analysis of echographic signal. Proc IMACS Congress OSLO.

[6] Cennamo G, Daponte P, Savastano M. 1986. Retinal biometry by RF signal analysis. Proc 11th SIDUO Congress, Capri (Italy).

[7] Childers D G, Skinner D P, Kemerait R C. 1977. The Cepstrum: a guide to processing. Proc of IEEE, vol. 65, No. 10.

[8] Daponte P, Savastano M. 1986. Noise problems in ophthalmic echography. Proc of 1st IMEKO Symposium on Measurement of Electrical Quantities 'Noise in Electrical Measurement', Como (Italy), pp. 39–44.

[9] Harris F J. 1978. On the use of windows for harmonic analysis with the Discrete Fourier Transform. Proc of the IEEE, vol. 66, No. 1. pp. 51–83.

[10] Kemerait R C, Childers D G. 1972. Signal detection and extraction by Cepstrum techniques. IEEE Trans. on Inform. Theory, vol. IT-18, No. 6, pp. 745–759.

[11] Rabiner L R, Shafer R W, Rader C M. 1969. The Chirp z-transform algorithm and its application. The Bell System Technical Journal.

[12] Seggie D A, Leeman S. 1987. Deterministic approach towards ultrasound speckle reduction. Proc of IEE, vol. 134, No. 2.

[13] Tseng F I, Sarkar T K, Weiner D D. 1981. A novel window for harmonic analysis. IEEE Trans. on Acoustics, Speech and Signal Processing, vol. ASSP-29, No. 2, pp. 177–188.

[14] Tseng F I, Sarkar T K. 1982. Enhancement of poles in spectral analysis. IEEE Trans. on Geoscience and Remote sensing, vol. GE-20, No. 2, pp. 161–168.

21. Eye size of the premature infant around presumed term

HANS C. FLEDELIUS

Summary

Seventy-three premature infants were born at conceptional age 25–37.5 weeks (birth weight 728–2620 g) and examined ophthalmologically, including ultrasound oculometry, at conceptional age 36–54 weeks (mean 41.9 weeks). Axial length averaged 17.08 in girls (n = 33) and 17.38 mm in boys (n = 40).

With axial length on ordinate and conceptional age at examination on abscissa, the regression line was given by y = 12.40 + 0.116 × (r = 0.60). Using this measure for adjusting axial length to a 40 week value, the estimated mean term-value for girls became 16.90 mm and for boys 17.14 mm. This is close to previous results published for full-term infants, as reviewed for instance by Francois and Goes (1981).

Those having had signs of retinopathy of prematurity did not significantly differ from the rest of the sample except for a trend to more negative refractive values. Nine ROP girls had an adjusted 40 weeks axial length mean value of 16.75; in 10 boys with ROP it was 17.23 mm.

For the whole sample, thicker lenses and more shallow anterior chambers have contributed to the predominantly negative refractive values encountered. In most cases emmetropia or hypermetropia ensued, after weeks or months. Thus we are not dealing with the entity of myopia of prematurity in such cases.

As a consequence of the more foetal proportions of the eye, the marked correlation between axial length and refraction, so well-known from children and adults, could not be demonstrated in the present sample.

Summing up, the aim of the study is (1) to re-evaluate eye size in infants around term, and (2) to investigate the influence of short gestational age, low birth weight, and retinopathy of prematurity on eye size around presumed normal term. For the above purposes full-term infants are being included for comparison, but these results are not ready yet.

Hillerød, Denmark

R. Sampaolesi (ed.), Ultrasonography in Ophthalmology 12, 165–172.
© 1990. Kluwer Academic Publishers, Dordrecht

In ophthalmic literature there are indications of smaller eye size being a feature of children surviving the hazards of premature delivery (Fledelius, 1976, 1982).

Firstly, eyes with blinding cicatricial retinopathy of prematurity (ROP) are deep-set and small (Francois and Goes 1971; Bertenyi and Fodor, 1981). This is due to a combination of arrested growth and secondary involution. Many such eyes have axial lengths of 13–15 mm (Fledelius, 1988), which means a return to the size they had at the time of the premature birth.

Next, some infants show almost complete regression of their ROP, eventually to leave an eye with fair vision and 'myopia of prematurity'. Such eyes are shorter than expected from degree of myopia when compared to subjects of the same age with ordinary juvenile myopia (Fledelius 1976; 1977; Tane et al., 1979).

Finally, also seemingly normal eyes of low-birth weight children have shown features of arrested growth when compared to full-term controls, both at the age of ten years (Fledelius, 1976) and at follow-up 8 years later (Fledelius, 1982). This implies that premature birth as such may be regarded a trauma even for eyes that develop normally. Apparently, the ex-prematures never quite catch-up, a view at variance, however, with previous observations by Grignolo and Rivara (1968). Except for the publications quoted only little has been published about eye size and low birth weight.

Accepting a general eye size deficit in those prematurely born, the question is: How early does it happen? How early can we state it? One might assume it to be associated with—and possibly get apparent already after—the first few stormy months of life, so very decisive for survival of the immature infant. Examining eye size in such infants around their scheduled (normal) term might give a clue hereto.

The present paper is a report on such recordings. As part one of an ongoing investigation it is to be followed by oculometry findings in a control sample of full-term infants.

Material and methods

In the neonatal unit of the County Central Hospital premature infants have regular ophthalmic controls up to the age of 10–12 weeks when (1) gestational age at delivery is < 35 weeks; (2) birth weight is < 1800 g; or (3) infants above these limits, but having required oxygen therapy for more than 24–48 hours.

After discharge the infants are controlled in the eye clinic. Here it is possible to supplement the serial evaluations by ophthalmoscopy (after Mydriacyl 0.5% twice, with Phenylephrine 5% added in cases of poor dilatation) with retinoscopic and ophthalmoscopic determination of refractive value, and to perform axial ultrasound oculometry (Sonometrics 400 DBR, 12.5 Mc solid-tip transducer) provided the infant is not too agitated. With

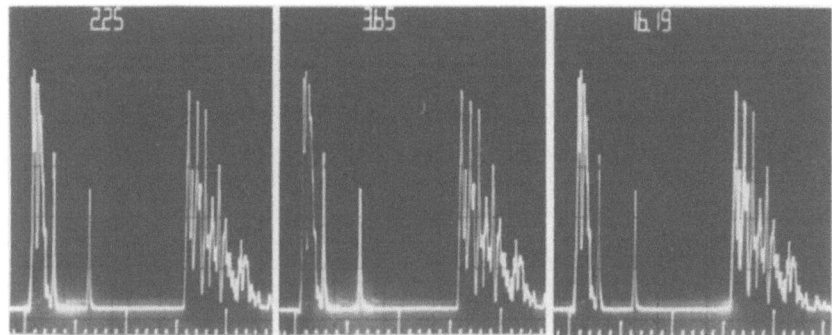

Fig. 1. Axial echogram from a premature infant, frozen on the screen. Uncorrected digital readings are shown for anterior chamber depth (left), lens thickness, and full axial length (right), with reference to the standard velocity setting 1550 m/sec of the equipment, cf. text.

some patience one may freeze suited axial echograms on the screen (Fig. 1) and make recordings with fair reproducibility.

The digital ultrasound recordings have been adjusted for the differences between the equipment's standard mean velocity setting of 1550 m/sec and the established values of 1532 m/sec for anterior chamber and vitreous, and 1641 m/sec for the lens.

The present sample comprises the 73 prematurely born infants in whom satisfactory ultrasound measurement could be performed, in the period from November 1985 to April 1988. Gestational age at delivery (Finnström score, range 25–37.5 weeks) is shown in Table 1 for the 33 girls (mean 32.5 weeks,

Table 1. Conceptional age (in weeks) at delivery (= gestational age, left, shown for the two sexes) and at the oculometric evaluation (right, with the two sexes pooled).

Gestational age, in weeks	All, n = 73	girls, n = 33	boys, n = 40	Conceptional age at examination, in weeks All, n = 73
24–25.9 w	1		1	
26–27.9	6	3	3	
28–29.9	9	2	7	
30–31.9	8	4	4	
32–33.9	27	11	16	
34–35.9	13	7	6	
36–37.9	9	6	3	5
38–39.9				19
40–41.9				20
42–43.9				13
44–45.9				4
≥ 46 w				12

Table 2. Birth weight distribution in the material.

	All, n = 73	girls, n = 33	boys, n = 40
BW up to 750 g	1	1	1
751–1000	6	1	5
1001–1250	6	1	5
1251–1500	14	6	8
1501–1750	13	8	5
1751–2000	12	8	4
above 2000 g	21	8	13

Table 3. Refractive distribution in the sample.

Refraction	−8	−7	−6	−5	−4	−3	−2	−1	0	+1	+2
n = 73	1	0	4	1	7	7	6	11	21	10	5

Table 4. Gestational age, birth weight, age at examination, refraction, and ultrasound measurements, given by mean value, standard deviation (in parenthesis), and range. The sample is subdivided by sex (left) and by the presence of retinopathy of prematurity (right;* selection, see text).

	girls n = 33	boys n = 40	with ROP n = 19	No ROP n = 19*
Gestational age	32.5 (2.93)	31.7 (2.97)	28.6 (2.14)	31.2 (1.48)
(weeks)	26–37	25–37.5	25–32	28–33
Birth weight	1725 (400)	1626 (488)	1222 (317)	1602 (311)
(g)	728–2620	757–2480	728–1850	995–2086
Age at examination				
(weeks from concept.)	41.5 (3.46)	42.1 (4.01)	41.7 (5.17)	40.1 (1.33)
	37.5–49	36–54	36–54	37.7–43
Refraction	−1.33 (2.25)	−1.24 (2.28)	−2.55 (2.37)	−1.18 (2.12)
(in D)	−8.0 – +2.0	−6.0 – +2.0	−6.0 – +1.0	−6.0 – +2.0
Ant.ch. depth	2.41 (0.26)	2.43 (0.27)	2.36 (0.34)	2.42 (0.19)
(mm)	1.80–2.96	1.77–2.95	1.8–2.95	2.0–2.8
Lens thickness	4.01 (0.13)	3.98 (0.19)	4.05 (0.13)	3.98 (0.13)
(mm)	3.84–4.40	3.55–4.67	3.87–4.40	3.80–4.25
Vitr. length	10.66 (0.61)	10.97 (0.62)	10.79 (0.90)	10.81 (0.49)
(mm)	9.15–12.55	9.87–12.89	9.15–12.89	9.97–11.62
Axial length	17.08 (0.71)	17.38 (0.72)	17.20 (1.08)	17.20 (0.51)
(mm)	15.35–19.0	16.05–19.85	15.35–19.85	16.25–17.97
Ax. length at term	16.90 (0.63)	17.14 (0.52)	17.00 (0.70)	17.19 (0.52)
(AL 40w, mm)	15.64–18.22	15.93–18.23	15.64–18.25	16.20–18.22

SD 2.93) and 40 boys (mean 31.7 weeks, SD 2.97) of the sample. With the two sexes pooled, the table further shows the conceptional age when actually examined. In girls, the range was 37.5–49 weeks, in boys 36–54 weeks; mean values were 41.5 (SD 3.46) and 42.1 (SD 4.01) respectively.

Table 2 gives the birth weight distribution (mean BW in girls 1752 g, SD 400; in boys 1626 g, SD 488; total range 728–2620 g).

Nineteen infants had early ROP changes up to stage 2–3, however with regression in all. Thus there were no cases of cicatricial RLF, or other major eye abnormalities, included.

Results

Refractive range was −8.0 to +2.0D. The mean value in boys was −1.33D (SD 2.25) and in girls −1.24 (SD 2.28). The refractive value distribution at examination is shown in Table 3.

In Table 4 (left columns) the ultrasound measurements in the two sexes are given by mean value, SD and range. For the right half of Table 4 a selection had been made of the 19 infants with ROP, 9 girls and 10 boys. As controls, a similar number of girls and boys were included, namely those of the whole sample with the shortest gestational age and no evidence of ROP when serially examined. Except for shorter gestational ages and lower birth weights, the 19 ROP infants and the 19 controls without ROP did not differ

Table 5. Correlation coefficients between gestational age, conceptional age at examination (both in weeks), birth weight (in g), refraction (in D), some axial ultrasound distances (ACD, LT, AL, in mm) and axial length adjusted to term value (AL40w, cf text).

			All n = 73	Female infants n = 33	Male infants n = 40
Age at examination (weeks after conception)	and	AL (mm)	0.60***	0.47**	0.70***
Axial length, at 'term', AL40w (mm)	and	GA (w.)	0.29**	0.52**	0.10
	and	BW (g)	0.15	0.07	0.28
Gest. age (weeks)	and	BW	0.69***	0.74***	0.65***
	and	Refr. (D)	0.24*	0.13	0.33*
	and	LT (mm)	−0.12	−0.36*	−0.01
Birth weight (g)	and	Refr. (D)	0.33**	0.27	0.39*
	and	ACD (mm)	0.23*	0.34*	0.17
	and	LT (mm)	−0.25*	−0.43*	−0.10

r ≠ zero, p < 0.05*, < 0.01**, < 0.001***

much. Only the mean refractive value difference — more myopia in the ROP group — came close to significance (t = 1.88).

Table 5 and 6 show results from correlation analyses including the various parameters under study.

Table 6. Correlation coefficients between refraction (in D) and axial eye distances (in mm). ACD = anterior chamber depth, LT = lens thickness, VL = vitreous length, AL = axial eye length.

		All n = 73	girls n = 33	boys n = 40
Refraction (D)	and ACD (mm)	0.40***	0.61***	0.23
	and LT (mm)	−0.27*	−0.55***	−0.11
	and AL (mm)	0.07	0.35*	−0.16
Ant. ch. depth	and LT	−0.49***	−0.68***	−0.39*
	VL	0.42***	0.45**	0.41**
	AL	0.62***	0.63***	0.62***
Lens thickness	and VL	−0.31**	−0.32	−0.30
	and AL	−0.22	−0.35*	−0.14
Vitr. length	and AL	0.95***	0.96***	0.93***

r ≠ zero, p < 0.05*, < 0.01**, < 0.001***

Discussion

As an initial step in the evaluation the correlation between conceptional age when examined and axial length has been evaluated (Table 5, top). With a correlation coefficient (r) of 0.60 a positive correlation is obvious. The regression line calculated for all 73 infants is y = 12.40 + 0.116 x. The equation signifies that within the age range under study (36–54 weeks from conception) there is an estimated axial length increase of 0.116 mm for every extra week of age attained by the infant before coming to the eye clinic for ultrasound oculometry.

Using this figure it has been possible to adjust all axial length measurements to a fictive 40 week value (AL 40 w), i.e. an estimate of eye size at normal term. Mean values and SD are 16.90 (0.63) and 17.14 (0.52) mm, for girls and boys respectively (Table 4). The correlation between adjusted term value on the one side and gestational age (at delivery) and birth weight on the other side appears in Table 5. There is a trend to suggest a longer axial length term value the higher the gestational age, particularly in girls. The weakness of the trend, however, is underlined by the fact that there are no r-values significantly different from zero when substituting gestational age with birth weight, in spite of the close correlation between these main prematurity parameters.

Table 6 shows the correlation coefficients calculated for refraction and refractive components, here given by the values actually measured. Adjustment to term-values was desisted from due to the far less unambiguous associations to conceptional age than demonstrated for axial length (above).

Commenting only part of the associations, focus will be on anterior eye segment structures. It appears that the shorter the gestational age—and the lower the birth weight—the more negative the refractive value, and the thicker the lens. This shall be weighed against our knowledge of intraocular proportions during the later months of foetal life, with a spheroid lens and a shallow chamber as main features. Subsequently proportions normalize during the first years of life; the anterior chamber gets deeper and the lens gets flatter and of larger diameter.

The lens thus occupies a much larger part of the (shorter) axial distance in the eye of the prematurely born; myopia is encountered more frequently (cf. Grignolo and Rivara, 1968) than in eyes of full-term infants, where positive refractive values predominate (Goldschmidt, 1969; Hosaka, 1988). This is reflected by the mean refractive values given in Table 4. Repeated examinations of premature infants often show that such myopia is fluctuating (Fletcher and Brandon, 1955). This feature may be a combined result of the spheroid lens shape and the difficulty in securing cycloplegia, since strong cycloplegics should not be used in the frail premature infant. There are reports to indicate that even cyclo-pentolate may imply cardiovascular risks (Havener, 1978).

In this context it should be stressed again that the above myopia in prematures is mainly a consequence of the optical geometry at that early age, and that the rule is emmetropia or physiological hypermetropia when seen even a few months after birth. Thus we are not dealing with 'myopia of prematurity' proper, an entity considered a permanent sequel to retinopathy of prematurity having otherwise regressed. Accordingly, this diagnosis can only be made after securing that the early myopia does *not* disappear; from my experience this requires 10–12 months' observation. As mentioned in the introduction, the oculometry findings in 'myopia of prematurity' indicate some arrest of normal eye growth: the axial length is shorter than expected from degree of myopia, the cornea is more curved, the anterior chamber a little flatter and the lens thicker. Oculometrically, all these features suggest that such eyes have retained more of the foetal proportions, in spite of a post-natal growth phase seemingly normal and a good or fair visual acuity.

A final remark about the important role for refraction played by fluctuations in lens thickness and other early anterior segment change. This is reflected also by the poor correlation demonstrated between axial (or vitreous) length and refractive value (Table 6), otherwise the most established correlation in oculometry materials comprising subjects on later age levels.

References

Bertényi A, Fodor M. 1981. A-mode ultrasonography in cases of leukokoria. In: Thijssen J, Verbeek A M (eds) Docum Ophthal Proc Ser 29: 97–102.

Fledelius H C. 1976. Prematurity and the eye (thesis) Acta Opthalmol (Copenh) Suppl 128.

Fledelius H C. 1977. Myopia of prematurity, oculometric considerations. In: White D & Brown R E (eds) Ultrasound in Medicine 3A, Plenum, New York and London, pp. 959–963.

Fledelius H C. 1982. Ophthalmic changes from age of 10 to 18 years, part III anterior eye segment, IV posterior eye segment. Acta Ophthalmol (Copenh) 60: 393–402, 403–411.

Fledelius H C. 1988. Ultrasound imaging in stage 5 ROP. Paper read at SIDUO XII Conf, Aug 1988, Iguazu, Argentina.

Fletcher M C, Brandon S. 1955. Myopia of Prematurity. Am J Ophthalmol 40: 474–81.

Francois J, Goes F. 1971. Ultrasonography in pediatric ophthalmology. J Ped Ophthal 8: 221–33.

Francois J, Goes F. 1981. Ocular biometry. In: Thijssen J, Verbeek A M (eds) Docum Ophthal Proc Ser 29: 135–64.

Grignolo A, Rivara A. 1968. Observation biometriques sur l'oeil des enfants nés a terme et des prématurés au cours de la premiere année. Ann Oculist 201: 817–26.

Goldschmidt E. 1969. Refraction in the human newborn. Acta Ophthalmol (Copenh) 47: 570–78.

Hosaka A. 1988. The growth of the eye and its components. In: Fledelius H C. Goldschmidt E (eds) Myopia workshop Fredensborg 1987, Acta Ophthalmol (Copenh) Suppl 185: 65–68.

Tane S, Ito S, Kushiro H, Kohno J. 1979. Echographic biometry in myopia of prematurity. In: Gernet H (ed) Diagnostica Ultrason in Ophthalmol, Remy Verlag, Münster, pp. 190–94.

22. Choroidal nevi: diagnosis with standardized echography

KARL C. OSSOINIG* and MAREN LOHMEYER**

Introduction

Elevated benign choroidal nevi are among the most frequently encountered 'pseudomelanomas' which clinically mimic malignant choroidal melanomas. These tumors call for an examination with Standardized Ophthalmic Echography in order to safely differentiate them from the malignant melanomas. While there are features typical of choroidal nevi noted ophthalmoscopically, the vast majority of these lesions, when elevated, cannot be differentiated safely from malignant melanomas with ophthalmoscopy, fundus biomicroscopy and fluorescein angiography alone.

Standardized Echography is an important diagnostic tool for the differentiation between benign elevated nevi and malignant melanomas of the choroid. This differential diagnosis all started with a case of an elevated choroidal nevus seen in the Department of Ophthalmology at the University of Iowa in the late 1970s. Because of a highly elevated P32 test, the eye in that patient was enucleated and the diagnosis of a benign elevated choroidal nevus was established histopathologically. Standardized Echography had been obtained prior to enucleation and had produced an echographic pattern clearly different from that of malignant melanomas. This was the starting point for using Standardized A-scan to diagnose elevated benign nevi, to differentiate them from malignant melanomas, and to monitor them carefully through echographic follow-up examinations.

In the Department of Ophthalmology at the University of Iowa, Standardized Echography is applied routinely in all cases of pigmented and non-pigmented choroidal tumors. Since more than a decade, Standardized Echography has now been successfully used to diagnose, differentiate and follow elevated benign choroidal nevi. Many of these elevated benign nevi have not changed in either structure or size over the follow-up period ranging from 1 to 10 years. However, some of the nevi were observed to change into

* Iowa City, USA
** Essen, FRG

R. Sampaolesi (ed.), Ultrasonography in Ophthalmology 12, 173–180.

malignant melanomas echographically. Sofar Standardized Echography has not been found to mislead in this differential diagnosis in a single case.

Differential diagnosis

Elevated choroidal nevi typically provide an echographic pattern in Standardized A-scan echograms, which sets them clearly apart from their malignant counterparts. Table 1 lists these echographic criteria of benign nevi contrasting them to the long established Standardized A-scan criteria of small malignant melanomas as indicated in Table 2. Most significant is the predominantly high internal reflectivity of elevated nevi as evidenced by high internal lesion spikes which are obtained at the Tissue Sensitivity setting of the Standardized A-scan instrument. There are typically one or two small areas within the elevated nevi (often superficially within the tumors) which show clearly decreased reflectivity rendering these tumors' internal structure 'irregular'. This is in contrast to malignant melanomas which have a regular internal structure with persistently low reflectivity, and also to choroidal hemangiomas which have a regular internal structure with persistently high reflectivity.

Table 1. Standardized A-scan criteria of elevated benign choroidal nevi as opposed to malignant melanomas.

Internal Structure:	IRREGULAR
Internal Reflectivity:	PREDOMINANTLY HIGH; one or two small areas of decreased reflectivity near tumor surface are common.
Vascularity:	NON-DETECTABLE

Table 2. Standardized A-scan criteria of small malignant choroidal melanomas as opposed to benign nevi.

Internal Structure:	REGULAR HOMOGENEOUS
Internal Reflectivity:	PERSISTENTLY LOW
Vascularity:	DETECTABLE in more than 95% of the cases

Figure 1 illustrates the classical Standardized A-scan echograms in the case of an elevated choroidal nevus. Figure 2 contrasts these by the standardized A-scan echograms obtained from a small malignant melanoma. Figure 3 shows the B-scan echograms obtained in the case of the elevated choroidal nevus, which, however, cannot be distinguished from the B-scan echograms of the small malignant melanoma (Fig. 4; same case as shown in Fig. 2). The echographic differential diagnosis between benign nevi and malignant melanomas is usually based on the Standardized A-scan findings only.

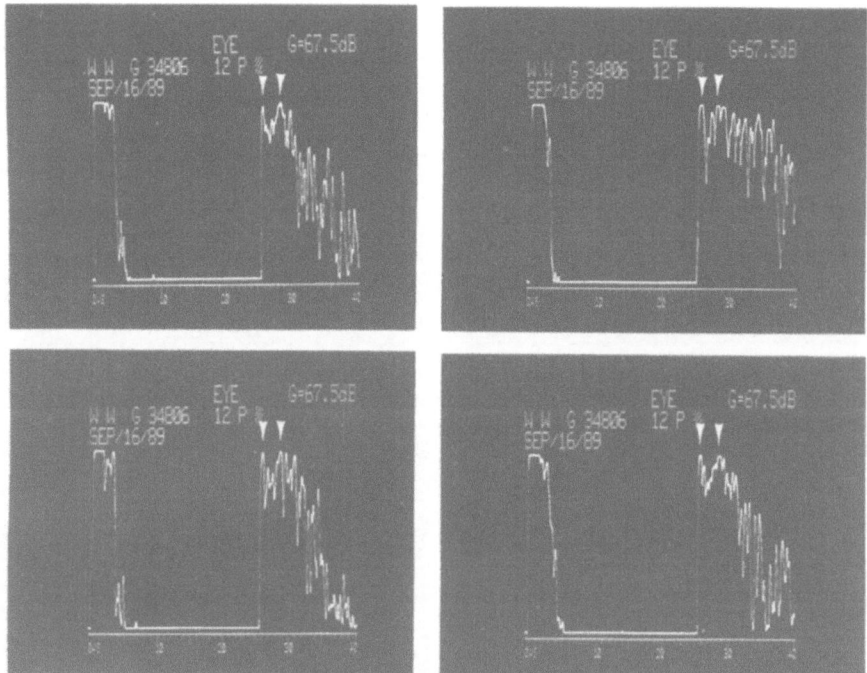

Fig. 1. Four representative Standardized A-scan echograms from a maximally 2.3 mm elevated benign choroidal nevus. The arrows indicate the surface signals obtained from the inner retinal (left) and inner scleral (right) surfaces. Note the high internal reflectivity of the nevus (high spikes between the surface signals). Also note the minor dip in inner lesion spike height near the retinal surface spike in the top right echogram (commonly obtained from one or two small areas of the tumor).

Change into malignant melanomas

In addition to making the diagnosis of benign nevus, Standardized Echography also helps to detect early signs of a change into a malignant tumor during follow-up: a decrease in reflectivity together with a more homogeneous internal structure are usually the earliest signs of a nevus turning into a malignant melanoma. These signs can be found before actual growth in height or in lateral dimensions occurs. At the same time vascularity may be noted for the first time. Once such a change into a malignant melanoma is documented, follow-up examinations at intervals not exceeding 3 months should be performed to early detect growth which should prompt treatment.

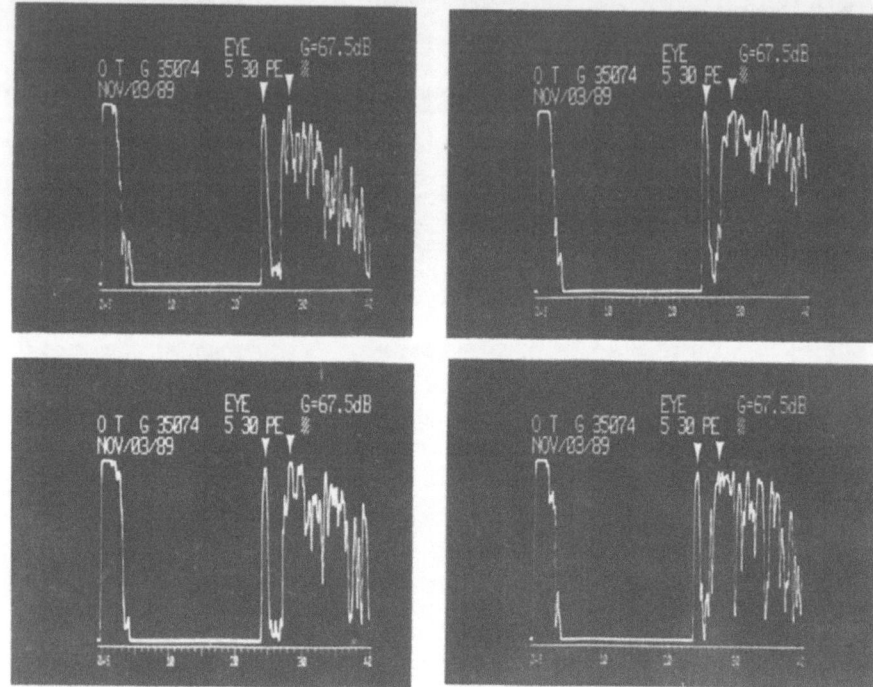

Fig. 2. Four representative Standardized A-scan echograms from a maximally 3.4 mm elevated malignant choroidal melanoma. The arrows indicate the surface signals obtained from the inner retinal (left) and inner scleral (right) surfaces. Note the low internal reflectivity as expressed by the low spikes between the surface signals. The single higher spike immediately preceding the inner scleral surface signal is the so-called posterior tumor spike representing the interface between the densely infiltrated choroidal remnants and the plain tumor cells in front of this layer.

Growth

An accurate and reliable measurement of the maximal tumor height requires the A-scan probe to be placed opposite the tumor location. This implies that a tumor at the posterior pole be measured with the probe placed on the appropriate region of the cornea. This is in contrast to the quantitative evaluation of internal tumor reflectivity, which requires a probe placement behind the limbus even in tumor locations at the posterior pole, in order to avoid sound penetration of the lens which through absorption and refraction would cast acoustic shadows falsifying the quantitation.

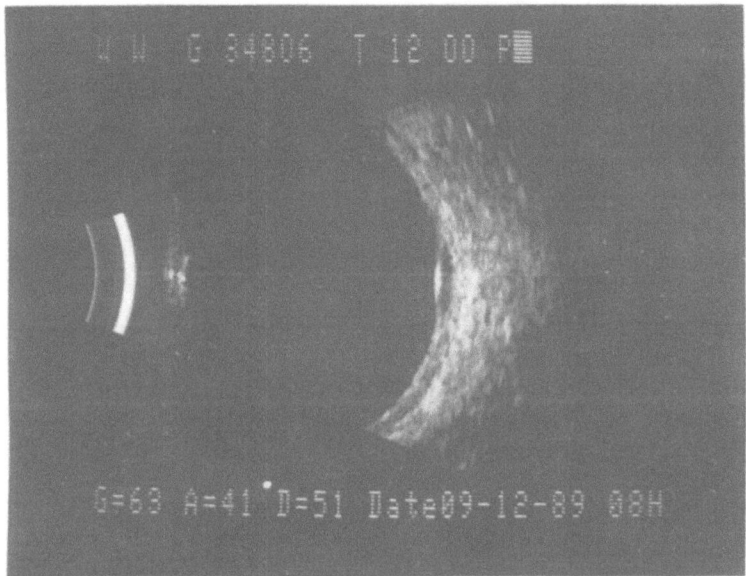

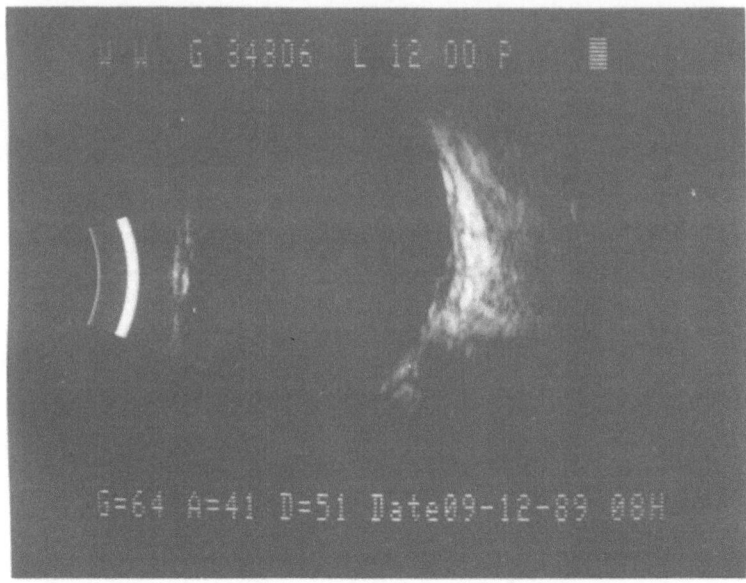

Fig. 3. Transverse (top) and longitudinal (bottom) B-scan echograms from elevated choroidal nevus (same case as in Fig. 1) showing the topographic situation as well as the lateral extent (across the 12:00 meridian in top echogram; along the 12:00 meridian in bottom echogram).

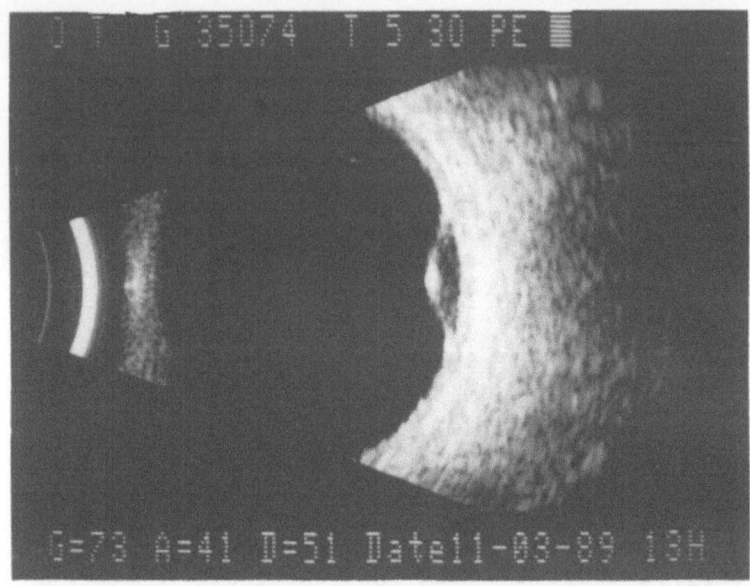

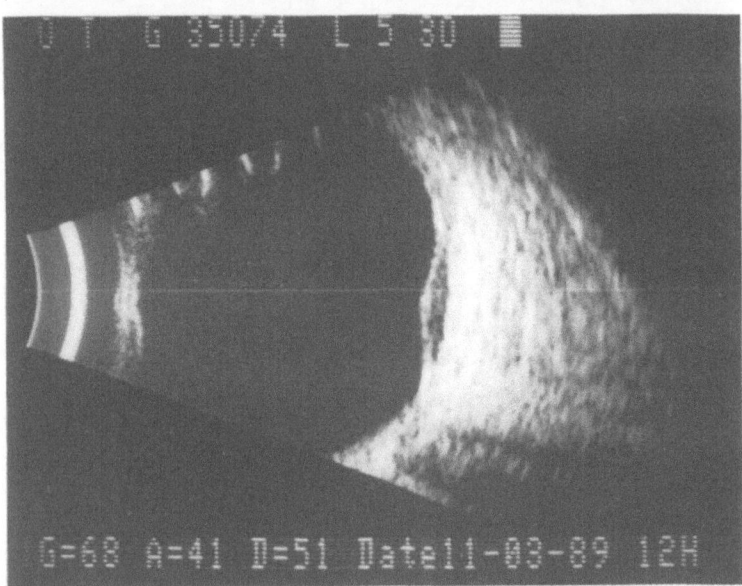

Fig. 4. Transverse (top) and longitudinal (bottom) B-scan echograms from small choroidal melanoma (same case as in Figure 2) demonstrating its topographic relationship and lateral extent.

Unless metastatic carcinoma is suspected or needs to be ruled out, the first repeat examination is done 3 months after the primary examination. If no change is observed, the next follow-up examination is done 6 months thereafter. If again no change is noted the following repeat examinations are performed in yearly intervals. This schedule is followed in all cases of clear ocular media. Naturally, the echographic follow-up examination is done sooner whenever the ophthalmoscopic picture changes suggesting growth of the tumor. It is recommended to follow fundus masses in no longer than 6-month intervals, if reliable ophthalmoscopy is not possible due to opaque ocular media or a fixed narrow pupil.

When following the maximum elevation of an elevated choroidal nevus with Standardized A-scan, one usually has to include the thickness of the overlying retina since only a clear separation of the retina from the tumor by fluid would allow the measurement of the tumor height proper. The retina overlying a choroidal nevus, however, undergoes a variety of changes affecting its thickness. Therefore it is quite common, that the maximal elevation of a choroidal nevus fluctuates over time by up to 0.5 mm. An increase of 0.5 mm or less in height therefore does not necessarily indicate tumor growth and should not alarm the examiner. Most of the time such a lesion will show again a decrease in maximal height during the next regular follow-up examination. Since, however, a slight increase in maximal tumor height may also signal real tumor growth, the examiner is advised to temporarily shorten the interval to the next examination from 1 year to 6 or even 3 months and to carefully check the ophthalmoscopic appearance in the meantime.

Most elevated choroidal nevi and small malignant melanomas are visible ophthalmoscopically. If sufficiently pigmented, these tumors can clearly be classified by Standardized Echography as either benign nevi or as malignant melanomas.

If a choroidal tumor is poorly pigmented or non-pigmented, or if its pigmentation cannot be evaluated due to opaque ocular media, a malignant melanoma can still be either diagnosed or ruled out with Standardized Echography. In the latter case, however, a positive diagnosis of a benign nevus is not possible during an initial examination. Early metastatic carcinoma and atypical (because irregularly structured) disciform lesions must also be considered. (Choroidal hemangiomas have a regular internal structure and thus differ from elevated choroidal nevi by not showing areas of decreased internal reflectivity, see above under *Differential Diagnosis*). Follow-up examinations usually clarify the diagnosis in these cases: disciform leasions tend to flatten out over time, while metastatic carcinomas quickly grow and spread, and early develop exudative retinal detachment (all findings absent in elevated choroidal nevi). Thus even in cases which lack clear pigmentation or where pigmentation cannot be evaluated ophthalmoscopically due to opaque ocular media, elevated choroidal nevi can be positively identified when observed over time.

Thus careful follow-up examinations of elevated tumors with Standardized Echography are important not only to detect the early change from a benign nevus into a malignant melanoma, or to establish growth of a nevus or melanoma, but also to further differentiate poorly pigmented or non-pigmented, non-melanomatous tumors or non-melanomatous tumors in eyes with opaque media thus diagnosing or ruling out elevated nevi under these circumstances.

Extraocular extension

Standardized Echography involving both A-scan and B-scan techniques also is a highly sensitive method for the detection of massive scleral infiltration and of even smallest extraocular growth. Any episcleral tumor growth exceeding 1 mm in size can be detected and identified reliably. Single tumor cells or very small tumor cell aggregates cannot be detected with echography, however. Extraocular growth smaller than 1 mm cannot be distinguished from dilated vessels with certainty. Such minor findings make careful follow-up examinations very important.

Conclusion

Standardized Echography is an important diagnostic tool for the management of elevated benign choroidal nevi: Standardized A-scan helps to diagnose a benign nevus and to differentiate it from malignant melanomas and from other choroidal tumors. The maximum height of the tumor is measured with great precision. Most importantly, a change from benign nevus to malignant melanoma is detected early even before growth occurs. The sclera and episclera behind the tumor are monitored for cellular infiltration with both A-scan and B-scan techniques. The lateral extent of the tumor can be followed with B-scan in case of opaque ocular media.

Acknowledgements

This research was supported in part by an unrestricted grant from Research to Prevent Blindness.

23. Echometry in congenital glaucoma: long-term results after 10 to 17 years of surgery

ROBERTO SAMPAOLESI

Abstract

We have controlled 61 eyes belonging to 44 children, who underwent surgery, with echometry, tonometry, optic disc and visual field with automatic perimetry (Octopus). The follow-up of this group allowed us to distinguish 3 clinical types with a different echometry pattern.

A first one, with complete healing and binocular vision which results in a normal eye. The axial length remains normal for the age.

A second one, at the end looks like an open angle glaucoma with a pathological cupping of the disc and visual field defects. The intraocular pressure was apparently regulated, but the axial length of the eye continued to grow.

And a third group divided into a) where the children came to the ophthalmologist late with a very enlarged eye; and b) where, although at the time they came the axial length was not so big, the time elapsed between the first visit and surgery taking place was so long, that the eye continued to enlarge. In both groups, in spite of having a normal optic disc, they have a macula alteration due to the ocular elongation, and the visual field may show either a central scotoma or a diffuse decrease of the mean sensitivity.

Introduction

When there are symptoms of congenital glaucoma in children from birth until the age of 2, the measurement of the intraocular pressure under anesthesia is often unreliable. For this reason in 1972 we began to measure the AL of the eye as a new parameter for the diagnosis of congenital glaucoma. This is because different anesthetics change the intraocular pressure by either increasing or decreasing it. On the other hand, it is impossible to perform a diurnal pressure curve for a baby [1].

Department of ophthalmology, University of Buenos Aires, Parana 1239–74, 1018 Buenos Aires, Argentina

R. Sampaolesi (ed.), Ultrasonography in Ophthalmology 12, 181–191.

I explained the importance of echometry: 1) in the diagnosis of congenital glaucoma during the VIIIth SIDUO in Nijmegen [2, 3] and 2) in the follow-up [4].

Now I present the results of surgery in connection with echometry, tonometry, visual field, cupping of the disc, etc., in a group of 61 children operated on in the first 2 years of life and whom I followed up during a period of 10 to 19 years. In all of these patients it was possible not only to check the echometry and tonometry but also the visual field with the Goldmann and Octopus perimeters and cupping of the disc.

During the last 30 years we have operated on more than 500 cases of congenital glaucoma.

Seventeen years ago we changed our surgical procedure. Until 1970 we had performed goniotomy and since then [5] trabeculotomy or combined surgery (trabeculotomy + trabeculectomy) according to 2 types of clinical forms:

Type 1

Chamber angle with mesodermal pathological remnants. Axial length up to 23 mm during the first two years of age.

Type 2

Chamber angle with high insertion of the iris and axial length over 23 mm during the first two years of age. The corneal diameter in these cases was over 13.5 mm.

In the first type we performed trabeculotomy and in the second, trabeculotomy plus trabeculectomy (combined surgery).

Material

Sixty one eyes belonging to 44 children, 26 males and 18 females.
– unilateral cases: 14 males, 13 females
– 17 bilateral cases: 12 males, 5 females
– 43 eyes with chamber angle type 1
– 18 eyes with chamber angle type 2.

We performed 32 trabeculotomies and 29 combined surgeries (trabeculotomy plus trabeculectomy).

Follow-up

During the follow-up we studied:
– Date on which signs and symptoms appeared (days or months).

- Time elapsed between the beginning of symptoms and date of surgery (days or months).
- The axial length was measured in milimeters before surgery and throughout the follow-up.
- intraocular pressure was measured with applanation tonometry before surgery and during the follow-up.
- With gonioscopy the chamber angle was classified as: type 1, mesodermal pathological remnants; type 2, high insertion of the iris.
- The corneal diameter was measured horizontally because the lymbus is diffuse both above and below in congenital glaucoma.
- The tears in Descemet's membrane and the endothelium were drawn and classified as central and peripherical.

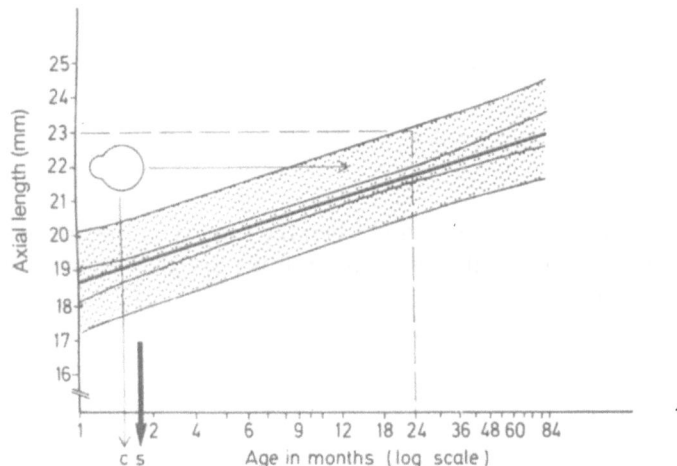

Fig. 1a.

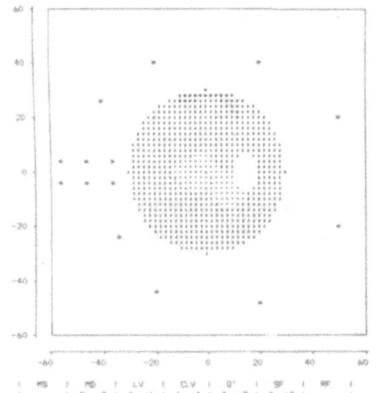

Fig. 1b.

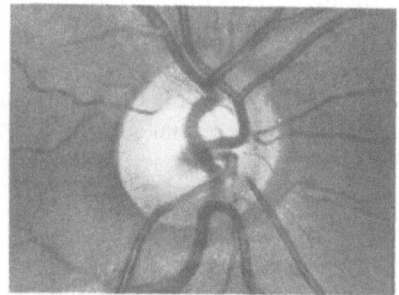

In the follow-up we studied the anatomical and functional results in the optic disc, the macula, the visual field, the vision and the binocular vision.

We compared the refraction (with cycloplegic agents) and the optic correction with the axial length.

Three types of clinical evolutions

It is necessary to bear in mind that the group we are dealing with is not older than 24 months, and at the age of 24 months the maximum normal axial length is 23 mm and the maximum intraocular pressure is not more than 7 to 14 mmHg [6, 7, 8, 9, 10].

Type I

The first type belongs to a group of infants who came during the first 6 months of age. The most important thing is that the parents brought the infant to the ophthalmologist as soon as symptoms appeared, and that the time between the consultation and the surgery was very short, only days or a week (Fig. 1).

Prognosis in cases like these is very good when the surgery normalises the intraocular pressure. The intraocular pressure until the age of 24 months is not more than 14 mmHg.

When we examine the same patient later, between the ages of 10 and 18, we find a normal optic disc, a normal visual field, vision 8–10/10, good binocular vision and stereopsis.

The pathology was ocular hypertension and a small elastic elongation of the eye. When surgery normalises the intraocular pressure, it becomes a normal eye.

Summing up, surgery was performed very early. There was only one functional disturbance: the ocular hypertension due to the congenital mesodermal remnants in the chamber angle which carried out a light enlargement of the eye.

In some cases, whose evolution belongs to type I, the vision is very poor owing to tears of Descemet and endothelium that go across the corneal optic centre.

Although on the corresponding fig. it is showed a normal visual field, in most of the patients of this group there appears a little diffuse depression of the light differential sensitivity.

Type II

The second type corresponds to a group of congenital glaucoma in which, though the diagnosis and surgery were made very early, surgery failed to

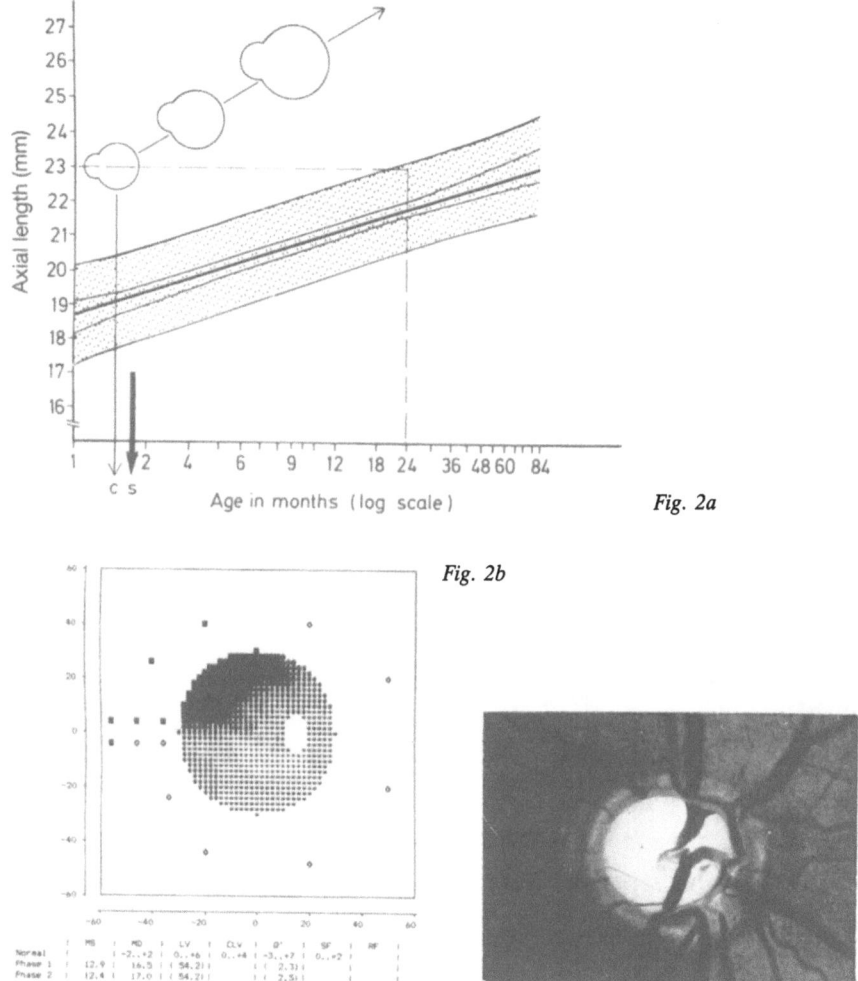

Fig. 2a

Fig. 2b

regulate the intraocular pressure and the length of the eye continued to grow (Fig. 2). Again, if we examine the same patient later, between the ages of 10 and 17, we find a glaucomatous cupping of the disc (6/6), large glaucomatous field defects, a vision between 0.5 and 0.7 or more, generally no binocular vision, and stereopsis. The evolution is similar to that of the open angle glaucoma in adults.

Because the intraocular pressures were not regulated, we sometimes re-operated on these cases. The mistake is to believe that the intraocular pressure at which these eyes remain, 15 to 22 mmHg in the first year of age, is normal. Here it is very important to bear in mind that the maximum normal intraocular pressure at this age is 7 to 14 mmHg.

When we made this mistake, it was in those cases where the child had a 35–40 mmHg pressure before surgery, corneal edema and photophobia, and

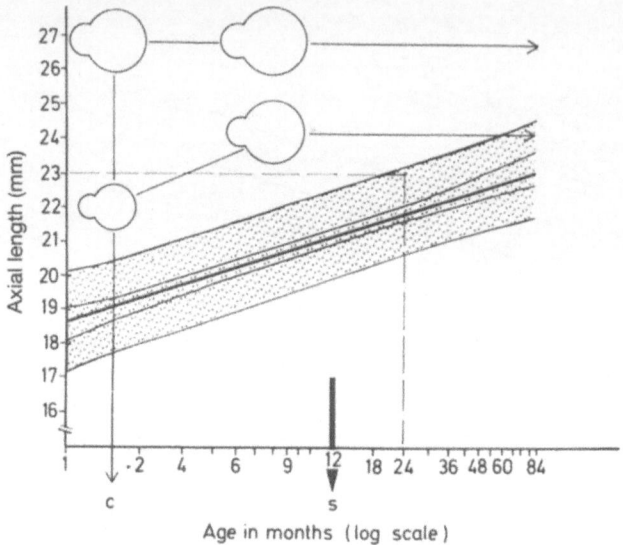

Fig. 3a

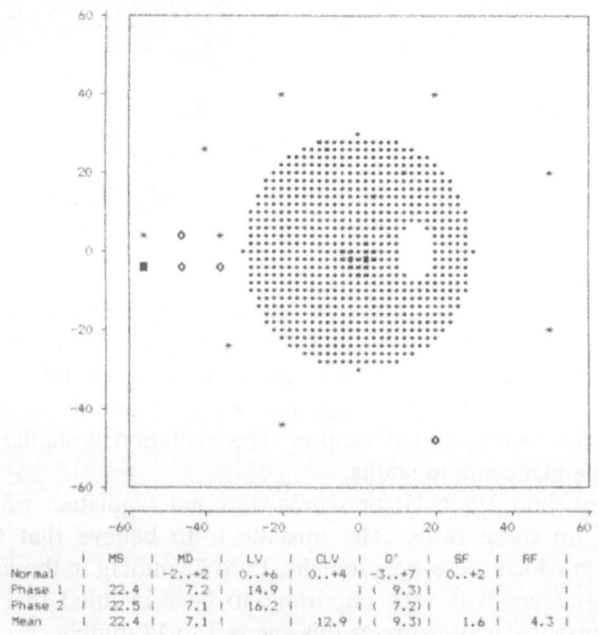

	MS	MD	LV	CLV	D'	SF	RF
Normal		-2..+2	0..+6	0..+4	-3..+7	0..+2	
Phase 1	22.4	7.2	14.9		(9.3)		
Phase 2	22.5	7.1	16.2		(7.2)		
Mean	22.4	7.1		12.9	(9.3)	1.6	4.3

Fig. 3b

after surgery the intraocular pressure remained at 20 mmHg, without any corneal edema or photophobia. The family was very happy with the results and the ophthalmologist, who knows that 20 mmHg is not a normal intraocular pressure, was flattered with the apparent success.

All these children must be re-operated on whenever medical treatment has not regulated the intraocular pressure. (Ocusert is of great help).

Although the visual field observed on the fig. presents a scotoma, this is so because this is a very evolutioned case in which, in spite of having been operated on several times, the pressure was not regulated. Normally, in this group there appears a very big diffuse depression of the light sensitivity, but no scotomas.

Type III

The third type of clinical evolution is divided into two groups: a and b: a corresponds to a group of congenital glaucoma who came late to the ophthalmologist when the eye was already enlarged with an abnormal axial length, 26, 28 or more milimiters; and b, a second group in which, at the time they came, the axial length was not so big, but the time between the first visit and surgery was very long and during that period the eye continued to grow (Fig. 3.)

If we examine these same patients later, between the ages of 10 and 17, we shall find a normal disc, a normal visual field, but the vision is fingercount, there is no binocular vision and no stereopsis. And when we look at the macula, there is no foveal reflex or it is altered, and the perifoveal reflex is anomalous and severely altered. Sometimes there is a posterior staphyloma. In the visual field it is observed a central scotoma with a diffuse depression of the light diffuse sensitivity.

In Table 1 are ensigned: the type of evolution, the number of eyes and the corresponding percentage:

Table 1.

Type of clinical evolution	Number of eyes	%
I	28	45.90
II	11	18.03
III	22	36.07
Total	61	100.00

We have seen these 3 different types of evolution and now let's go back to the second type which is the most interesting one if we wish to preserve both the vision and the visual field of the child.

In Fig. 4a is the evolution of the intraocular pressure and on Fig. 4b the evolution of the axial length. In this child we performed 3 operations. It is a

188

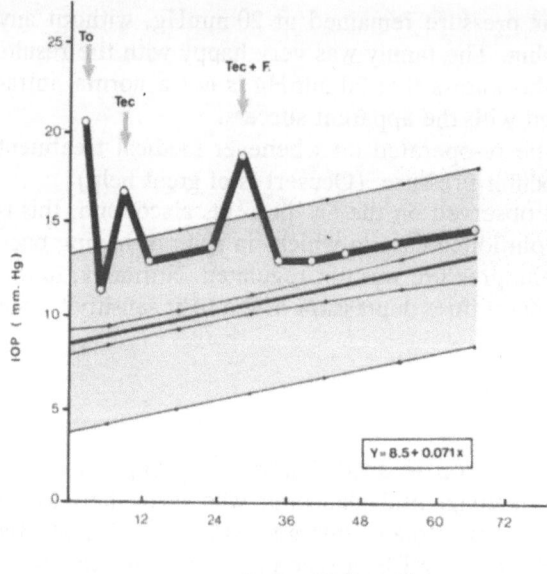

(a) Evolution of the intraocular pressure

To: TRABECULOTOMIE
Tec: TRABECULECTOMIE
Tec + F: "   + FLUOROURACIL

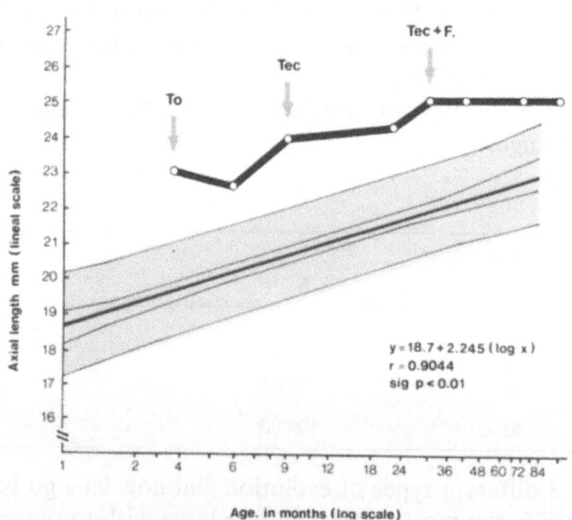

b Evolution of the axial length

Fig. 4.

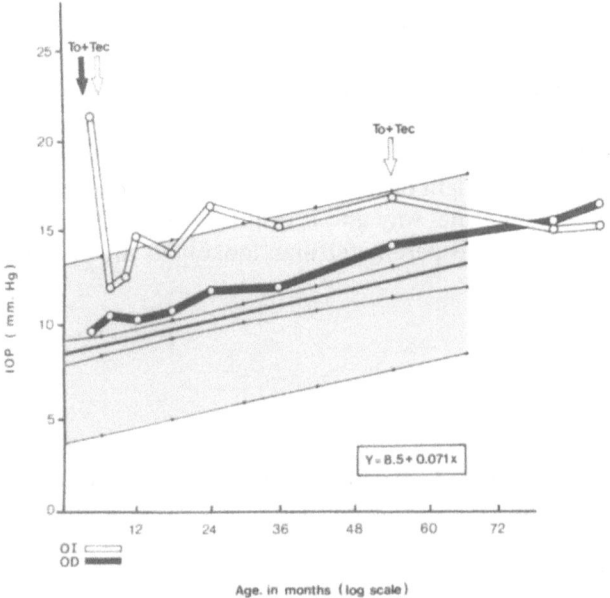

(a) Evolution of the intraocular pressure

To: TRABECULOTOMIE
Tec: TRABECULECTOMIE
Tec + F: "   + FLUOROURACIL

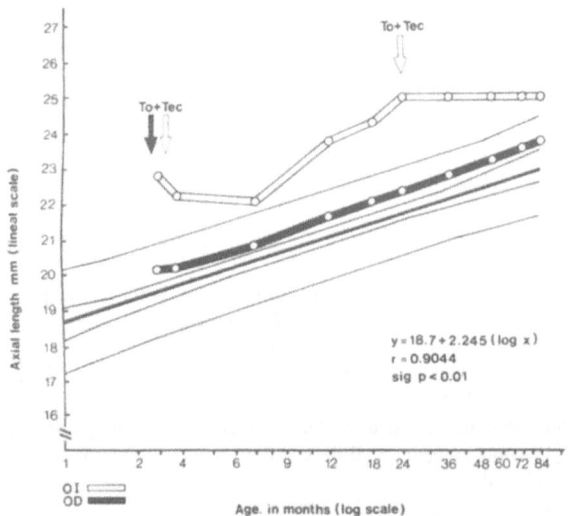

(b) Evolution of the axial length

Fig. 5.

very simple case because when the intraocular pressure rises the axial length rises too. It is not a problem to decide new surgery. On Fig. 5 is on the left the evolution of the intraocular pressure of another case. In this one the intraocular pressure remained always just at the upper level of the normal values, it is very difficult to decide whether to operate again or not. On Fig. 5b, is the evolution of the axial length of the same case. It's evident that the axial length increases in an abnormal way and it is much easier to decide to indicate new surgery looking at this parameter than looking at the evolution of the intraocular pressure.

Discussion

The axial length of the eye is a very useful parameter in the diagnosis and follow up of congenital glaucoma. As we can see it was very useful in the follow up of the 3 different types of evolution of 61 eyes of operated congenital glaucoma.

The most important type is type 2. Of the cases included in this type the axial length continued to grow in spite of surgery. In some cases the intraocular pressure and the axial length are correlated and show surgical failures. In other cases it is very difficult to judge the results of surgery via the intraocular pressure because the values are in the upper limits of the zone of normality, and are therefore unreliable.

In these cases it is the axial length that indicates if it is necessary to reoperate. Of our 61 eyes, 11 required reoperating on between 1 and 3 times (18.03%). Of the rest the intraocular pressure was regulated and axial length growth halted after the first surgery (81.97%).

References

[1] Sampaolesi R. 1974. Oculometría en el diagnóstico del glaucoma congénito. De: Glaucoma Panamericana, Buenos Aires, pp. 653–661.
[2] Sampaolesi R. 1981. Ocular Echometry in the Diagnosis of Congenital Glaucoma. Docum Ophthalm Proc Series, Vol. 29, J M Thijssen, and A M Verbeek (ed) Dr. W. Junk Publishers, The Hague, pp. 177–189.
[3] Sampaolesi R, Caruso R. 1902. Ocular Echometry in the Diagnosis of Congenital Glaucoma. Arch Ophthalmol 100: 574–577.
[4] Sampaolesi R. 1984. Echométrie oculaire, un nouveau parametre dans le diagnostic et le controle de l'évolution du glaucome congénital. Bull. et Mém. S.F.O., 95e, pp. 401–409.
[5] Sampaolesi R. 1971. Die Trabekulotomie als erste Operation fürs kongenitale Glaukom bei Kindern bis zum ersten Lebensjahr. Bericht D Ophthal Ges LXXI: 358–372.
[6] Sampaolesi R, Reca R, Carro A. 1967. Presión ocular en el niño normal hasta los 5 años. Arch Oftal B Aires XLII: 180–185.
[7] Sampaolesi R. 1969. La pression oculaire et le sinus camerulaire chez l'enfant normal et dans le glaucome congenital au dessous de l'age de 5 ans. Doc Ophthalm 26: 497–515.
[8] Sampaolesi R, Reca R, Carro A, Armado A. 1974. Normaler intraokularer Druck bei

Kindern bis zu 5 Jarhen mit und ohne Allgemeinnarkose. Seine Wichtigkeit fur Fruhdiagnose des angeborenen Glaukoms. Glaukom-Symposium Wurzburg 1974. Herausgegeben von W. Leydhecker. Ferdinand Enke Verlag Stutgart, pp. 278–289.

[9] Ratdke N D, Cohan B E. 1974. Intraocular pressure measurement in the newborns. Amer J Ophthal 78: 501.

[10] Ytterborg J. 1960. On scleral rigidity. Oslo University Press.

[11] Reibaldi A. 1982. Biometric ultrasound in the diagnosis and follow-up of congenital glaucoma. Annals of Ophthalmology 707.

[12] Tarkkanen A, Uusitalo R, Mianowicz J. 1903. Ultrasonographic biometry in congenital glaucoma. Acta Ophthalmol 61: 618–623.

[13] Uusitalo R J, Tarkkanen A. 1987. Ultrasonographic Biometry in Infantile glaucoma. A prospective follow up study glaucoma. Update III. G K Kriegelstein (ed.) Springer Verlag Berlin Heidelberg pp. 142–148.

24. Long-term biooculometry of developmental glaucoma

H. LERCHNER and B. VIDIC

Developmental glaucoma is a severe eye disease, where there is till now no sufficient medical treatment available. There are better diagnostic criterias and there is an improvement of the microsurgery technique, but there are still cases, which carry a grave prognosis. They often require more than one surgery and can nevertheless lead to a visual handicap. Developmental glaucomas need a good compliance between patients, parents and ophthalmologists and an intensive long term control.

Since the introduction of echography in ophthalmology, there is a number of clinical studies, concerning the measurement of eyeball length. Sampaolesi has stressed the clinical important value of echooculometry, especially in cases with borderline or even normal intraocular pressure. There is a great variable of intraocular pressure during the day, and it is impossible to perform a diurnal pressure curve of a child. The increasing of axial length is an effect of too high IOP over a period of weeks and months, and this we can easily recognize by ultrasound biometry.

The aim of our retrospective study was to determine characteristics of juvenile or adult eyes with developmental glaucoma after surgery.

Material and method

In the last twenty years, 45 children suffering from developmental glaucoma underwent different surgical procedures at our clinic. They were invited to come to an examination. Eighteen patients followed our call.

A complete ocular examination with aplanation tonometry, gonioscopy and fundoscopy, refraction and visus, measurement of corneal diameter and ultrasound echometry was performed. For that we used the immersions technique with a liquid filled scleral shell, fitted between the lids. Our ultrasonography unit is the 7200 MA Kretz with a focussed 8 Mhz transducer. We took polaroid photos and converted the microseconds into

Universitäts-Augenklinik Graz, Austria

R. Sampaolesi (ed.), Ultrasonography in Ophthalmology 12, 193–198.
© *1990. Kluwer Academic Publishers, Dordrecht*

194

milimeters by considering the different sound velocities in the various parts of the eye. The measurement was taken in non mydriatic state.

Our long term study was made on 18 patients with developmental glaucoma: 12 with primary congenital glaucoma (9 with bilateral, 3 unilateral = 20 eyes, because one of the bilateral glaucomatous eyes had to be enucleated), 6 patients with secundary glaucoma, 3 patients with Sturge-Webers Syndrom (1 bilateral, 2 unilateral = 4 eyes), 1 patient with bilateral Riegers Syndrom and 2 patients with bilateral juvenile glaucoma. 13 male and 5 female patients from 4 to 33 years old took part. All of them underwent antiglaucomatous surgery, 1 to 28 years ago. The bilateral Sturge-Weber — and the juvenile glaucom patients had only one eye operated on.

Intraocular pressure, measured by aplanation tonometry, was normal in 24 eyes (80%), 2 eyes (6.7%) were functionally blind and had a high IOP with 42 and 58 mmHg. Elevated tension existed in 4 eyes (13.3%). In spite of surgery 11 patients had to continue antiglaucomatous treatment.

Results

There is a great variable in the biometric parameters:

Figure 1 shows all the patients with the length of anterior chamber and the totally axial length. Anterior chamber depths range from 1.5 to 4.9 mm. According to former biometrical studies, eyes with developmental glaucoma

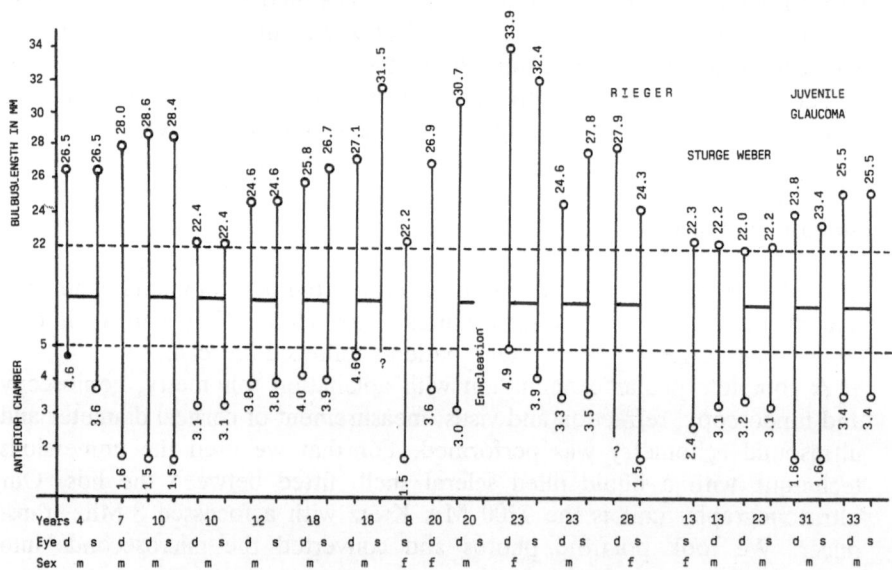

Fig. 1. Anterior chamber and bulbuslength in mm (n = 18 patients with 30 eyes).

have also a deeper anterior chamber than normal ones, the shallow anterior chamber seems to us to be the result of surgery. In two cases of athalamia the anterior chamber could not be measured.

According to the time and success of surgery the total axial length varies from 22.0 to 33.9 mm. 20 eyes with primary congenital glaucoma underwent surgery. 11 eyes (55%) longer than 24.6 mm needed more than one operation to normalize the intraocular pressure. On the other hand 2 eyes (10%) with an axial length of 26.5 mm were regulated by one operation. 1 eye (5%) remained the normal size with 24.6 mm in spite of multiple operations. Due to the late onset all the operated eyes with Sturge-Weber glaucoma and juvenile glaucoma were of normal size between 22.0 and 25.5 mm (emetropia between 20.12 and 25.94 mm). The female patient with Riegers's Syndrom developed a high myopia with bulbuslength of 27.9 mm and 24.3 mm, resulting in the bad, prognosis and 6 operations on the right and 5 operations on the left eye.

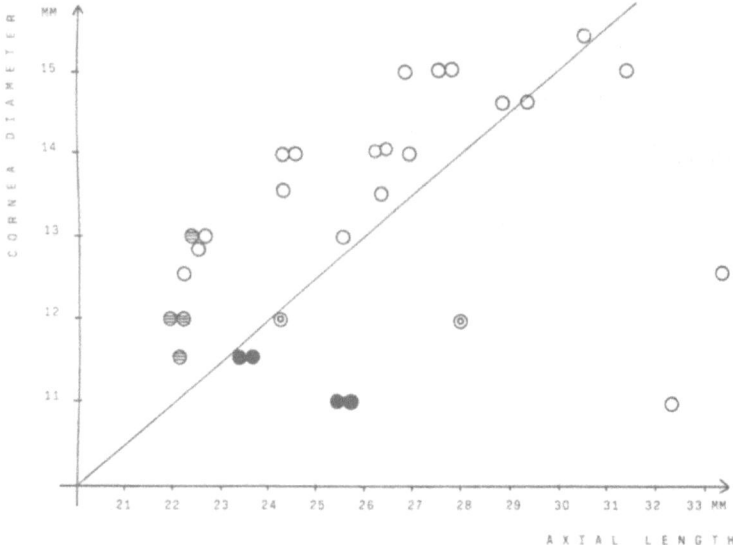

Fig. 2. Correlation between axial length to corneal diameter.
(○) primary congenital glaucoma, (⊖) Sturge Weber Syndrom,
(◎) Rieger's Syndrom, (●) juvenile glaucoma.

Figure 2 shows the correlation between axial length to corneal diameter. We plotted the axial length against the corneal diameter with the known restriction that we have only few patients with different age and primary and secundary glaucomas. A linear correlation with a factor of 1.99 (standard deviation σ = 1.5) resulted. Only one patient with a high myopia was far from average (right eye: CD 12.5 mm, AL 33.9 mm, left eye: CD 11.0 mm, AL 32.5 mm).

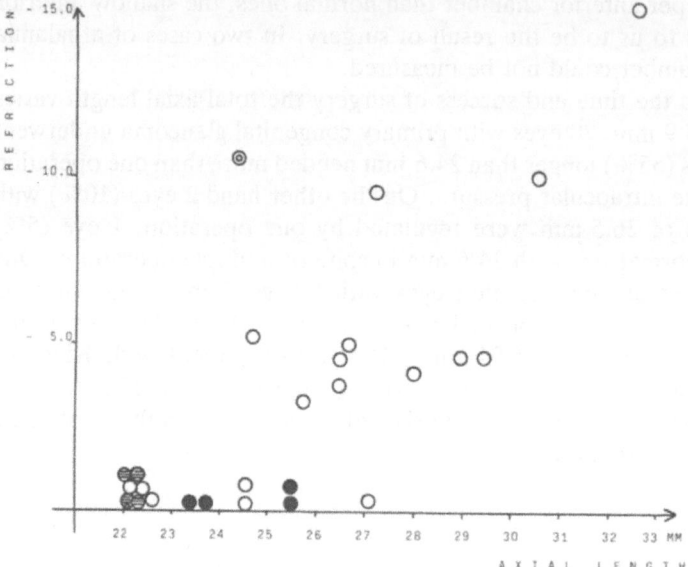

Fig. 3. Correlation between axial length to refraction.
(O) primary congenital glaucoma, (⊜) Sturge Weber Syndrom,
(◎) Rieger's Syndrom, (●) juvenile glaucoma.

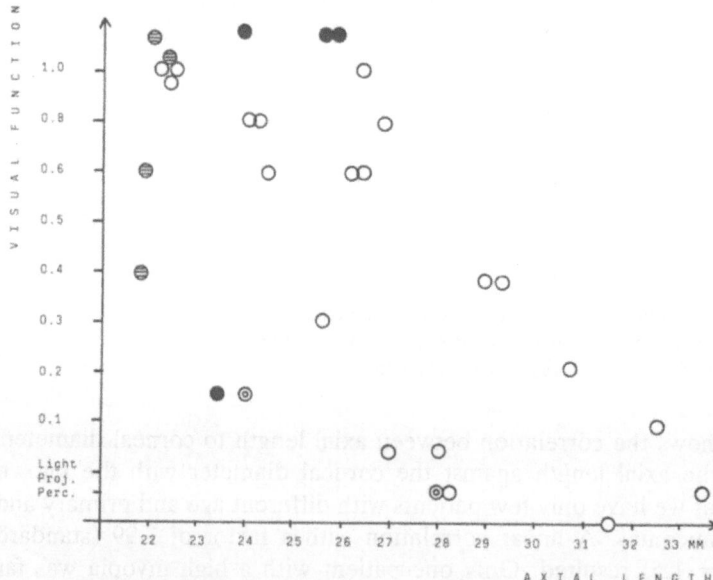

Fig. 4. Correlation between axial length to visual acuity.

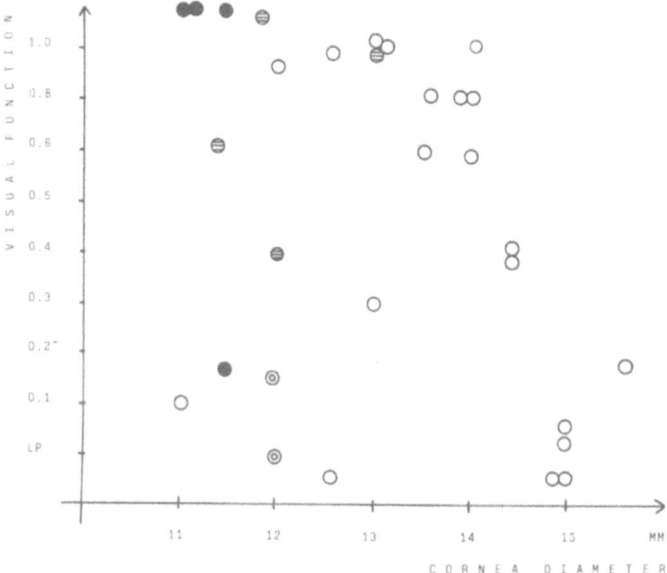

Fig. 5. Correlation between corneal diameter to visual acuity.

Axial length and refraction see Fig. 3. The large dimension of the eyeball lead to a myopia. It is reduced by the simultaneous growth of the cornea, inducing the increasing of the corneal curvature and therefore less dioptric power. No patient of our study is hypermetropic. High myopia with more than —9 dptr. was found only in 4 eyes (= 13.3%). This rate might be higher, because another 4 eyes could not be refractioned due to an opaque cornea.

The correlation of visual acuity and axial length and corneal diameter is indicated in Figs. 4 and 5. The visual acuity of eyes with developmental glaucoma depends on various factors, such as the clarity of cornea and lens, anisometropia and optic nerve function. Eyes up to an axial length of 27 mm can have normal visus, all of the longer eyes of our study have a reduced visual acuity with a maximum of 0.4. There is no correlation between corneal diameter and visual function. Only corneas larger than 15 mm have a visual loss.

Conclusion

Ultrasonographical measurement of the axial length has become clinical routine examination, which is one of the best parameters for the success of treatment for developmental glaucomas. Our aim is to avoid large eyes, as it has been known since Hippocrates, Celsius and Galen and is described 1573

198

by Parè as "oeil de boeuf". At the moment, when the eyeball is extremely large no therapy can help and a poor visual acuity results. There is a good chance for the visual function when the discovery of developmental glaucoma is early enough and therapy begins immediately.

References

Bluth K. 1984. Ultrasonic biometry in congenital glaucoma. Ophthalmic Ultrasonography, Docum Ophthal Proc Series 38: 267–275.

Buschmann W, Bluth K. 1974. Regelmäßige echograph. Messung der Achsenlänge des Auges zur Kontrolle der Druckregulierung bei Hydrophthalmie. Klin Monatsbl Augenheilkunde 165: 878–886.

De Carvalho C A, Betinjane A J. 1983. Ultrasonographie echometry in the control of congenital glaucoma. Glaucoma Update II, 169–174.

Draeger J, Wirt H. 1988. Klassifizierung und Therapie des Glaukoms im Kindesalter. Fortschr Ophthalmol 85: 63–69.

Francois J, Goes F. 1981. Ocular biometry, Ultrasonography in Ophthalmology. Docum Ophthal Proc Series 29: 135–164.

Gernet H, Hollwich F. 1969. Oculometrie des kindlichen Glaukoms. Ber Zusammenkunft Dtsch Ophthalmol Ges 69: 341–348.

Hoskins Jr. H D, Shaffer R N. 1983. Developmental Glaucoma. Glaucoma Update II, Springer Verlag, pp. 109–193.

Larsen J S. 1971. The sagittal growth of the eye. Acta Ophthalmol 49: 873–886.

Massin M, Pelatt B. 1984. Ultrasonic biometry in congenital glaucoma. A clinical study. Ophthalmic Ultrasonography, Docum Ophthal Proc Series 38: 261–266.

Sadanao Tane, Junko Kohno. 1984. Ultrasonic biometry of the sagittal growth of eyes in children. Ophthalmic Ultrasonography, Docum Ophthal Proc Series 38: 227–293.

Sampaolesi R. 1983. Ocular echometry and the diagnosis of congenital glaucoma and its evolution. Glaucoma Update II, Springer-Verlag, pp. 175–184.

Sampaolesi R. 1981. Ocular echometry in the diagnosis of congenital glaucoma. Ultrasonography in Ophthalmology, Docum Ophthal Proc Series 29: 177–189.

Vidic B, Pongratz E, Lerchner H. 1988. Langzeitergebnisse nach Glaukomoperationen im Kindesalter, Spektrum Augenheilkde, in 2/5: 218–220 press.

25. Relation between axial length and refraction in eyes with congenital glaucoma

ALBERTO J. BETINJANE and CELSO A. CARVALHO

Summary

The purpose of the present communication was the evaluation of the frequency of refractive error in 107 patients with congenital glaucoma which had their intra-ocular pressure surgically controlled. Those findings were correlated to the respective biometric values of the axial length of the eye. The biometric study was obtained by ultrasonography. The biometric findings and its respective refractive error in the congenital glaucoma group were compared to the same parameters of a group of normal eyes in three different age groups up to the age of 15 years.

Introduction

Myopia is frequently observed in cases of congenital glaucoma since it is directly related to the size of the eyeball or its axial length, which is usually enlarged in that disease (Kwitko, 1973; Sampaolesi, 1974; Betinjane, 1982).

The refraction of an eye, on the other hand, is not only dependent on the axial length but also on the characteristics of other eye structures as those of the cornea and lens. So, any condition that can change the anatomy of those structures will alter or affect the ocular refraction.

Therefore, although myopia is commonly presented in eyes with congenital glaucoma, it is not always found in the expected proportion to the axial length of the eyeball. The aim of the present study is to correlate axial length and ocular refraction of eyes with congenital glaucoma.

Method

In the present work, 107 eyes with controlled congenital glaucoma were studied and distributed in three age-groups up to the age of fifteen years old.

Rua Prof. Arthur Ramos 96–8° Sao Paulo, Brazil

R. Sampaolesi (ed.), Ultrasonography in Ophthalmology 12, 199–204.

All of them had a clinical picture of congenital glaucoma defined by applanation tonometry, measurements of the horizontal corneal diameter, biomicroscopy, gonioscopy and ophtalmoscopy. All of them had a stable, controlled intra-ocular pressure obtained through anti-glaucomatous surgeries (trabeculotomy or trabeculectomy).

A group with normal eyes was established as a control group. Those normal eyes demonstrated eyeballs without signs of pathology in it or its annexes.

The normal eyes were characterized by showing emmetropia or hyperopia as well as absence of abnormalities related to any type of eye pathology.

All patients (normal and with congenital glaucoma) were submitted to refraction and ultrasonographic biometry. The Kretz echograph, 7200 MA with 10 MHz probe, was used for the ocular biometry (making use of an interposition method).

In younger children the examinations were performed under general anesthesia (pentrane), and both ocular refraction and biometry were carried out with mydriasis and cyclopegia (tropicamide and cyclopentolate were used).

The refraction of normal and glaucomatous eyes were classified according to the following criteria:
– Group I: eyes with emmetropia and low hyperopia (up to + 2.00 SD).
– Group II: eyes with low myopia (up to −3.00 SD).
– Group III: eyes with high myopia (higher than −3.00 SD).

All the individuals (normal ones and those with congenital glaucoma), according to the age, were sub-divided into the following sub-groups:
– up to 18 months old
– between 19 months and 3 years old
– more than 3 years old and less than 15 years old.

In this way, an attempt was made to appraise the incidence of the refraction observed in the eyes with congenital glaucoma and its relationship to the normal ones according to age-groups, as well as its correlation with the biometric axial length.

Results

The Table I shows the frequency of the type of refraction observed in eyes with congenital glaucoma, which were studied according to the established age-groups.

In all studied age-groups, it was found that eyes with myopia (low and high) were more common than emmetropic and hyperopic eyes.

So, about 3/4 of them revealed themselves as being myopes (low and high) and 1/4 of them as having either emmetropia or low hyperopia.

The Table II shows the axial length values found in the normal eyes and in those with congenital glaucoma (in the three refraction groups) according

Table 1. Refraction in eyes with controlled congenital glaucoma.

Age \ Refraction	Emmetropes and hyperopes (till +2)	Low myopia (till −3)	High myopia (more than −3)	Number of eyes
Till 18 months	6 eyes (22.22%)	11 eyes (40.74%)	10 eyes (37.03%)	27
19 months till 3 years old	8 eyes (27.58%)	8 eyes (27.58%)	13 eyes (44.82%)	29
More than 3 years old & less than 15 years old	12 eyes (23.52%)	16 eyes (31.37%)	23 eyes (45.09%)	51
Total %	26 eyes (24.29%)	35 eyes (32.71%)	46 eyes (42.99%)	107

to the age-groups. The corresponding graph (Fig. 1) shows the relationship among those same values.

Except for Group I (emmetropic and low hyperopic eyes) and for the age-group up to 18 months, it was noticed that eyeball axial length values actually expressed themselves as being larger in the eyes with congenital glaucoma than in the normal ones of the same age-groups.

Table 2. Antero-posterior length congenital glaucoma and normal eyes.

Age \ Refraction	Controlled congenital glaucoma			Normal hyperopia
	Hyperopia	Low myopia	High myopia	
Till 18 months	20.15 ± 2.1	21.84 ± 1.72	23.98 ± 1.29	20.09 ± 2.0
19 months till 3 years old	23.06 ± 0.82	23.87 ± 1.11	25.3 ± 1.8	21.72 ± 1.10
More than 3 years old & less than 15 years old	23.37 ± 1.57	24.86 ± 2.6	26.72 ± 1.9	22.7 ± 1.24

Hyperopia   : till + 2.00 SD.
Low myopia : till − 3.00 SD.
High myopia : more than − 3.00 SD.

202

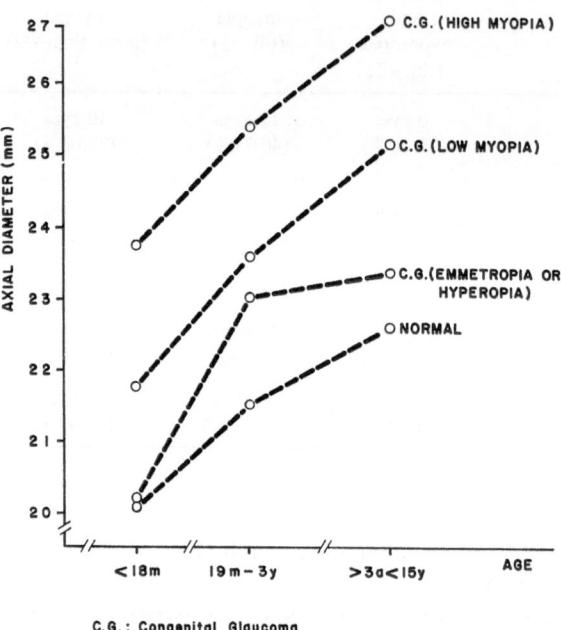

REFRACTION
AXIAL DIAMETER X AGE

C.G.: Congenital Glaucoma

Fig. 1. Relationship between axial length values found in normal eyes and those with congenital glaucoma (in the three refraction groups) according to the age groups.

Comments and conclusions

Four factors influence the ocular refraction: the eyeball axial length, the cornea curvature, the lens refrigent power and the anterior chamber depth. Undoubtly the axial length is the most important of all those parameters.

Several authors have been able to demonstrate correlation between axial length and ocular refraction (Jansson, 1963; Rivara et Cambiaggi, 1964; Luycks-Bacus and Weekers, 1966; Franceschetti et al., 1968; Gernetih, 1969; Larsen, 1971; Machekhin, 1972).

In the majority of cases, eyes with increased axial diameter are myopes, being the magnitude of myopia directly related to its axial length. So, there is a significant correlation between axial length and the nature of the ammetropia (François and Gois, 1973).

As regards to ocular growth, according to some authors, in normal condition the eyeball grows up to an age that can vary from 11 to 15 years old (Sorsby et al., 1961; Larsen, 1971; Delmarcelle and Luycks, 1971).

In this stage, in order to reduce the ammetropia and sometimes to avoid its development, the eyeball is suffers the so-called emmetropization which is constituted by an harmonization among the different parameters that have influence on ocular refraction and which are also interdependent.

In the particular case of congenital glaucoma, although myopia is a common find, its magnitude does not always reaches the expected values due only to the exaggerated enlargement of the eyeball. The final refraction will be also influenced by other changes induced by the disease in other eye structures, so as:

1) A more flattened cornea (the eyeball enlargement and the corneal growth will cause its flattenning);
2) Decrease of the lens axial diameter (at the same time that the eyeball enlargès, the scleral ring adjacent to the ciliary body also increases its diameter, causing stretching of the zonular fibers, and so decreasing the lens axial diameter);
3) The relative backward positioning of the lens is another factor that influences the refraction of the congenital glaucoma eyes, which is also commonly seen in these kind of eyes (Kwitko, 1973).

As it was expected, with regard to the ocular biometry we could notice clear differences in the dimensions of the axial length in the three refractional groups considered. So, the eyes of Group I (emmetropes and hyperopes) showed smaller dimensions if compared to Group II (low myopia) and the difference being much bigger if compared to Group III (high myopia).

However, it was observed that in despite of the refractory nature, all the eyes with congenital glaucoma showed an enlargement of their axial length in relation to the normal eyes of the same age-group.

These findings are similar to those mentioned in a previous publication (Betinjane, 1982) in which there was a study of the ocular biometry in eyes with congenital glaucoma, but without taking into account the ocular refraction and the control or not of the disease.

However, in the younger group we were able to observe that the dimensions of the axial length of the eyes of Group I (with congenital glaucoma, emmetropes and hyperopes) were similar to those values of the normal eyes. This could be explained as a consequence of the fact that those eyes would stop growing at an abnormal rate when the intra-ocular pressure is early controlled (Betinjane, 1982). So, the dimensions attained by those eyes would not reach values sufficiently altered so as to show no significant differences in enlargement when compared to normal eyes of the same age-group. The opposite would happen in those cases on which the effective control of the disease was reached only after a very late period of time. In this way, the eyeball dimensions would be largely altered and so quite different of the normal eyes at the same age.

Through these results we can conclude that although myopia (low and high) is the most frequently found type of refractive defect encountered in the congenital glaucoma, hyperopia can also occur with some periodicity so being refraction closely related to the axial length of the eye in cases of congenital glaucoma, similar to the normal eyes (Luyckx-Bacus and Weekers, 1966; Gernetih, 1969; Machekhin, 1977). However, we can admit the existence of an important emmetropization mechanism that influences the final refraction of these eyes, since the emmetropia and the hyperopia were observed in eyes with enlarged axial diameter in relation to normal ones.

References

Betinjane A J. 1982. Contribuição ao estudo da biometria ultrasonográfica no glaucoma \congênito. Tese Doc. Li-vre, — Fac. Med. USP. 1982.
Ceschetti A. 1968. New results concerning the problem of axial lengths of the eye in anisometropie. Dans: Vanysex J., Diagnostica Ultrasonica in Ophtalmologia. Brno. pp. 235–238.
Delmarcelle Y, Luyckx-Bacus J. 1971. Evolution biometric de la chambre anterieure chez l'enfant etude de 1960 globes. Bull Soc Belge Ophthal 158: 451–465.
Franceschetti A Th, Linder A, Fraceschetti A. 1968. New results concerning the problem of axial lengths of the eye in anisometropie. Dans: Vanysex J., Diag nostica Ultrasonica in Ophthalmologia. Brno pp. 235–238.
François J, Gois F. 1973. Biometric de la myopic ophthalmologica, Basel, 147: 49–65.
Gernetieh 1969. Datensammlung in der Klinischen Oculometrie. Doc Ophthal 27: 42–47.
Jansson F. 1963. Measurements of intraocular distances by ultrassound. Acta Ophthal Kbh Suppl 74: 1–51.
Kwitko M. 1973. Meredith Corporation, New York.
Larsen J S. 1971. The saggital growth of the eye. Acta Ophthal Kbh 49: 239–262.
Luyckx-Bacus J, Weekers J F. 1966. Estude biometrique de l'oeil humain par ultrasonographie ire parte: les ametropies. Bull Soc Belge Ophthal 552–567.
Machekhin V A. 1977 Ultrasehalbiometrie bei Augen mit Unterschiedlicher Refration Oftal., 24: 204–207.
Rivara A, Cambiaggi A. 1964. Rapporto fra entita della refrazione lunghezza dell'asde oculare antero-posteriore e gravita delle alterazioni corloretinicho in soggetti miopi. Atti Dez XLVIII Congr Soc Oft Ital XXII: 2–4.
Sampaolesi R. 1974. Glaucoma. Buenos Aires, E. Medica Panamericana pp. 653–665.
Sorsby A, Benjamin B, Sheridan M. 1961. Refraction and its components during the growth of the eye. Secre. Rep. Serv. Med., Res. Coun., London, 301 HMSO.

26. Biometric study of eyes with angle closure glaucoma

J. I. YANKELEVICH, G. IRIBARREN and R. SAMPAOLESI

Introduction

With A-scan standardized ultrasonography we examined 29 eyes of 16 patients with angle closure glaucoma. The aim of this study was to determine on one hand the biometric characteristics of glaucomatous eyes and on the other to see if we could find a difference between those eyes that had developed acute angle closure glaucoma.

Material and methods

We examined 29 angle closure glaucoma eyes which we divided into 2 groups.

Group A

Consisted of 16 eyes with angle closure glaucoma of 9 patients (7 female, 2 male), mean age: 71.6 ± 3.08 years, mean ocular refraction: +0.92 +0.24 diopters, mean I.O.P.: 18.3 ± 1.4 mm. Hg.

Group B

Included 13 eyes of 7 patients (5 female and 2 male) that had developed acute glaucoma at least in one eye, mean age: 68.3 ± 5.33 years, mean ocular refraction: ± 1.23 ± 0.72 diopters, mean I.O.P.: 16.2 ± 1.45 mmHg.

All patients were under miotic therapy which was discontinued two days before examination so as to be able to dilate the pupil with tropicamide 1%.

All of the acute angle closure glaucoma patients had been previously operated on (Trabeculectomy).

University of Buenos Aires, Argentina

R. Sampaolesi (ed.), Ultrasonography in Ophthalmology 12, 205–208.

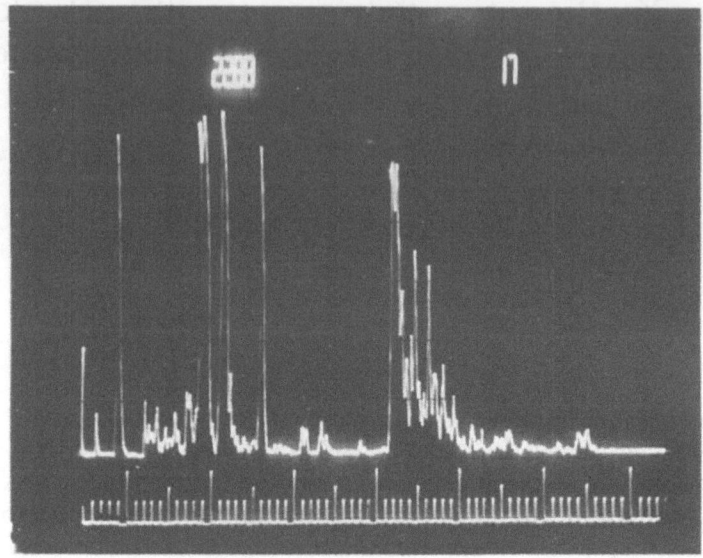

Fig. 1. Echogram obtained with a Sonokretz unit with inmersion technique.

We used a Sonokretz unit with a standard probe. We preferred the inmersion technique using plastic scleral contact shells filled with saline solution.

Measurements of anterior chamber, lens, vitreous and axial length were taken directly from the screen, measuring with gates from peak to peak. Ultrasound velocity was changed according to the ocular parameter measured.

Results

We know that angle closure glaucoma has definite biometric findings.

First the shallow anterior chamber, second the lens thickenning which is associated with an abnormal forward position and third, the axial length is reduced. The disease is more frequent in hypermetropic eyes and female patients.

Our results are shown on Table 1.

For the first group;

axial length: 22.20 ± 0.74 mm.

anterior chamber depth: 2.46 ± 0.65 mm.

lens: 3.84 ± 0.65 mm.

vitreous: 15.17 ± 0.79 mm.

The second group shows;

axial length: 22.20 ± 0.73 mm.

Table 1.

	Angle closure glaucoma (N: 16)		Acute angle closure glaucoma (N: 13)			
	media (mm)	DS	media (mm)	DS	t	significance
Axial length	22.20	0.74	22.20	0.73	0.00	NS
Anterior chamber depth	2.46	0.65	2.17	0.72	1.14	NS
Lens thickness	3.84	0.65	4.31	0.41	2.27	p < 0.05
Vitreous	15.17	0.79	14.80	0.62	1.38	NS

Anterior chamber depth: 2.17 ± 0.72 mm.
lens: 4.31 ± 0.41 mm.
vitreous: 14.80 ± 0.62 mm.

Comparing both groups we found that all eyes were shorter than normal and that findings for axial length and vitreous length were almost the same.

The most striking difference was found in the anterior chamber and lens values, showing the acute angle closure glaucoma eyes a shallower anterior chamber and a thicker lens.

Using the Wilcoxon test there was a significative difference only for the lens thickness for a p value < 0.05.

Conclusions

We already know from previous papers that ultrasound biometry brings important information in relation with the different glaucoma forms.

In our study, comparing acute angle closure with chronic angle closure patients we could only find a significative difference in relation with the lens thickness, stressing the point that this papameter may be one of the most important causative factor in the development of acute angle closure glaucoma.

References

Cennamo G, Rosa N. 1987. Biometric evaluation of the lens in glaucomatous and normal eyes. Documenta Ophthalmologica Proceedings Series 48: 117.

Delmarcelle Y, Emllignon J, Luyck J, Weekers R. 1971. Etude biometrique du globe oculaire dans le glaucome a angle fermé. Bull Soc Franc Ophtal 84: 449.

Gabai R, Calabrese D, Cennamo G. 1983. Lens ultrasonographic biometric evaluation in Acute angle closure glaucoma. International Simposium on Glaucoma, Jerusalem, Israel.

Goes F, Francois J, Benozzi J. 1981. Ultrasonographic study of the ocular parameters after Glaucoma Surgery. Documenta Ophthalmologica Proceedings Series 29: 171.

208

Lowe RF. 1969 Causes of shallow anterior chamber in primary angle closure glaucoma. Ultrasonic biometry of normal and angle closure glaucoma eyes. Amer J Ophth 67: 87–93

Luyckx-Bacus J, Weekers J F. 1967. Contribution a l'étude des glaucomes par ultrasonographie. Ann Oculistique 200: 489–504.

Vitreoretinal diseases

Vitreoretinal disease

27. Correlation between echography, vitreous surgery findings and follow-up

J. POUJOL, A. CANTALLOUBE and M.–C. CHAINTRON

Summary

The authors present a series of 100 cases of vitreous disorders. The correlation between the echographic statements such as posterior vitreous limit detachment or retinal detachment was verified by surgery or follow-up.

Introduction

The major therapeutic problem in cases of vitreous hemorrhage is to determine the indication and time of the vitrectomy. Echography provides essential prognostic data when the hemorrhage is too dense to evaluate the condition of the posterior segment by optical means. Ultrasound detection of a retinal detachment usually leads to immediate vitrectomy with associated treatment of the retinal detachment. However it is not always possible to confirm the existence of a retinal detachment and to differentiate it from a posterior vitreous detachment or from vitreous membranes, even with the improved quality of the pictures provided by modern B-mode ultrasound.

This article presents a retrospective study of 100 successive cases of vitreous hemorrhage examined in the Ultrasound Laboratory of the Quinze-Vingts Hospital over a period extending from March to October 1987. Every patient's file was reviewed several months after the echographic examination to verify the findings. Agreement or disagreement between the ultrasonic diagnosis and the vitrectomy or the follow-up was established. In this study we did not take into account patients referred from other hospitals as reviewing their files was practically impossible.

Ultrasound Laboratory, Quinze-Vingts National Centre for Ophthalmology, 28 rue de Charenton, 75012 – Paris, France

R. Sampaolesi (ed.), Ultrasonography in Ophthalmology 12, 211–216.

212

Material and methods

Equipment and techniques

All the patients in this study were examined with an OPHTHASCAN from
Biophysic Medical with a 64 level gray scale and a 10 Mhz sector-scan
contact tranducer. B-scans were performed in transverse, sagittal, coronal

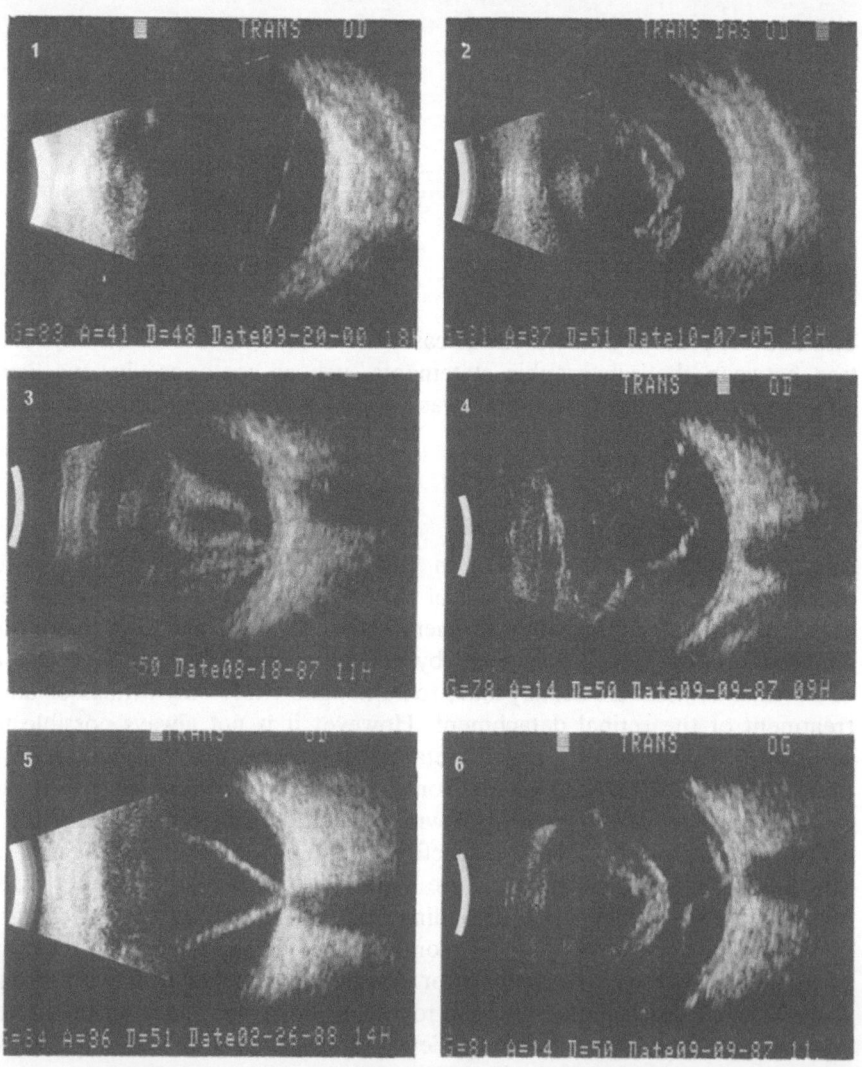

Fig. 1. (1) Vitreous tractional detachment. (2) Vitreous hemorrhage with total posterior
vitreous detachment. (3) Vitreous hemorrhage with posterior limit attachment in the
macular area. (4) Vitreous hemorrhage with vitreous posterior limit far from the
optic disc. (5) Total retinal detachment. (6) Associated posterior vitreous detachment
and retinal detachment.

and oblique planes. The axial length of the eye was systematically measured with A-scan. Diagnostic A-scan was not performed as we abandoned its use in 1982.

Case selection

We have taken into account patients referred for an ultrasonic examination for opaque vitreous hemorrhage. We eliminated from this series any eye which had undergone total vitrectomy, with or without silicone oil injection.

Results

- A normal posterior segment was found in 33 eyes. Vitrectomy was performed within a few days in nearly half of these cases (15 out of 33). It confirmed the echographic diagnosis of flat retina and in most cases made it possible to learn the cause of the vitreous hemorrhage. In the other cases (18 out of 33), the decision was follow-up until the hemorrhage disapeared; the diagnostic results were the same.
- A posterior vitreous detachment was detected in 23 eyes. It was confirmed later in 21 out of 22 eyes, but in 2 eyes an isolated or associated retinal detachment was present.
- Echography detected other abnormalities of the posterior segment in 33 eyes (Table 2) without any associated picture of retinal detachment.

Table 1. Causes and circumstances of the vitreous hemorrhages.

Traumatic 27	IOFB (7 extracted)	12
	perforating injuries	8
	ocular contusions	3
	windshield injuries	2
	traumatic rupture of cataract incision	2
Immediate 13 post-op.	after cataract extraction	6
	after retinal detachment surgery	7
Spontan. 60 vitr. hemorrhages (4 patients with anticoag. therapy)	retinal tears	17
	diabetic retinopathy	10
	retinal vein occlusion	9
	age related macular deg.	4
	vitreous retraction without retinal tear	3
	hemoglobinopathies	2
	Eales disease	2
	other vascularitis	1
	choroidal melanoma	1
	choroidal osteoma	1
	post-op. of a cerebral aneurism	1
	unknown cause	9

214

Table 2. Different echographic appearances of the posterior segment with flat retina.

Diffuse intra-vitreal echoes	13
Intra-vitreal hematoma	5
Thickened choroid	8
Intra-ocular foreign bodies	4
Choroidal hematoma	1
Choroidal melanoma	1
Choroidal osteoma	1
Scleral indentation	1
Retinitis proliferans	2
Total	38

(total exceeds 33, as in traumatized eyes other disorders are often associated).

Table 3. Ultrasound accuracy in the diagnosis of vitreous hemorrhage associated disorders.

Ultrasonic diagnosis	No.	Correct Dg.	Erron. Dg.
Normal post. segment	33	33	0
Post. vitreous det. with flat retina	23	21	2
Varied disorders of the post. segment with flat retina	33	31	2
Retinal detachment	8	8	0
Doubtful retinal det.	3	2 RD	1 FR
Total	100	93 or 90%	7 or 10%
		(with and without the doubtful results)	

Follow-up confirmed this diagnosis of a 'flat retina' in 31 cases out of 33. In 2 cases the retina was detached.
– A retinal detachment was detected in 8 cases; all of them were verified by surgery.
– We had doubtful results in 3 cases where ultrasound was unable to differentiate a posterior vitreous detachment from a retinal detachment. Two cases out of the three were vitreous membranes.
– We compared the echographic diagnosis and the final diagnosis, so as to evaluate the reliability of ultrasound in this series (Table 3). We had 93 or 90 correct diagnoseses out of 100, depending on whether or not the doubtful cases were included.

Discussion

– Several authors published articles on vitreous hemorrhage and ultrasound. Among them (Table 4):
   Jack et al., 1974 [1] gave a diagnosis of retinal position with 85% accuracy in a series of 35 mainly diabetic patients. Jerneld et al., 1979 [2] had 78%

Table 4. Ultrasound accuracy according to different authors.

Authors	Accuracy	Number of eyes
Jack et al. (1974)	83 %	35 (24 diabetic)
Jernels et al. (1979)	78 %	49 diabetic eyes
Poujol et al. (1988)	90 %	100 eyes (10 diabet.)

accuracy for the diagnosis of retinal detachment in 49 eyes in diabetic patients.
– In this series we had 90% accuracy in 100 mainly traumatic eyes with only 10 diabetic patients. Several difficult cases were included:

In three cases the differential diagnosis between a total retinal detachment and a highly reflective membrane was not possible. The study of after-movements was of no use.

In two cases (one normal, one Eale's disease) the echographic diagnosis of posterior vitreous detachment was erroneous: these eyes presented a total retinal detachment with rather low reflectivity which was more evocative of a vitreous detachment. These were in fact long standing detachments, which explains the low reflectivity.

In one case, ultrasound diagnosed intra-vitreal membranes in a twelve month old vitreous hemorrhage in an aphakic eye. In fact, vitrectomy discovered a total, ancient, retinal detachment.

In another case, echography revealed only vitreous hemorrhage echoes. Vitrectomy performed eight days later showed a retinal detachment. However, three days prior to the operation, the patient had observed a loss of light perception on this eye and this allows us to date the occurence of the retinal detachment to after the echographic examination and before the surgery.

In eight, ultrasonically diagnosed, retinal detachments, four were limited and four total, of which two were associated with a posterior vitreous detachment.

In our study, one should remark the diversity of causes for these vitreous hemorrhages (Table 1), with 40% traumatic cases and only 10% diabetic retinopathies. Moreover, 5% of these spontaneous vitreous hemorrhages were caused by, or associated with an isolated vitreous detachment. Morse et al., 1974 [3] had nearly the same results (3.7%).

Conclusion

The diagnostic accuracy, mainly between flat retina, posterior vitreous detachment and retinal detachment has improved. It appears to be due to the development of better echographic instruments, especially with an increased gray-scale.

However comparisons between different publications remain difficult as the series are made up of very differents kinds of patients.

216

References

[1] Jack R L, Hutton W L, Machemer R. 1974. Ultrasonography and vitrectomy. Am J Ophthalmol 78: 265.

[2] Jerneld B, Algvere P, Singh G. 1980. An ultrasonographic study of diabetic vitreo-retinal disease with low visual acuity. Acta Ophthalmol 58: 193–201.

[3] Morse P H, Aminulari A, Scheie H G. 1974. Spontaneous vitreous hemorrhage. Arch Ophthalmol 92: 297–298.

28. Power spectrum analysis of ultrasonic radio-frequency signals in vitreous diseases

SADANAO TANE, TATSUHIRO KAKEHASHI, MASAYA HIRATA,
TAKEMITSU HASHIMOTO, MARIKO HASHIMOTO,
HIROSHI KOGAKURA and AKIRA KOMATSU

Although A-scan and B-scan images of ocular diseases are clinically important for differential diagnosis, much useful diagnostic information is not yet
available through these procedures. However, wave spectral analysis by
computer can gather much of the missing information, thereby providing
material effective for diagnosis. Table 1 shows a diagram of the experimental
conditions.

In this study, we conducted spectral wave analysis of ultrasonic information from the eye by using a computerized wave form analyzer and
attempted to make a differential diagnosis by wave form analysis, which is
regarded as acoustic staining in the living body. B-mode images of ocular
diseases were first obtained by a 10-MHz probe using the immersion
method, and an A-mode beam was applied to the portion showing the most

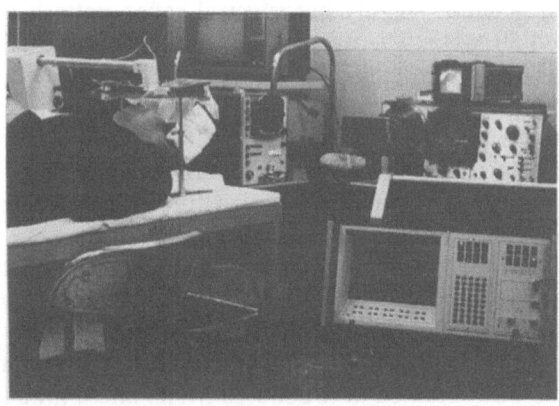

Fig. 1. The experimental apparatus (DATA-6000 Universal wave-form analyzer).

Dept. of Ophthalmology, St. Marianna University, School of Medicine, 2095 Sugao, Miyamae-
ku, Kawasaki, Japan

R. Sampaolesi (ed.), Ultrasonography in Ophthalmology 12, 217–223.
© *1990. Kluwer Academic Publishers, Dordrecht*

marked lesion. The radio-frequency signal of this portion was captured by oscilloscope and was then submitted to wave spectral analysis with a DATA-6000-Universal wave form analyzer (Fig. 1).

According to the results of basic experiments on rabbit eyes, analysis of the reflected spectral echo-wave range of experimental retinal detachment revealed a convex pattern with the maximum point of reflected spectral waves at 10 MHz, the same frequency as that of the transducer used. In the subsequent range, 20–50 MHz, there was also a weak and relatively flat spectral echo-wave reflex of less than −30 dB between 10 and 50 MHz.

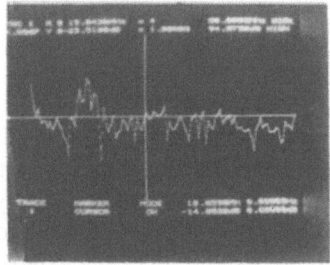 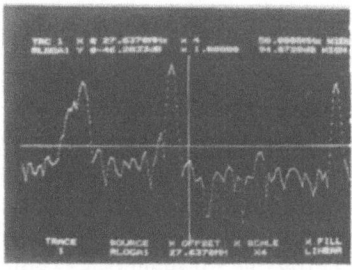

Fig. 2. The spectral echo-wave analysis of the A-scan ultrasonograms of the experimental vitreous hemorrhaage (left) and vitreous opaque due to experimental uveitis (right) in rabbit eyes.

Figure 2 shows the results of reflected spectral echo-wave analysis of rabbit eyes with experimental vitreous hemorrhage and experimental uveitis. The vitreous hemorrhage case on the left shows the maximum peak at about 10 MHz and a general, slightly flat spectral reflex pattern around −30 dB between 10 and 50 MHz. The uveitis case on the right shows marked peaks at about 10, 25 and 50 MHz in the whole range of reflected spectral echo-waves, which is due to the presence of multiple vitreous membrane formation inside the vitreous body.

Next we examined human eyes with various ocular diseases. We examined 22 eyes with retinal detachment, 34 with vitreous hemorrhage and 16 with other ocular diseases, totaling 72 eyes.

As in the analysis using animal eyes, an analysis of human retinal detachment shows a convex pattern with the maximum point at around 10 MHz (the frequency of the transducer used), and a slightly flat pattern at the other frequencies. Similar to previous cases, the maximum point of reflected waves was obtained at around 10 MHz, and a gradually increasing pattern was seen in the spectral range higher than 10 MHz (Fig. 3). Eyes with vitreous hemorrhage were examined as controls. There were no marked variations in the intensity of reflected spectral echo waves throughout the entire range higher than 10 MHz. Thus, the spectral refles pattern shown is flat with intensity −30 dB.

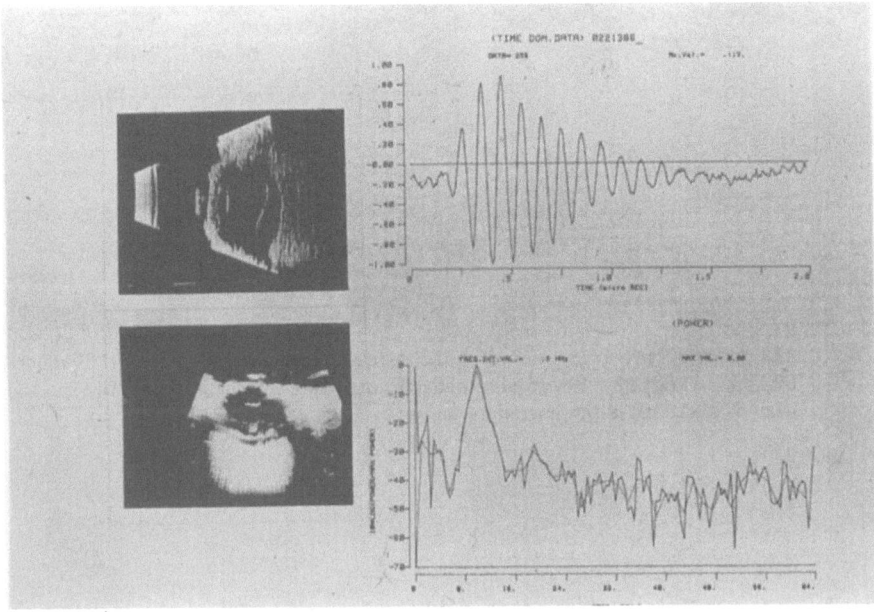

Fig. 3. An analysis of the spectral wave of echogram of the human retinal detachment.

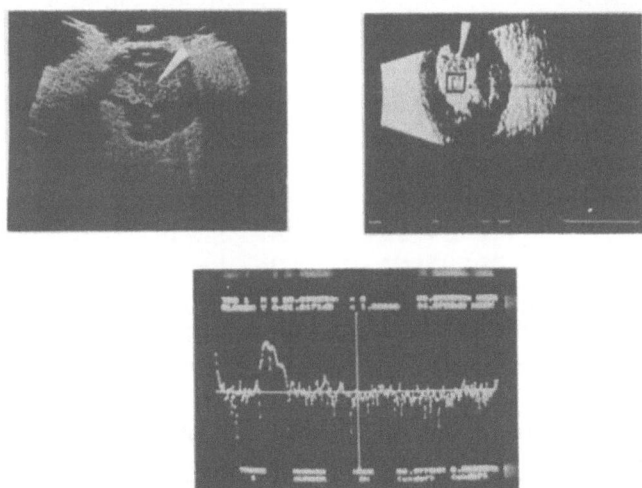

Fig. 4. An analysis of the spectral wave of ultrasonogram of a massive preretinal hemorrhage with funnel-shaped vitreous membrane. (The upper part) The B-scan ultrasonogram of massive vitreous hemorrhage: (The lower part) The spectral analysis of A-scan ultrasonogram of this case.

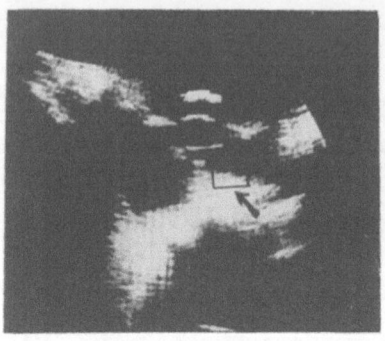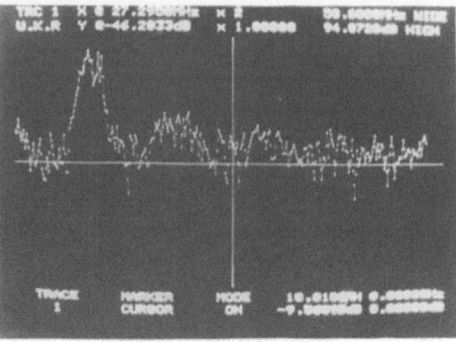

Fig. 5. The spectral wave-form analysis of the A-scan ultrasonogram of a case of retino-blastoma. (Left) The B-scan ultrasonogram of retinoblastoma. (Right) The spectral analysis of A-scan ultrasonogram of this case.

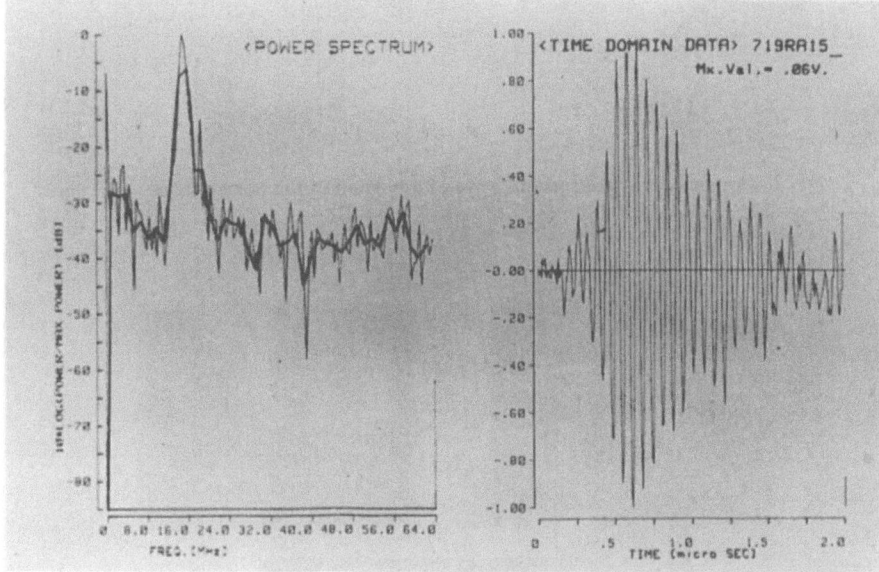

Fig. 6. Spectrum analysis of the ultrasonogram of the eye with retinal detachment. (Ultrasonic spectrum analysis of human retinal detachment shows a convex pattern with maximum point at around 10–15 MHz, the frequency of the transducer used, and slightly flat pattern of less than −30 dB at the other frequency (20–60 MHz).

Table 1. The experimental condition of the echographical spectral wave form analysis of vitreous diseases.

The Examination Method
A) St. Marianna's High-powered Ophthalmic Ultrasonic Diagnostic Equipment
B) Probe : 10MHz, 7mmφ, focused PZT transducer
C) Oscilloscope (Hitachi, V-650-F type)
D) Computerized Universal Wave Form Analyser (DATA 6000)

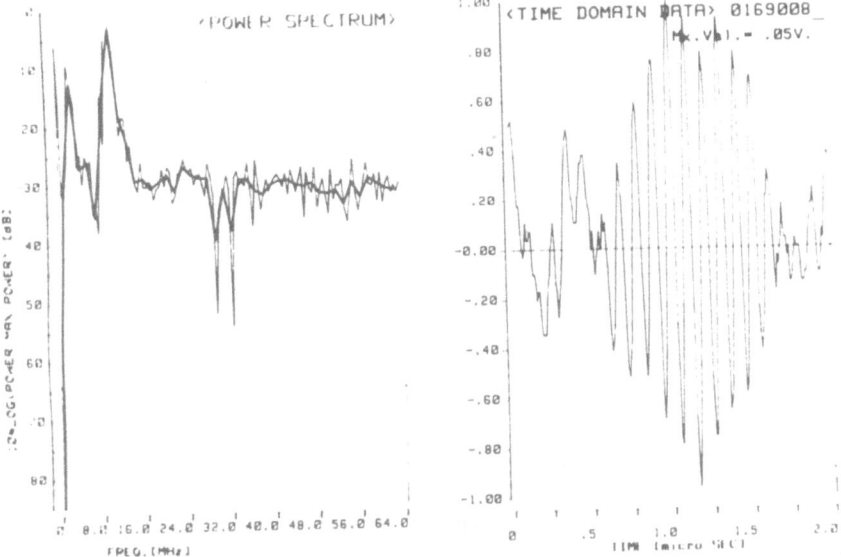

Fig. 7. Spectral analysis of the ultrasonogram of the eye with vitreous hemorrhage showed an approximately fixed and flat spectral reflex around −30 dB over the entire area in the frequency range of the reflex echo.

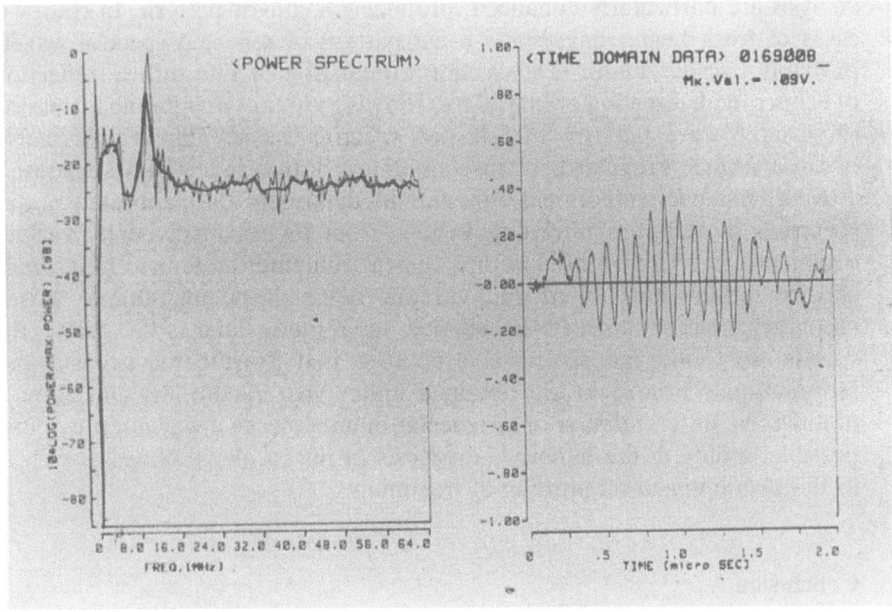

Fig. 8. Spectral analysis of the ultrasonogram of the eye with intravitreal membrane formation after absorption of vitreous hemorrhage. The small convex continuous waves of about −20 dB are followed after the large convex spike at 10–15 MHz.

Next, a case of massive preretinal proliferation showing vitreous hemorrhage accompanied by funnel-shaped proliferations of the vitreous membrane was examined. Large spectral waves with intensity of about −20 dB representing diffuse reflection seen throughout the entire range of reflected spectral echo waves in the area higher than 10 MHz (Fig. 4). Spectral analysis of a case of retinoblastoma showed a strong reflex at around 10 MHz.

A somewhat strong but multi-chevron pattern with −15 dB was obtained at the other frequencies.

The eyes with retinal detachment showed a peak spectral reflex in the frequency range of the reflex echo around 10 MHz of the transducer used, showing a convex pattern. In the subsequent range, 20–50 MHz, they showed a weak and relatively flat spectral reflex of less than −30 dB (Table 6). The eyes with vitreous hemorrhage showed an approximately fixed and flat spectral reflex around −30 dB over the entire area in the frequency range of the reflex echo (Fig. 7). By contrast, the eyes with intravitreal membrane formation after absorption of the vitreous hemorrhage were found by spectral analysis of the reflex waves to give small convex or flat continuous waves of about −20 dB (Fig. 8).

In cases of retinal detachment, echo-wave reflex is strongly oriented to one direction because the surface of the detached retina is smooth, and therefore echo waves around the frequency used in the wave spectral analysis are particularly enhanced, producing a convex pattern. In contrast, cases of fresh hemorrhage show a flat pattern of reflected spectral waves, probably because uniform absorption attenuation or fine diffuse reflection of echoes in all direction occurs. Cases showing vitreous membrane formation show large wave patterns of reflected spectral waves. This is presumably because surface irregularities cause an almost diffuse reflection of echoes.

Mathematical evaluation techniques to determine the calibrated power spectrum of reflected ultrasonic echoes from tissues involved by various ocular diseases can be used with a clinical computer system to objectively classify retinal detachment and vitreous hemorrhagic membrane. Tissue structures can be acoustically stained in B-mode images to define the specific anatomic and structural properties that provide the acoustic differentiation. These data are obtained under vivo conditions, and allow a noninvasive differentiation of intraocular membranes in a way not previously possible, aiding in the definitive diagnosis of intraocular diseases as well as in the planning and monitoring of treatment.

Conclusion

Spectral analysis of wave forms of A-scan radio-frequency signals by a computerized wave form analyzer has provided simpler differential diagnosis of tissues in living human eyes. Thus, this method, in addition to A-scan and

B-scan, has enabled us to conduct analytic diagnosis of ocular diseases more readily than before.

References

Coleman D J, Lizzi F L. 1983. Computerized ultrasonic tissue characterization of ocular tumor. Am J Ophthalmol 96: 165–175.

Tane S, Kohno J, Komatsu A, Horikoshi J. 1984. Tissue characterization by computerized ultrasonic spectral analysis of ocular diseases. Folia Ophthalmol Jpn 35: 2361–2365.

Thijssen J M, Cloostermans M, Bayer A L. 1981. Measurement of ultrasound attenuation in tissues from scattered reflections. In: Ultrasound in Ophthalmology, Proceedings of the 8th SIDUO Congress. Thijssen J M (ed) The Hague: Dr W Junk Publishers. pp. 431–439.

Trier H G, Lepper R D. 1981. Tissue characterization in ophthalmology. In: Ultrasonic Tissue Characterization. Thijssen J M (ed) The Hague: Martinus Nijhoff Publishers. pp. 74–86.

29. Vitreous membranes: update echographical diagnosis

A. REIBALDI, T. AVITABILE, G. CASCONE and L. FRANCO

Summary

Differential diagnosis of vitreous membranes with echography is still a problem.

Up to now the most used parameter to perform this differential diagnosis is reflectivity; the Authors in this study stress the usefulness to consider besides reflectivity, motility, topography and thickness. To obtain all these parameters together they have found out usefull B-scan and especially last generation equipments provided with rapid scansion, high resolution and possibility to perform tissue elaboration on frozen images.

Introduction

Biological membranes possibly occupying vitreous cavity are:
– Vitreous posterior detachment
– Retinal detachment
– Choroideal detachment
– Newly formed membranes

Echographic differential diagnosis among these, although has reached high quality standards thanks to the construction of new equipment with high resolution probes, represents actually a complex and delicate problem for any echographist; this is more evident in relation to the nearly daily use of vitrectomy which makes such diagnosis not academic, but essential (Cardia et al., 1979; Reibaldi et al., 1979, 1983; Avitabile et al., 1987).

Echography and particularly B-scan technique thanks to the chance of studying the vitreous expecially in cases of opaque media have revealed to be of great help for a further development of vitreous surgery (Coleman et al., 1973).

Also since the beginning of such surgical technique Our School has tried

Institute of Ophthalmology, Catania University, Catania, Italy

R. Sampaolesi (ed.), Ultrasonography in Ophthalmology 12, 225–231.
© 1990. Kluwer Academic Publishers, Dordrecht

to define echography as a valid support (Reibaldi et al., 1979, 1983), in fact all its indications are connected with all possible causes of formation of endovitreous membranes (Gallenga et al., 1979; Reibaldi et al., 1979).

Therefore by means of echography, apart from the transparent media, we are able to have quite a detailed picture of vitreous aspect so that it is possible to give informations to the operator about when, where, and which instruments to use for vitrectomy (Reibaldi et al., 1983).

One of the main problems for the echographist in this kind of pathology is to differentiate vitreous membranes, formed after haemorrhage or inflammation etc., from posterior vitreous detachment, from retinal or choroideal detachment.

Today in order to solve this question there are two proposals of different Schools.

The school of Coleman, using mostly B-scan technique, has focused its attention on the following parameters: localization, extension, and thickness (Coleman et al., 1973).

In fact B-scan technique allows us to evaluate these three parameters with multiple scansions with 2 mm gap from each other, starting above the superior limbus towards fornix.

Of course this is possible because such technique offers a bidimensional image of the examined bulbar section, so that we can evaluate at the same time localization, extension and thickness of different vitreous membranes.

On the contrary, the school of Ossoinig, appeals mostly to standardized A-scan technique, by which it is possible to measure reflectivity of a membraneous structure inside vitreous considering scleral reflectivity as a standard and it was noticed that retina has a higher reflectivity in comparison to a vitreous membrane (Ossoinig, 1979).

This classical technique offers good results and it is always valid, but it has the disadvantage of requiring two instruments, one for topography, and the other for differential diagnosis, and furtherly it can be performed only by highly experienced echographists and even in the hands of experts it presents some difficulties.

Such difficulties are connected to the loss of anatomical regularity due to formation of big haematic clots or big membranes; in these cases standardized A-scan technique, studying only reflectivity, appears to be not free from mistakes.

In this study we want to go on the same way outlined by Our School since 1983, to demonstrate how information about reflectivity detectable by standardized A-scan, are contained also in a B-scan image but are more difficult to be appreciated.

In the past a computerized false colour technique was used so that structures of different reflectivity appeared with different colours (Reibaldi et al., 1983, 1986, 1987; Avitabile et al., 1984). Nowadays thanks to the new equipments with highly differenced grey levels, with the possibility of tissue elaboration on frozen images, with the ability to present in false colours a black and white B-scan image, according to reflective characteristics, it is possible within certain limits to get some information on reflectivity also in B-scan, selecting all those points presenting same grey levels, or rejecting from a frozen image a series of grey levels.

Furthermore, with these instruments we can better define edges analyzing their regularity and then we can study image texture. For a correct echographic differencial diagnosis of endovitreous membranes we suggest considering besides reflectivity three other parameters: mobility, thickness, and topography, all obtenible by means of last generation B-scan equipment.

From an ecographic point of view the membranes occupying vitreous cavity are:
- posterior vitreous detachment
- retinal detachment
- choroideal detachment
- newly formed membranes (including post-haemorrhagic ones, post-inflammatory, proliferative retinopathy etc.).

At the Echography Center of the Institute of Ophthalmology, University of Catania, we have been using the following equipment:
- Ophthascan S, A- and B-scan; A-scan with S-curve standardized amplification;
- Storz Renaissance A- and B-scan, with electronic scanning probe and 64 grey levels;
- Sonomed B 3000 with tissutal elaboration of frozen images;
- Ocuscan 200 A with immersion apparatus, M-mode and visualization of signal in radio frequency.

Reflectivity

We have spoken diffusely about this diagnostic echographic parameter which is a hinge in A-scan standardized echography (Ossoinig, 1979). In our opinion, with modern echography, it can be studied also with B-scan echography. Higher reflectivity, in the considered pathology, is found in retinal detachment and choroidal detachment; on the contrary, vitreous membranes, have a lower reflectivity, if they are not old and fibrotic, and in these cases they have a higher and irregular reflectivity. Finally vitreous detachment has an even lower reflectivity, which can increase in cases of blood spreading on posterior hyaloid.

Motility

This parameter can be studied only roughly by A-scan, while most specifi technique is M-mode (Bonavolontá et al., 1983), which however is out of daily practice. So in our opinion the most reliable and practical technique to analyze this parameter is B-scan performed with instruments provided by electronic high speed scansion probes.

Obviously post movements of a structure are studied when the eye has stopped after a quick movement. Vitreous posterior detachment is the pathology endowed with the highest movement because it does not have any insertion, retinal detachment has an average motility, decreasing in old detachments, choroideal detachment lacks post movement because it is anchored to the four vorticous veins (Poujol, 1981) and finally vitreous membranes move together with the eye without post movement.

Topography

This kind of data is obtainable only with the B-scan which gives a bidimensional image of ocular structures allowing us to study the relationship of pathologic membranes.

Vitreous detachment never inserts on optic disk, while retinal detachment can inserts or not. Choroideal detachment inserts pathognomically to vorticous veins forming a characteristical angle with the scleral wall (Poujol 1981).

To study newly formed membranes the B-scan is required either to localize and to define them, otherwise difficult to obtain by means of A-scan (Coleman et al., 1974).

Occasionally new membranes are difficult to be recognized from a partial retinal detachment.

To locate membranes inserting points on ocular globe can be helpful; infact if they are attached in many points anteriorly to ora serrata it is usually a new membrane, on the other hand if they are attached to ora serrata and/or to the optic disk it is generally a retinal detachment (Coleman et al., 1974).

Thickness

This parameter is studied in A-scan, but even better in B-scan with high resolution power which gives information not only on thickness but also on regularity.

Vitreous detachment has the least thickness which can increase if blood is spread on posterior hyaloid.

Retinal detachment is thicker and regular, while even thicker but also regular is the choroideal detachment.

Finally, vitreous membranes being different from previous structures, newly formed and not anatomically preformed, have the peculiarity of an irregular thickness.

A and B-scan ultrasonography give us useful information regarding thickness and consistency of these membranes however information obtained with echography are hard to correlate with real consistency at surgery (Coleman et al., 1977).

Conclusions

We want to point out that according to us differential diagnosis of considered pathologies (vitreous posterior detachment, retinal detachment, choroideal detachment, vitreous membranes) has always been exclusively made by A-scan, based on the study of reflectivity, being a hard test even for experienced echographist.

According to our experience by means of new B-scan equipment available in commerce, we tried to emphasize the study of three other parameters other than reflectivity: motility, topography, and thickness, which are different in the various kinds of pathologies considered so that it is easier and safer to perform diagnosis based on four instead of one parameter (Table 1).

Table 1. Study of the parameters reflectivity, motility, topography and thickness.

Vitreous
Reflectivity: low (higher in the presence of blood stratification)
Motility: maximum
Topography: no insertion in the disk
Thickness: minimum, regular

Retina
Reflectivity: very high
Motility: medium
Topography: possible insertion in the disk
Thickness: medium, regular

Choroid
Reflectivity: very high
Motility: absent
Topography: insertion in the vorticous veins
Thickness: maximum, regular

Membranes
Reflectivity: very high
Motility: absent
Topography: multiple insertion (possible in the disk)
Thickness: irregular

Obviously the study of these parameters is possible thanks to B-scan on a frozen image which give us a lot of informations thanks to the numerous manipulations. To stress the usefulness of B-scan examination it is particularly important to give valid criteria in differential diagnosis among endovitreal membranes because this approach is surely an easier interpretation making this semeiological technique of good comprehension and diffusion requiring especially a short and simple training for the echographist.

References

Avitabile T, Guerriero S, Scuderi G L, Veneziani N, Distante A. 1984. Recenti acquisizioni nella diagnostica ecografica delle membrane vitreali. Atti LXIV Congr. Naz. SOI. pp. 307–311, Roman 29–11/1–12.

Avitabile T, Cacciato F, Bonaccorsi O. 1987. La diagnostica differenziale delle membrane vitreali up-date. Tavola Rotonda attualitá in tema di Strumentazione Diagnostica Ecografica II Congr. Naz. SIEO. Catania.

Avitabile T. Fichera M, Pappalardo A. 1988. L'ecografia nel follow-up della retinopatia diabetica. Comunicazione Giornate Mediterranee di Oftalmologia. Roma.

Bonavolontá A, Cennamo G. 1983. M-mode echography pattern study in retinal detachment. In: J S Hillmann, M M Le May (eds) Ophthalmic Ultrasonography Proceedings of the 9th SIDUO. Congress.

Cardia L, Reibaldi A, Sborgia C, Santoro F. 1979. Acquisizioni e limiti della vitrectomia via pars-plana. Atti XIII Congr. SOM. Chieti.

Coleman D J. 1972. Ultrasound in vitreous surgery. Trans Am Acad Ophth e Otol 76: 467–479.

Coleman D J. Jack R L. 1973. B-scan ultrasonography in diagnosis and management of retinal detachment. Arch Ophthalmol 90: 29–34.

Coleman D J, Franzen L A. 1974. Vitreous surgery. Preoperative evaluation and prognostic value of ultrasonic display of vitreous hemorrhage. Arch Ophthalmol 92: 375–381.

Coleman D J. 1975. Ultrasonic evaluation of the vitreous body. Ultrasonography in Ophthalmology. Bibl Ophthal 83: 86–90.

Coleman D J, Lizzi F L, Jack R L. 1977. Ultrasonography of the Eye and Orbit. Lea e Febiger Philadelphia.

Gallenga P E, Mazzeo V, Cennamo G, Reibaldi A. 1979. Moderni aspetti semeiologici per la chirurgia del vitreo. Atti XIII Congr. SOM. Chieti.

Ossoinig K C. 1979. Standardized echography: basic principles, clinical applications and results. Inter Ophthalmol Clin XIX: 127–285.

Poujol J. 1981. A characteristic echographic sign of choroidal detachment the appearance of the angle of junction with the ocular wall. In: J M Thijssen, A M Verbeek (eds) Ultrasonography in Ophthalmology Proceedings of the 8th SIDUO Congress, pp. 265–267.

Reibaldi A, Delle Noci N, Lorusso V V. 1979. La nostra esperienza sull'utilità della ecografia nella vitrectomia. Atti IV Congr. SISUM. Modena.

Reibaldi A, Di Pilato M, Avitabile T. 1983. Five years of ultrasonography diagnosis in combined surgery through the parsplana. In: J S Hillmann, M M Le May (eds) Ophthalmic Ultrasonography Proceedings of the 9th SIDUO Congress pp 115–119.

Reibaldi A, Avitabile T, Guerriero S, Distante A, Veneziani N L. 1983. Primi risultati sulla possibilità di differenziazione ecografica tissutale mediante falso colore. Comun. VIII Congr. SISUM. Bologna.

Reibaldi A. 1983. L'ecografia nelle membrane vitreali. Relazione Corso Aggiornamento Le Malattie del Vitreo. Roma.

Reibaldi A, Guerriero S, Avitabile T, Veneziani N, Pasquariello G, Pasquali F. 1986. Improvementes on computer assisted echography. Relazione XI Congr. SIDUO Capri.

Reibaldi A, Guerriero S, Avitabile T, Uva MG, Veneziani N, Pasquariello G, Pasquali F. 1987. Texture analysis di immagini ultrasonografiche in oculistica. Clin Ocul e Pat Ocul VIII: 17–25.

Reibaldi A, Avitabile T, Guerriero S, Uva MG. 1987 Possibility of Ocular tissue differentiation by means of false-colour assisted echography. In: K C Ossoinig (ed) Ophthalmic Echography Proceeding of the Xth SIDUO Congress pp. 201–206.

30. Reliability of standardized ultrasound in pre-operative diagnosis for vitreous surgery in diabetic patients

J. A. BADIA, W. DEGREGORI, G. IRIBARREN
and R. SAMPAOLESI

Summary

Thirty five patients with proliferative diabetic retinopathy were examined with ultrasound. The authors show the correlation found between echography and vitreous surgery findings.

Introduction

Vitreous surgery has made remarkable progress in recent years.

Diabetic retinopathy is one of the most common indication for echography in those eyes in which a correct visualization of the fundus is not possible because of lens opacities or vitreous hemorrage.

Interpretation of the findings is often difficult because of the complex vitreoretinal relationship. The interpretation depends both on B and A scan data.

The purpose of this paper is to show the correlation found between ultrasound and vitreous surgery findings in proliferative diabetic retinopathy patients.

Material and methods

Thirty-five patients with proliferative diabetic retinopathy were divided into two groups.

Group A included 18 patients with mild to massive proliferative retinopathy with or without vitreous traction.

Group B included 17 patients with moderate to massive proliferative retinopathy, evidence of vitreous traction and localized or total retinal detachment.

University of Buenos Aires, Argentina

R. Sampaolesi (ed.), Ultrasonography in Ophthalmology 12, 233–237.

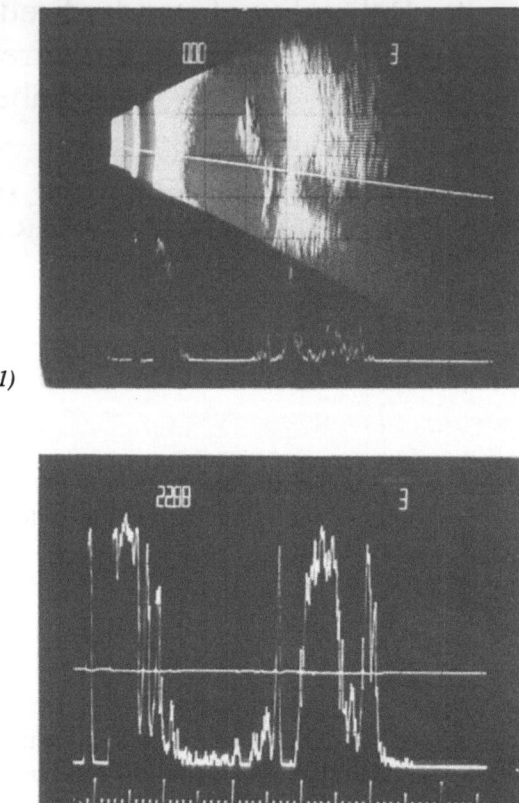

(1)

(2)

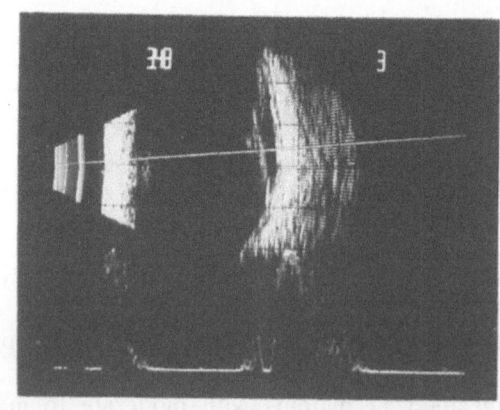

(3)

Figs. 1, 2, 3. Group A: mild to massive proliferative retinopathy with or without vitreous traction.

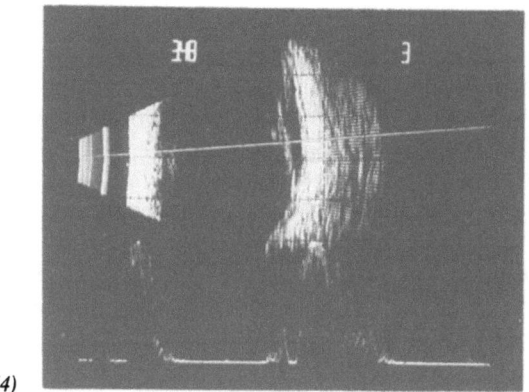

(4)

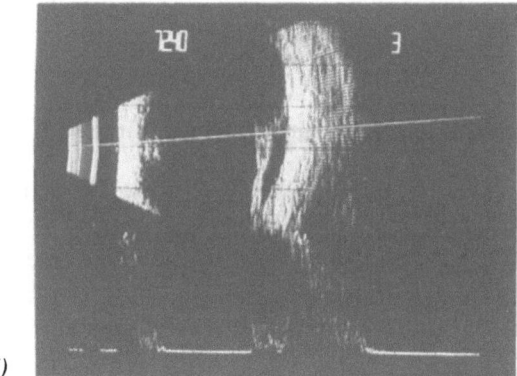

(5)

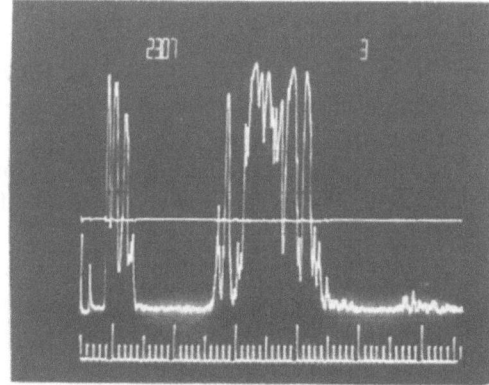

(6)

Figs. 4, 5, 6. Group B: mild to massive proliferative retinopathy, vitreous traction and localized or total retinal detachment.

The instrument used was a Sonokretz with 8 MHz and 10 MHz probes for A- and B-scan respectively.

All patients were examined on the days prior to surgery. Ultrasound was preformed in the horizontal, oblique and vertical planes with A- and B-scan, and Quantitative I and II techniques.

B-scan criteria was; shape, distribution and mobility.

A-scan criteria was; shape, distribution, mobility and the study of reflectivity.

Findings were plotted in the chart and finally a two dimentional drawing of the fundus was made in order to compare with vitreous surgery findings.

Results

In group A, 18 patients, the diagnosis was correct in 15 cases.

Two cases had localized retinal detachment considered as membranes, but they had borderline reflectivity.

One case showed a localized retinal detachment not diagnosed.

Mean reflectivity in relationship with quantitative II A scan was 22, 38 db.

In group B, 17 patients, 13 had a local or total retinal detachment.

One case was a proliferative membrane diagnosed as retinal detachment, another case was a retinal detachment considered as membrane; both cases showed borderline reflectivity.

Two cases had localized retinal detachment diagnosed as membrane.

Mean reflectivity for this groupw as 14.72 db.

Conclusion

The combination of standardized A- and B-scan shows to be a reliable method to give information of the status of diabetic retinopathy eyes that are ready to undergo vitreous surgery.

The borderline cases just mentioned show that sometimes it is very difficult to differentiate a dense proliferative membrane from a longstanding retinal detachment.

It is probable that the development of new A- or B-scan criteria can help us to solve this problem.

References

Bigar F et al. 1977. Combined A-B scan Echography. Preoperative evaluation of Vitrectomy patient. Mod Prob Ophthalmol 18: 2.

Muller-Breitenkamp R, Trier H G, Völker B, Mester U. 1983. Errors in Diagnostic ultrasound, a Critical review of 68 patients undergoing diagnostic ultrasound before vitrectomy. Documenta Ophthalmologica Proceedings Series 38–107.

Ossoinig K C. 1974. Quantitative Echography—The basis of Tissue differentiation. J Clin Ultrasound 2 (1): 33.

Ossoinig K C. 1979. Standardized Echography. Basic Principles clinical Aplications and results. Int Ophthalmol Clin 19 (4): 127.

Ossoinig K C, Islas G, Tamayo G E, Tamburrelli C. 1987 Detached Retina versus dense fibrovascular membrane. Standardized A-scan and B-scan criteria Documenta Ophthalmologica Proceedings Series 48: 275.

Reibaldi A, Di Pilato M. Avitabile T. 1983. Five years of ultrasonographic diagnosis in combined surgery trough the pars plana. Documenta Ophthalmologica Proceedings Series 38: 115.

Shimizu K, Minoda K. 1981. Preoperative evaluation of Vitreous surgery by ultrasonography. Documenta Ophthalmologica Proceedings Series 29: 33.

31. Ultrasound imaging in retinopathy of prematurity: retinal detachment in ROP stage 5 eyes and eye size as prognostic indicator

H. C. FLEDELIUS

Introduction

In principle, ultrasound evaluation of retinopathy of prematurity (ROP) may apply to two situations:

A) During the acute stages of retinopathy ultrasound could be used for diagnosing early retinal detachment, as discussed also at the workshop that led to the international classification of retinopathy of prematurity decided upon in 1984. Ophthalmoscopically it may be extremely difficult to establish the transition from ROP stage 3 to 4; often there are hazy media in such eyes, and the all-over examining conditions are far from optimal. Thus ultrasound might be useful, but the proposal was rejected, for three reasons. 1) To make it accessible for all ophthalmologists the new 1984-ROP classification should be based alone on ophthalmoscopy. 2) Objections against introducing ultrasound equipment were foreseen from those in charge of neonatal wards since no unnecessary strain, including risk of infection, should be applied to the frail immature infant. 3) The B-scan transducers in common use are not suited for the tiny anatomy to be examined.

B) The state of affairs is different when the infant with non-regressed severe ROP has reached the age of 4–7 months. The infant has grown and is clinically stable. Obviously ultrasound can now be used for clarifying intra-ocular morphology, as touched upon in the definitive 1987 classification of (late) stage 4 and 5 ROP. The item was further stressed in an impressive article by Jabbour et al. (Dec. 1987) summing up the experience from 184 consecutive patients with stage 5 ROP. Assessed against the eventual outcome of vitrectomy, ultrasonography proved to be the predictive method of choice, the shape of the funnel retinal detachment (FRD) being a so important prognostic feature.

Both articles showed beautiful drawings of eyes with various types of retinal detachment, all to suggest that the experienced ultrasonographer should meet no problems in depicting such morphology. Having examined

Department of Ophthalmology, Central Hospital, 3400 Hillerød, Denmark

R. Sampaolesi (ed.), Ultrasonography in Ophthalmology 12, 239–248.
© 1990. Kluwer Academic Publishers, Dordrecht

11 patients with severe ROP, however, my own findings appear less une-quivocal than apparent from the statements of Jabbour and coworkers.

At the 1984 SIDUO X meeting ROP and posterior eye segment ultra-sound anatomy was put under discussion through clinical series reported by groups headed by Mazzeo and Takao. Against the present background, including the increased knowledge gained by clinicians' use of the ROP classifications, I wanted to reconsider the topic in a SIDOU context.

Material and methods

Eleven children with a severe visual handicap due to ROP were evaluated ultrasonographically, all by the author. The age range at examination was 4½ months to 12 years.

Case No. 1 was seen in the University Eye Clinic at Rigshospitalet, Copenhagen 1978; equipment Bronson-Turner B-scan. The remaining 10 patients were seen in the County Hospital Eye Clinic 1982–1988; equipment Sonometrics DBR 400, A- and B-scan. Contact scans were used. When required, topical anaesthesia (oxybuprocaine as eye drops) was given.

Table 1 presents the data. In 7 subjects both eyes were blind. In cases No. 3 and 9 the better eye showed myopia of prematurity. Six were examined only once. Five had 2–5 examinations.

Regarding treatment, two eyes had cryotherapy, and two eyes had RD surgery with encircling band; eventually all 4 eyes ended in the ROP 5 category. One eye with ROP 4 had cataract extraction and pars plana vitrectomy, performed at the age of 10 years.

Results

Fifteen out of the 22 eyes had typically clear lenses and leukocoria and were classified as ROP stage 5. There was no light perception, and a funnel-shaped retinal detachment (FRD) was the anticipated posterior eye segment morphology.

The ultrasound findings are given in the last two columns of Table 1. B-scan showed FRD in 3 eyes,with what Mazzeo et al. (1987) described as a 'complete retrolental mass with a triangle-shaped or T-shaped retinal detachment'. In three eyes, the echopattern was compatible with funnel detachment, but far less conspicuous (FRD?). Echographically, the remain-ing 9 eyes showed no evidence of retinal detachment, and with an echo-pattern resembling that of synchysis scintillans the designation DVO (dense vitreous opacities) has been used in Table 1.

For the illustrations I desisted from showing the dense triangle- or T-shaped echocomplexes tapering towards the optic disc region, a pattern familiar to all. Instead, the figures demonstrate what here is called DVO.

Table 1. Clinical and ultrasound findings in 11 patients with severe ROP in one eye or in both eyes. Five had repeated ultrasound evaluations. FRD = funnel retinal detachment, PM posterior mass, DVO = dense vitreous opacities, SVO = slight vitreous opacities.

Case No	Sex	Birth year	Gest. age/birth weight	Age at US-exam	ROP stage r.e.	ROP stage l.e.	Ultrasound finding		Axial length (mm)	
1.	m	1968	27/1240	10 years	5	5	FRD	FRD	14	14
2.	f	1975	30/1100	12 years	5	4	DVO	PM	15	18.5
3.	m	1979	28/1240	5 years	2	5	normal	DVO	22.5	16.2
4.	m	1982	30/1100	12 months	5	5	DVO	DVO	12	12
5.	f	1984	29/1335	5–18 months	5	5	DVO	DVO	14.5	14.5
6.	m	1984	29/1520	5–30 months	5	5	FRD?	DVO	14	15
7.	f	1985	25/920	5 months	2	4	normal	SVO	19.2	17.7
8.	f	1986	27/728	4–7 months	4	2	PM?	normal	14	18
9.	m	1986	28/865	4–24 months	2	5	normal	DVO	19.8	16.9
10.	m	1987	25/920	5–14 months	5	5	FRD?	FRD?	14	14
11.	m	1987	27/920	4½ months	5	5	FRD	DVO	15	15.1

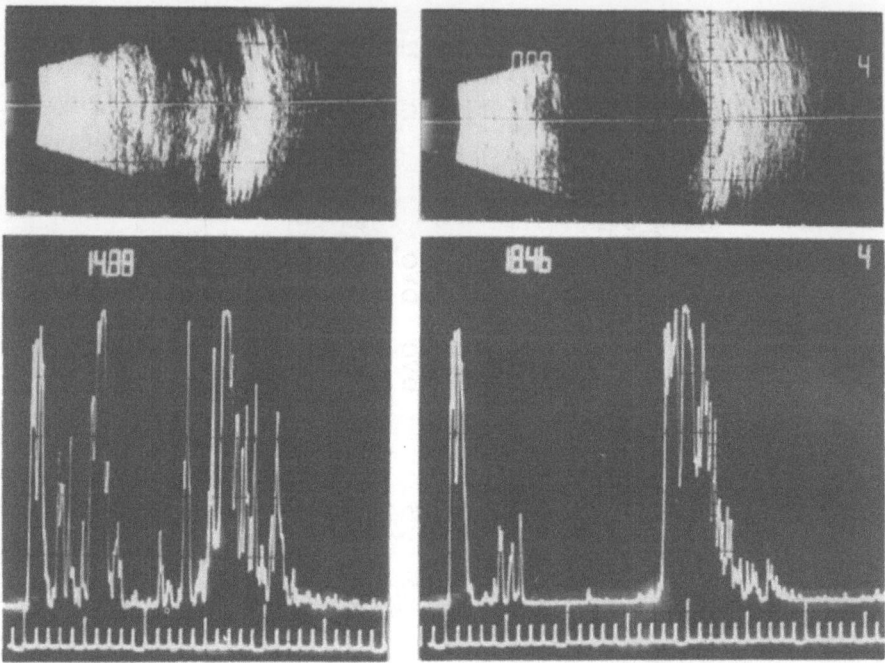

Fig. 1. A 12-year-old girl with ROP 5 of right eye (pictures to the left) and ROP 4 of left eye (right pictures). Case No 2, cf. table 1 and text.

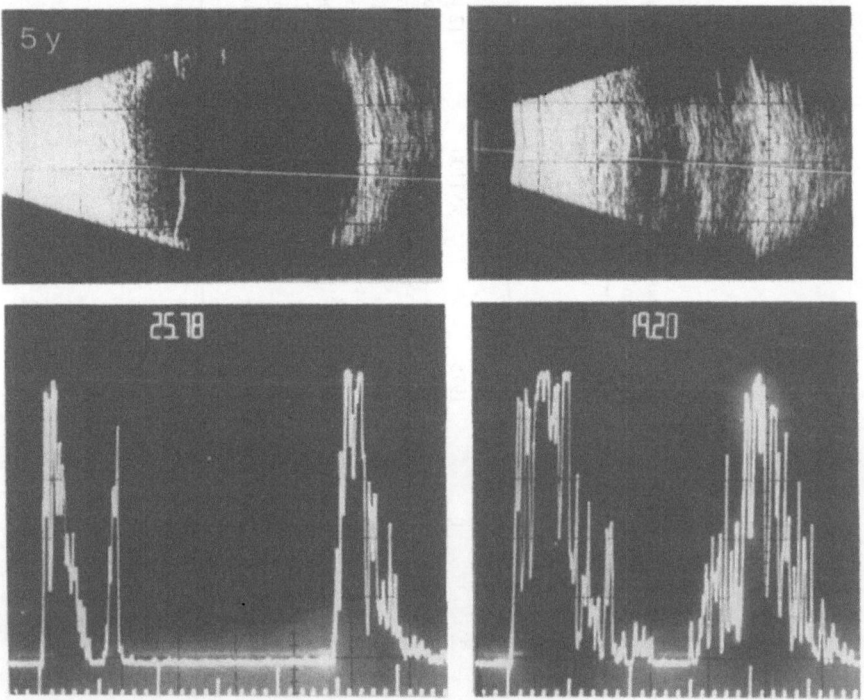

Fig. 2. A 5-year-old boy with myopia of prematurity of right eye (left pictures) and ROP 5 of left eye (pictures to the right). Case No 3, cf. table 1 and text.

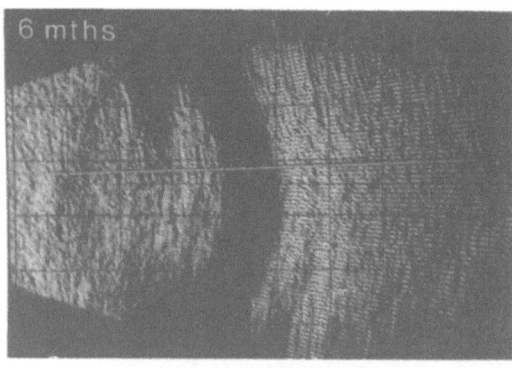
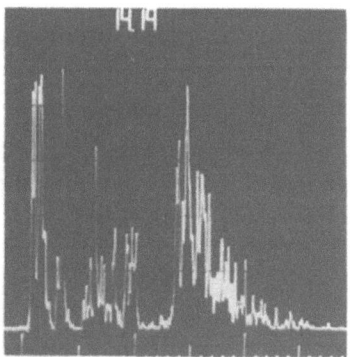
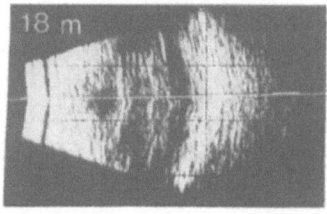
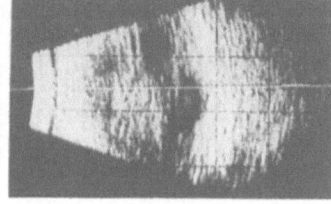

Fig. 3. Examinations at ages 6 and 18 months of a girl with bilateral ROP 5. Case No. 5.

Case No. 2 (Fig. 1). Blind right eye, ROP 5. Left eye ROP 4, with light perception; slight visual improvement was felt after cataract surgery and vitrectomy performed at the age of 10 years. Ultrasound evaluation at the age of 12 years was difficult because of deep-set eyes and coarse nystagmus. Right eye DVO pattern. Left eye echofree posterior compartment except a posterior mass. Axial lengths 14.9 and 18.5 mm.

Case No. 3 (Fig. 2). Right eye 6/12, myopia of prematurity (–10.0 sph × –1.5 cyl) when examined at the age of 5½ years. Blind left eye ROP 5, with DVO. The axial lengths shown are through-the-lid measurements.

Case No.5 (Fig. 3). The two ROP 5 eyes being identical, only the left eye is shown at top, examined at the age of 6 months, double size echogram. Below, the two eyes at the age of 18 months. Axial lengths about 14.5 mm.

Case No.6 (Fig. 4). A posterior DVO is seen at the age of 5 months in both ROP 5 eyes, with stronger echoes one month later. At bottom, the left eye at the age of 14 months and 30 months, now with condensated zones in the DVO-pattern, but without obvious RD resemblance.

Axial lengths

All stage 5 eyes were very short, a feature to indicate involution of the eye under study. In one patient (Fig. 4) the actual eye shortening could be demonstrated by serial measurements.

244

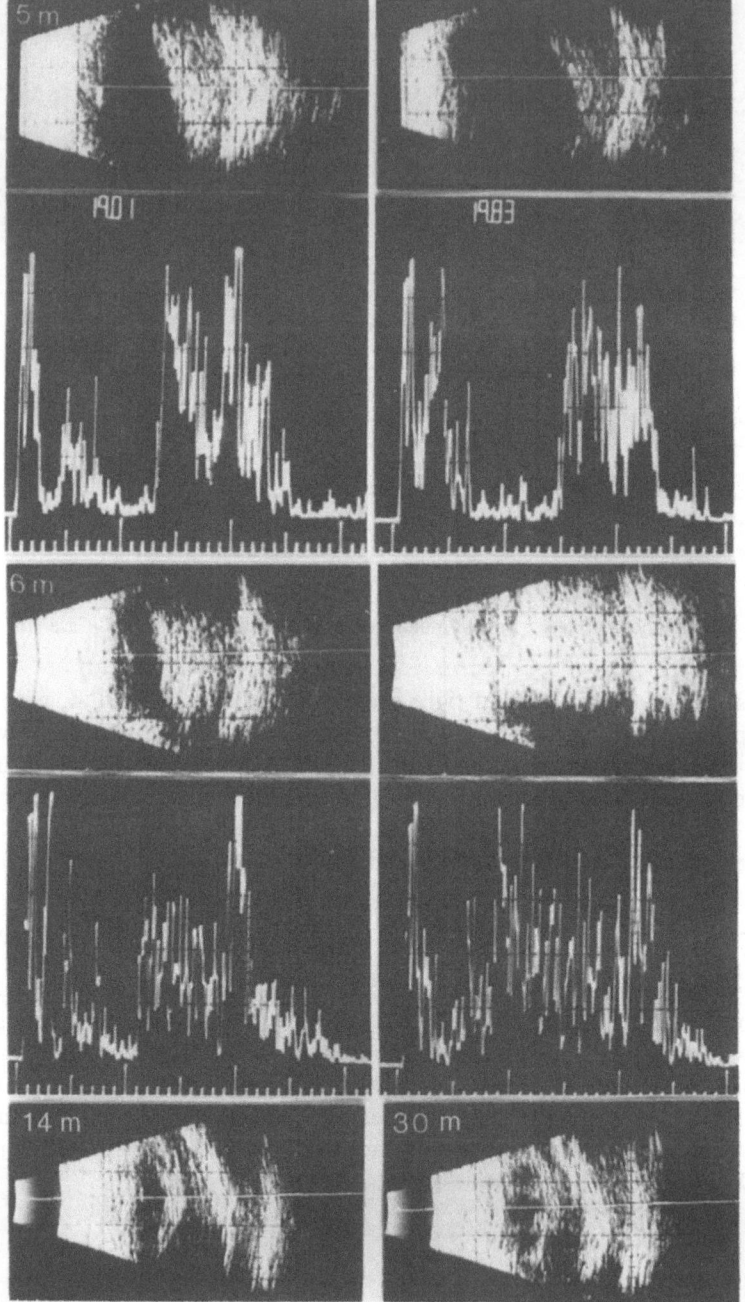

Fig. 4. Serial examinations, at the age of 5,6 14, and 30 months. Case No 6, a boy with
bilateral ROP 5.

Discussion

Statements from literature

So far, full consensus regarding ultrasound imaging of severe ROP has not been achieved. On the one hand, the already quoted statements of Jabbour et al. (1987) appear very clear-cut. Far less unequivocal are my own results, and other reports may be placed on a scale bridging the two views. Some quotations will be given:

On the 1984 SIDOU X session there were two papers dealing with the item. Analysing 11 ROP cases examined at the age of 3 months to 15 years, Mazzeo and coworkers stated that the echographic findings adhered well to the clinical staging. Apparent discrepancies between clinical and echographical classifications were, however, present in three of the 11 subjects. On repeated examinations, one ROP 5 eye thus showed only a retrolental echocomplex, 'a finding that cannot be explained since it is well known that cicatricial ROP is characterized by a partial or total retinal detachment'.

These authors further quoted a case by Shammas (1983) with exactly the same (negative) echopattern, and they summarized that 'on comparison of echographic findings with drawings published by vitreo-retinal surgeons, only partial agreement emerged'. Mention was also given of Trese (1984) for being 'unable to predict by ultrasound which eyes had a partially closed and which had a totally closed retinal detachment'.

On the same 1984-conference, Takao et al. described B-scan findings in 11 subjects with rush-type active ROP. An early membrane-like structure of wedge-shape demonstrated on B-scan was thought to represent extraretinal fibrovascular proliferation, the structure required for defining stage 3 ROP, but this could not be confirmed where the ocular media allowed inspection. Conversely, in eyes where such extraretinal proliferation was established ophthalmoscopically, the authors found no obvious counterpart on the ultrasound screen.

In 1985 Shapiro & Stone felt the need to publish ultrasound findings in 30 eyes from 20 patients, examined at age 5 months to 40 years, 'since there had been no previous in-depth analysis of the B-mode ultrasonic appearance of eyes with ROP exhibiting leukocoria'. After valuably having emphasized anterior segment changes, they reported that membraneous changes consistent with fibroproliferation in the vitreous could be seen as low-amplitude echoes in the vitreous of 63% of the eyes in the series and could be differentiated, in part, from the echoes of a totally detached retina in that the latter have higher amplitudes.

In 1987, the phrasing of the ROP retinal detachment classification committee appeared cautious: It was said that the more unusual configurations of the FRD in stage 5 ROP 'can sometimes be appreciated by ultrasonography'. Further, 'subretinal blood or exudate may be identifiable by ultra-sonographic examination but can be difficult to distinguish from one another by this modality; subretinal membranes may be present, but they are usually recognized only during surgery'.

Recently, then, there is the view of Jabbour et al. (1987), based on the vitrectomy outcome in the largest ROP sample analysed so far with respect also to ultrasound, cf. introduction. 'The most valuable preoperative examination tool proved to be ultrasonography, since it accurately gave us most of the information on posterior eye segment morphology (90–100% correct predictions), however with the exception of retinal vascularity (ultra-sound of no value at all) and some of the membrane morphology (57% correct).

Discussing the above paper, Tasman added (1987): 'also in our experience the most helpful preoperative diagnostic tool has been ultrasonography. However, we have been unable to duplicate the results where there is a narrow funnel both anteriorly and posteriorly'.

On lines with the Jabbour group and Tasman were comments by de Juan (of Duke University Center, Durham, US) forwarded during a 1986 Jeru-salem conference on ocular circulation and neovascularization, the occasion being a paper I gave on ROP blindness in Denmark. Here I put under discussion one of my above ROP 5 cases (Fig. 3, at top) where the B-scan DVO pattern seemed puzzling, considering that anatomically a funnel detachment was expected. After completing the present survey, the ultra-sonic experience of de Juan and coworkers has become available on print (1988). In a sample of 27 ROP infants the B-scans were interpreted mainly as some type of funnel detachment. In a few cases there were patterns corresponding to my DVO designation, however interpreted by the authors as subretinal echoes due to haemorrhage. My experience is that blood remnants do not reflect so strongly unless they have undergone organization, which is unlikely that early. Further, their illustration did not show evidence of retinal detachment as an anterior demarcation of the echo-complexes.

Comments

Against the overwhelming evidence presented in the recent US-materials, one should obviously hesitate before expressing reservation or doubt based on small material and retrospective evaluation. However, some points and questions may be forwarded:

1) From ultrasound experience in adolescents and adults a funnel-shaped retinal detachment is *always* easy to demonstrate by B-scan ultrasound.

2) Conversely, if a typical FRD B-scan configuration cannot be demon-strated, one may question the presumed or postulated presence of a funnel detachment.

3) Some of the ultrasonic DVO-patterns shown in my own series bear resemblance to what is found for instance in eyes with synchysis scintillans, a

finding to signify medium or strongly reflecting particles in the vitreous or in other ocular compartments. Undoubtedly, experienced ultrasonographers will agree that examining such eyes, a combination of changing transducer direction, gaze direction, and sensitivity setting, would separate an orderly RD-pattern from the diffuse echopatterns otherwise seen, provided RD is present.

4) Accordingly one may ask if the posterior eye segment morphology in advanced non-regressed ROP is more varied than apparent from the pathologic specimens and didactic drawings chosen for the quoted US 1987-publications, for instance. Per definition, the blind ROP 5 eye harbours a total retinal detachment, but could other morphology be conceived? An avascular retina with an atrophic optic nerve might thus explain the visual finding, for instance.

5) The paper of Jabbour et al. (1987) gave no details of the age of the infants when examined, ultrasonic equipment or equipments used, over-all examining condition including +/– general anaesthesia etc. Probably many were under general anaesthesia. In principle, this would allow the examiner to use forceps to change the eye position, for instance, with a better chance of demonstrating the strong reflecting anatomical surfaces and their connection to the posterior pole of the eye.

6) As a last point I would like to emphasize eye size proper, a parameter which has not gained due attention in the above materials. It is well-known that eyes blind because of ROP are usually microphthalmic (Francois and Goes (1971), Bertenyi and Fodor (1981), for instance). In general, however, axial length has not been employed as a prognostic indicator of its own right when trying to predict the result of surgical restoration of posterior eye segment anatomy, the ultimate goal of which should be some useful vision for the subject.

Undoubtedly, the material of Jabbour et al. (1987) makes such estimates possible. For the future this might be helpful in selecting the ROP-infants who could benefit from vitrectomy and other late surgical procedures. Knowledge about posterior eye segment morphology on B-scan certainly is required, but axial length may prove of equal importance. Probably, an eye size under a certain limit, depending on the infants age, is an obstacle to restoring vision of any practical importance.

References

Bertényi A, Fodor M. 1981. A-mode ultrasonography in cases of leukokoria. In: Thijssen J, Verbeek A M (eds) Docum Ophthal Proc Ser 29: 97–102.

Committee for classification of ROP. 1984. An international classification of retinopathy of prematurity. Arch Ophthalmol 102: 1130–34.

Committee for classification of the late stages of ROP. 1987. An international classification of retinopathy of prematurity II, the classification of retinal detachment. Arch Ophthalmol 105: 906–12.

Fledelius H C, Hansen S E. 1987. Retinopathy of prematurity, past and recent experience in

Denmark. In: BenEzra D, Ryan SJ (eds) Docum Ophthal Proc Ser 50: 169–73. Discussion by deJuan E.

Francois J, Goes F. 1971. Ultrasonography in pediatric ophthalmology. J Ped Ophthal 8: 221–33.

Jabbour NM, Eller AE, Hirose T, Schepens CL, Liberfarb R. 1987. Stage 5 retinopathy of prematurity. Prognostic value of morphologic findings. Ophthalmology 94: 1640–45.

deJuan E, Shields S, Machemer R. 1988. The role of ultrasound in the management of retinopathy of prematurity. Ophthalmology 95: 884–88.

Mazzeo V, Ravalli L, Falco L, Scorrano R. 1987. B-scan in retinopathy of prematurity (SIDUOX 1984). In: Ossoinig KC (ed) Docum Ophthal Proc Ser 48: 431–35.

Shammas J. 1983. Atlas of ophthalmic ultrasonography and biometry. CV Mosby, St. Louis.

Shapiro DR, Stone RD. 1985. Ultrasonic characteristics of retinopathy of prematurity presenting with leukokoria. Arch Ophthalmol 103: 1690–94.

Takao Y, Hayashi H, Oshima K, Kitagawa Y. 1987. B-scan ultrasonographic findings in eyes with rush-type ROP. In: Ossoinig KC (ed) Docum Ophthal Proc Ser 48: 437–41.

Tasman WS. 1987. Discussion to Jabbour et al., Ophthalmology 94: 1646.

Trese MT. 1984. Surgical results of stage V RLF and timing of surgical repair. Ophthalmology 91: 461–66.

32. Gas retinal detachment treatment and echography

A. REIBALDI, T. AVITABILE, A. PAPPALARDO and L. FRANCO

Summary

It is well known that in last years retinal detachment surgery is changing expecially thanks to the use of gases.

One of the main problem is to monitorize these patients before and after the surgery considering that owing to gas presence it is difficult to utilize classic ophthalmoscopy.

The authors present their surgical case report and their echographic follow up especially based on the use of B-scan which allows bubble localization, its measurement (area with new equipementes), and its relation with residual detachment.

Introduction

Pneumatic retinopexy is a surgical technique used in the treatment of selected cases of retinal detachment, it was first performed 15 years ago (Norton, 1973; Vygantas, 1973), but only recently has been greatly diffused since the discover of new gaseous substances had demonstrated the efficiency to tampon (Dominguez, 1985; Hilton et al., 1986).

Among most commonly used gases: air, FS6, C3F8, our choice dropped on perfluoropropane (C3F8), due to its greater expanding attitude, infact its volume multiplies four times in 96 hours, and due to its extented period inside the eye before reabsorbing (30 days). So that it guaranties a better and longer tamponade effect in comparison to air, and to sulfur hexafluoride (FS6), which expands 1,5 times and it is able to stay inside the eye for 10–15 days. (Reibaldi et al., 1987, 1988, 1988).

The aim of this paper is to try to answer by means of echography to many unsolved questions.

Catania University, Institute of Ophthalmology, Catania, Italy

R. Sampaolesi (ed.), Ultrasonography in Ophthalmology 12, 249–255.

Role of echography

Ocular echography has a well determined role in the treatment of retinal detachment by means of a pneumatic retinopexy, before and after operation. (Avitabile et al., 1987)

Before surgery every eye that has to be treated undergoes, to: A-scan ecobiometry, measuring anter-posterior and latero-lateral diameters to evaluate eye dimensions, in order to establish the amount of gas to use (0,4 or 0.5 cc of C3F8), and to the B-scan to overview clinical feature.

After surgery we will perform a B-scan echography daily for 7 days, and then once a week for 1 month, to monitorize the gas bubble expansion, its topographic connection with retina and the amount of eventual residual detachment.

Expecially for this purpose, echography, has shown to be particularly effective, because in these cases ophthalmoscopy is not easy due to optical phenomena like reflexion, diffusion and diffraction of light, caused by the surface of gas bubble; so we will not be able to well evaluate retina conditions behind the bubble.

Furtherly the evaluation of gas bubble in ophthalmoscopy would be subjective and rather uncertain; on the contrary by means of echography we are able, to perform accurate measurements and to calculate the area of a section of the same bubble.

In fact experimentally, echography has proved to be of great help to perform mathemathic calculations enabling us to get the approximate volume of a gas bubble, so that we can evaluate how much it expands in the follow up.

Parver and Lincoff (1978) on mathematical and experimental model outlined how it is possible to calculate exactly the volume of an intraocular gas bubble which assumes the shape of a polar cap on the base of the ray of glass model of vitreous cavity and on the contact arc between bubble and glass wall. On the other hands those evaluations in human eye under direct observation would be affected by parallatic mistakes giving us unreliable values.

Material and methods

In our Echography Center at the Institute of Ophthalmology of Catania University, we have been using a last generation A- B-scan computerized instrument, able to perform accurate measurements of eye dimension by A-scan, which is provided with an acquiring automatic system of the image when the probe is perfectly perpendicular to retina. The equipment gives us, then, immediately, in mm, the antero-posterior value and the depth of the anterior chamber. From these two data we can easily get eye ray value, which will be used to calculate the gas bubble volume. By means of B-scan, using markers on a frozen image it is possible to measure the distance between the anterior part of the bubble and posterior profile of the eye, recording daily the movements of the anterior face of the bubble while it is expanding, and besides, we can define by means of a poligonal line, the edge of the bubble and calculate the area of the maximal section. Since, as we know, gas, like air, is not crossed by ultrasounds, from an echographic point of view, it will appear like a foreign body, with a typical shape both in the A-scan and B-scan.

In the A-scan we shall notice the presence of a high reflectivity peak inside vitreous cavity, followed by a shadowing of posterior structure.

In the B-scan, the anterior face of the bubble will present a high reflectivity interface, followed by a shadowing of retina, choroid, sclera and of retrobulbar structures.

While the A-scan examination is performed with patient in supine position before surgery, to establish the amount of C3 F8 to inject according to eye dimensions, the B-scan is used to monitorize the eye after surgery, and it is performed with seated patient, upright head and eyes in primary look position.

We pointed out a particular protocol providing a series of 4 scansions obtained putting the probe on eyelids both horizontally and vertically on upper and inferior lid, nasally and temporally; so that we can have eye images respectively of inferior, superior, temporal and nasal quadrants.

In this way we will obtain a real map of the eye, and we could evaluate relationship between gas bubble and retina, visualizing at the same time both and allowing us to appreciate progressive bubble expansion and flat retina under the bubble. Then at the end of the test, aligning probe perfectly we will freeze the image which can better show bubble shape and we will perform on it, measurements of distance between front wave and posterior complex, establishing the edge of the bubble by means of a poligonal line, in order to evaluate the maximal obtainable section area.

Of course to make these measurements reliable, it will be necessary to perform them by putting the probe always in the same position and taking as a referring point always the same sections where the bubble appears of maximal dimensions; it would be remarkable, then, if it could be performed by the same operator to reduce chances of mistakes [to a minimum].

In this way we will get maximal section surface bubble in mm^2 and we will calculate the volume of the bubble which geometrically assumes the shape of polar cap.

Referring to the mathematic model of Parver and Lincoff (1978), it is possible, to know the eye ray, and the surface of maximal section data obtained echographically, we will be able to calculate the bubbles volume.

The surface 'S' corresponding to the maximal section of the bubble, is obtained by the following formula:

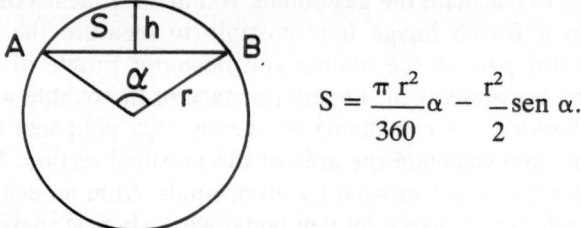

$$S = \frac{\pi r^2}{360}\alpha - \frac{r^2}{2}\,\text{sen}\,\alpha.$$

Where alfa is the angular extension expressed in degrees, of the contact arc between bubble and internal surface of the eye.

Knowing both area S and ray r, because previously determined by means of echography, it is possible to obtain mathametically the alfa value, and with that one we can, then calculate height h.

$$h = r\left(1 - \cos\frac{\alpha}{2}\right).$$

At this point we can calculate the volume 'V' of polar cup.

$$V = \frac{\pi h^2 (3r - h)}{3}$$

In order to evaluate and monitorize bubble volume variations, we performed a first measurements one hour after gas injection inside the eye and then daily after 24, 48, 72, 96 hours.

Case report

Since December 1986 till today in the Institute of Ophthalmology of Catania University we have been using a pneumatic retinopexy in 24 eyes affected by retinal detachment, in patients between the age of 45 and 77, 11 males 13 females; all of them had a retinal detachment in one eye only.

Corrected visual acuity in affected eye was 10/10 in 2 cases, 9/10 in 1 case, and between 6/10 and hand movements in the remaining cases.

Detachment extended to 1 quadrant in 7 cases, 2 quadrants in 13 cases, and 3 quadrants in 4 cases. (Table 1).

Table 1.

1 Quadrant	7 Cases
2 Quadrants	13 Cases
3 Quadrants	4 Cases

Results: in 14 patients retina reattached, within 24 hours, in 8 patients in 48 h, while in 2 patients, a man and a woman respectively 72 and 74 years old, who were not able to keep the correct position, reattachment did not take place (Table 2).

Table 2. Results.

Retinal reatchment within 24 h	14 Cases
Retinal reatchment within 48 h	8 Cases
No retinal reatchment	2 Cases

In these two patients who were then surgically treated with traditional encircling and buckling technique, evacuative puncture and criopexy, retina was perfectly reattached.

Only in 1 case, on the first day after surgery, gas came out and we had to repeat the injection.

In this case by means of the B-scan echography we detected a reduction instead of an increase of gas bubble.

After treatment, visual acuity was 10/10 in 3 patients, with an increase of 1/10 in a patient with 9/10 visual acuity; in 14 cases visual acuity was between 5/10 and 8/10 and in the remaining 5 cases between 3/50 and 2/10. The 2 patients operated with the tradictical technique reported a final visual acuity of 1/10 and 2/10 respectively.

Correlation between initial and final volume was studied in our report. Smaller eyes, with diameters of about 18 mm, had the first day a maximal section of 33 mm^2 with corresponding volume of 285 mm^3; while on 4th day a maximal section of 94 mm^2 surface, with a 1057 mm^3 volume with an average rate between first and 4th day of about 1 : 3.70.

In the bigger eyes, (24.5 mm of diameter) we had, on the first day an area of 60 mm^2 with a volume of 695 mm^3 and a 161 mm^2 area and then a 2434 mm^3 volume at 4th day and a rate of about 1:3.56. (Table 3)

Table 3. Volume calculation.

Diameter	1st day		4th day		1 day/ 4 day
	Area	Volume	Area	Volume	
18 mm	33 mm^2	285 mm^3	94 mm^2	1057 mm^3	1 : 3.70
24.5 mm	60 mm^2	695 mm^3	161 mm^2	2434 mm^3	1 : 3.56

We can state, then, on the base of experimental data, now gas can expand itself reaching a 4 times volume in about four days, as it has already been proved.

Conclusions

In our experience pneumatic retinopexy resulted as a very effective technique and at the same time simple to be performed; we can state that in certain selected cases it represents a valid alternative to traditional surgery of retinal detachment; furthermore it has the advantage to be performed in local anaesthesia, even if it must be outlined that a good result is always related to a good patient compliance.

Validity and effectiveness of this technique is related to the complete respect of anatomical structures without apposition of surgical buckling or external circling that deforming the eye morfology, affect patient's refraction and visual acuity.

We think that echography is an essential aid for the amount of gas to be used, and to monitorize post-surgery follow-up. It gives us precious informations that ophthalmoscopy is not able to do, especially concerning that area of retina beyond gas bubble.

B-scan technique allows a daily evaluation of position, volume, and bubble connections with eye and detached retina, pointing out when it reaches maximal dimensions and when the retina is flat.

Our results encourage us to keep going on this way to study closely certain aspects: for instance if the tamponade effect on retina occurs on retina directly from bubble, or if vitreous is between retina and gas bubble.

In the end it looks clear that up today contribution given by echography to evaluate parameters concerning pneumatic retinopexy, appears to be essential to measure gas inside the eye; we wish in the future, on the base of new experiences and new echobiometric data, to know more precisely, the amount of C3F8, to be used especially in relation to eye dimensions, in order to provide a higher success rate.

References

Arpa P, Zenomi S, Vinciguerra M, De Molfetta V. 1987. Valutazione del tamponamento episclerale dopo vitrectomia ed espansione della camera vitrea con gas. Atti LXVII Congresso SOI. Roma.

Avitabile T, Pappalardo A. Reibaldi A. 1988. Il ruolo dell'ecografia nella retinopessia pneumatica. Atti II Congr. Naz. SIEO. Catania 7 Nov. 1987, In: Clinica Oculistica e Patologia Oculare IX, 4: 276–278, Luglio-Agosto.

Bonnet M, Aracil P, Pekold C, Dacol E. 1987. Etude de 130 decollement de retine ayant necessite un tamponnement interne par un gas expansif. Bull Soc Ophthal Franc. LXXXVII, 5: 693–696.

Bonnet M, Santamaria E, Mouche J. 1987. Intraoperative use of pure perfluoropropane gas in the management of proliferative vitreoretinopathy. Graefe's Archive Clin Exp Ophthalmol 225, 299–302.

Borgioli M, Cona F, Lambertucci D. 1988. Pneumoretinopessia e fotocoagulazione argon laser nel trattamento di casi selezionati di distacco regmatogeno di retina. IV Congresso Società Italiana Laser in Oftalmologia. Cortina D'Ampezzo 20–22 Gennaio.

Constable I J. 1974. Perfluoropentane in experimental ocular surgery. Invest Ophthalmol 13: 627–629.

Costandines G, Hochart G, Vanhullebusch A, Aracil P, Ribiere L, Castier P. 1986. Le traitment des dechirures retiniennes superieures avec decollement de retine par la seule injection intra-vitreenne de gas associèe la crioàpplication. Bull Soc Ophthal Franc LXXXVI 6–7: 883–886.

Critteden J J, De Juan E, Tiedeman J. 1985. Expansion of long-acting gas bubbles for intraocular use. Principles and practice. Arch Ophthalmol 103:831–834.

Dominguez D A. 1985. Cirugia precoz y ambulatoria del despriendimento de retina. Arch Soc Espan Oftal 48: 47–54.

Grance J D. 1985. Utilisation du gaz dans la tecnique de tampònnement interne du decollement de la retine. J Fr Ophtalmol 8, 11: 749–755.

Hilton G, Grizzard W. 1986. Pneumatic retinopexy: a two-step outpatient operation without conjunctival incision. Ophthalmol. 93: 626–641.

Hilton G, Kelly N, Salzano T, Tornambe P, Wells J, Wendell R. 1987. Pneumatic retinopexy: a collaborative report of the first 100 case. Ophthalmology 94: 307–314.

Lincoff A, Haft D, Liggett P, Reifer C. 1980. Intravitreal expansion of perfluorocarbon bubbles. Arch Ophthalmol 98: 1646.

Lincoff A, Kreissig I. 1981. Intravitreal behavior of perfluorocarbons. Dev Ophthal 2: 17–23.

Lincoff H, Mardirossian J, Lincoff A, Liggett P, Iwamoto T, Jakobiec F. 1980. Intravitreal longevity of three perfluorocarbon gases. Arch Ophthalmol 98: 1610–1611.

Lincoff H, Coleman J, Kreissig I, Richard G, Chang S, Wilcox L M. 1983. The perfluorocarbon gases in the treatment of retinal detachment. Ophthalmology 90: 5, 548–551.

Lincoff H, Horowitz J, Kreissig I, Jakobiec F. 1986. Morphological effects of gas compression on the cortical vitreous. Arch Ophthalmol 104: 1212–1215.

McAllister I, Zegarra H, Meyers S, Gutman A. 1987. Treatment of retinal detachment with multiple breaks by pneumatic retinopexy. Arch Ophthal 105: 913–916.

Mathis A, Camuzet F, Bertrand E, Arne J L, Bec P. 1983. Decollement de retine bulleux superieur: interet de l'injection intravitreenne d'hexafluorure de soufre. J Fr Ophthalmol 6: 11, 889–893.

Menchini U, Scialdone A, Davi' G, Introini U L. 1987. Trattamento di casi selezionati di distacco di retina regmatogeno mediante pneumoretinopessia. Atti LXVII Congresso SOI. Roma.

Norton E W D. 1973. Intraocular gas in the management of selected retinal detachments. Tr Am Acad Ophth & Otol 77: 85–98.

Parver L M, Lincoff H. 1978. Mechanics of intraocular gas. Invest. Ophthalmol. Visual Sci 17: 1, 77–79.

Poliner L, Grand M, Shoch L, Olk R, Johnston G., Okun S, Boniuk I L. 1987. New retinal detachment after pneumatic retinopexy. Ophthalmology 94: 315–318.

Reibaldi A, Randone M, Caccamo M. 1987. La chirurgia del distacco di retina oggi. Congr. Internazionale 'La prevenzione della cecità e la problematica degli ipovedenti' Catania.

Reibaldi A, Avitabile T, Caccamo M. 1988. La retinopessia pneumatica. XIII Congresso SOSi. Siracusa Febbraio.

Reibaldi A, Avitabile T, Lanzafame F. 1988. Il nostro orientamento nel trattamento di alcuni casi particolari di distacco di retina. Congr. Internazionale 'Giornate mediterranee di oftalmologia' Roma.

Scialdone A, Visconti C, Giuliani V, Locatelli A, Menchini U. 1988. La pneumoretinopessia nel trattamento del distacco di retina con foro maculare. VI Congresso Società Italiana Laser in Oftalmologia. Cortina D'Ampezzo.

Stucchi S, Cassina A, L O Votrico A, Magnocavallo M. 1987. La retinopessia pneumatica. Un trattamento ambulatoriale? XLII Congr. Soc. Oftalmologica Lombarda. Milano.

Vygantas C M, Peyman G A, Daily M J, Ericson E S. 1973. Octafluorocyclobutane and other gases for vitreous replacement. Arch Ophthalmol 90: 235–236.

Yed J, Vidaurri-Leal J, Kreissig I, Jakobiek F. 1986. Morphological effects of gas compression on the cortical vitreous. Arch Ophthal 104: 1161–1163.

Zenzilla M, Buoso S. 1987. Uso del gas SF6 in casi selezionati di distacco retinico regmatogeno. Atti LXVII Congr. SOI. Roma.

33. Echographically driven extraction of foreign bodies

T. AVITABILE, M. FICHERA, F. CACCIATO, L. FRANCO
and A. MONTAGNA

Summary

In this study we want to show the possibility of echographically to drive the surgeon in the extraction of intraocular foreign bodies. For this reason we used 40 bovine eyes in which we introduced a foreign body via pars plana and then pulled out only with ultrasound guide.

We found that difficulties increase the more the foreign bodies were closer to retina. For foreign bodies localized in middle vitreous such technique has been reliable enough.

Introduction

Bulbar traumatology has always been considered a great problem for all ophthalmologists expecially in case of perforating trauma with retained foreign bodies.

They often provoke anatomical changes and frequent opacifications of dioptric media. Causes of such traumas are of different nature, from traffic to ergophthalmology, to sport, to violence, etc.

Ocular traumatology is to be considered with growing interest either for severe lesions in children (Holland, 1964), in subjects in working age (Saraniti et al., 1987), with subsequent high social costs, and for an increase of 7% of ocular traumas yearly (Boles Carenini et al., 1981).

In our opinion then anything concerning semiological and therapeutical approach in such patients is to be considered with great interest.

Echography has surely a primary role in the approach to the traumatized eye (Reibaldi et al., 1980, 1981; Rossi et al., 1981). Particularly in a patient with retained intraocular foreign bodies, ultrasound allows an exact localization related to anatomical structures whatever X-rays opaque or transparent (Reibaldi et al. 1980), furtherly they can predict whether they could be treated by the magnetic probe or not (Penner et al., 1971).

Institute of Ophthalmology, Catania University, Catania, Italy

R. Sampaolesi (ed.), Ultrasonography in Ophthalmology 12, 257–260.

It has also been stated by our school that through experimentation it is possible to recognize their nature according to some echographic peculiarity (Reibaldi et al., 1981).

It has also been stated by our school that through experimentation it is possible to recognize their nature according to some echographic peculiarity (Reibaldi et al., 1981).

But where ultrasound appears to be particularly useful is in the exact evaluation of concomitant lesions (Reibaldi et al., 1982) and in setting the proper surgical approach by means of single or combined techniques like vitrectomy and/or lensectomy (Reibaldi et al., 1979; Cardia et al., 1986).

So echography is of primary importance both in diagnosis and therapy. In this paper we planned to conduct an experimental study concerning the chance to use ultrasounds to echo-drive the surgeon in the surgical extraction of endobulbar foreign bodies.

A similar but technically different study had been conducted by Bronson in 1964–65, who used an ultrasonic A-scan extractor, built for this purpose, to pull out non magnetic intraocular foreign bodies.

Materials and methods

In order to perform this study we have used 40 bovine eyes. Conjunctiva and sclera were opened at about 4 mm from limbus while a metallic plain, circular, 5 mm diameter foreign body was introduced through the wound. Later after an exact localization by means of 10 MHz probe in B-scan, the echographist by a two hands technique and using only ultrasounds as a guide, tried the extraction of the foreign body. We used B-scan image, because it allows the localization and visualization of the foreign body and at the same time the forceps, the latter recognizable by means of little opening and closing movements of its branches.

Results

Different problems in the extractions of foreign bodies were correlated to different localizations.

So that we formed subsequently three groups: foreign bodies in middle vitreous, foreign bodies localized next to retina (not closer than 3 mm), and those placed on retina.

Foreign bodies were localized as follows: 27 in middle vitreous, 4 next to retina, 9 on retina. 13 out of the 27 localized in middle vitreous were pulled out at first attempt, 4 at the second, 7 at the third, 3 at the fourth. We considered as an attempt the closure of the forceps.

One out of the 4 foreign bodies localized next to retina was pulled out at first attempt, 1 at the third attempt, while in the other two cases, we tweezed retina in 1 case, and lifted retina in another, so that we considered both as a failure.

Foreign bodies on retina were 9; retina was tweezed 7 times trying extraction, and twice we obtained extraction at first attempt.

Conclusions

To confirm and improve the diagnostic and therapeutic usefulness of ultrasounds, in patient with ocular traumas, expecially with a retained foreign body, we considered the use of this experimental research.

Such experimental study has showed us first that test must absolutely be conducted by a two hands technique concerning either surgical aspect and echographic one.

Probe has to be placed at the opposite side of the foreign body in order to localize forceps.

Extraction was easy in all cases where foreign bodies were in middle vitreous, and proportionally difficult closer to retina. In fact when foreign bodies were placed on retina, probably except 2 cases, we have always caused retinal lesions, by tweezing or perforation by foreign bodies.

In our opinion this technique was absolutely reliable only in those cases where foreign bodies were localized in middle vitreous. Reliability of this technique is to be considered absolutely poor when foreign bodies are localized on retina, for the easily caused trauma following its entrance or its extraction.

We want anyway to outline that until now it is only an experimental technique which needs further research and improvement, both from the surgical technique and from an echographic point of view. In order to have some hope of applying it to human eyes in future where foreign bodies are not extraible with any technique, including the most advanced where those eyes would be enucleated anyway.

References

Avitable T, Fichera M, Cascone G. 1987. 'Il ruolo della ecografia in ergoftalmologia'. Comun. Congr. Intern. su La prevenzione della cecità e la problematica degli ipovedenti. Catania.

Avitabile T, Fichera M, Bonaccorsi O. 1987. L'ecografia nella chirurgia vitreo-retinica dell' occhio traumatizzato. Comun, al LXVII Congresso SOI, Roma.

Bellone G, Gallenga P E. 1970–1971. Diagnostica ecografica dei corpi estranei in oftalmologia, Parte III: corpi estranei localizzati all'orbita. Rass Ital Ottalmol 1: 122–129.

Boles Carenini B, Grignolo F M, Giovenale R, Lombardo L. 1981. Epidemiologia dei traumi oculari. Atti LXI Congr. SOI, pp. 9–42, Roma.

Bronson N R. 1964. Nonmagnetic foreign body localization and extraction. Am J Ophthalmol 58: 133.

Bronson N R. 1965. Techniques of ultrasonic localization and extraction of intraocular and extraocular foreign bodies. Am J Ophthalmol 60: 596.

Cardia L, Sborgia C, Micelli Ferrari T. 1986. Traumatologia vitreoretinica e vitrectomia. Attı XX Conv. SOM. Bari. pp. 109–121.

Holland G. 1964. Hanalyse von 2309 verletzungen der augenund liden. Klin Mbl Augenheilk 145 (915).

Penner R, Pasmore J W. 1971. Magnetic U.S. non magnetic intraocular foreign bodies. An ultrasonic determination. Arch Ophthalmol. Chicago 76: 676–677.

Reibaldi A, Delle Noci N, Lo Russo V V. 1979. La nostra esperienza sull'utilità dell'ecografia nella vitrectomia. Com. IV Congr. Naz. SISUM, Modena.

Reibaldi A, Gallenga P E, Cennamo G, Mazzeo V. 1980. L'ecografia nei corpi estranei endobulbari. Atti XIV Congr. SOM, Formia.

Reibaldi A, Lorusso V V, Cantatore F. 1980. L'ecografia nei traumi oculari. Comun. Congr. SISUM, Milano.

Reibaldi A, Persio A, Scuderi G L, Tritto M. 1981. Possibility of recognizing the nature of èndobulbar foreign bodies. Comun. 4th European Congr. on ultrasonic in medicine, Dubrovinic Cavtat.

Reibaldi A, Cantatore S, Di Pilato M. 1981. La diagnosi precoce nei traumi bulbari. Comun. VI Congr. Naz. AIMPS, Pugnochiuso, 18–20 giugno 1981. Giornale med. d'emergenza n. 8, pp. 13–16.

Reibaldi A, Lorusso V V, Di Pilato M. 1982. Le possibilità diagnostiche dell'ultrasuonografia nel riconoscimento di corpi estranei endobulbari e lesioni concomitanti. Atti III congr. interegionale in ergoftalmologia e traumatologi oculare. Torino.

Reibaldi A, Di Pilato M, Avitabile T. 1983. Five years of ultrasonographic diagnosis in combined surgery through the pars-plana. Relazione IX SIDUO, Leeds 20–23 luglio 1982, Ophthal. Ultrasonography. Hillman J. (ed) pp. 115–118.

Reibaldi A, Gallenga P E. 1986. L'ecografia bulbare oggi. Relaz. LXVI congr. SOI, Roma.

Rossi A., Mazzeo V. 1981. L'ecografia nei traumatismi oculari. Atti LXI congr. SOI, pp. 79–86.

Saraniti G, Avitabile T, Fichera M, Pappalardo A. 1987. Menomazioni visive e loro cause nella traumatologia oculare da infortuni sul lavoro: 10 anni di esperienze cliniche. Comun. Congr. Intern. su La prevenzione della cecità e problematica degli ipovedenti. Catania.

34. A case with a macular granuloma seropositive for *Toxocara canis* examined with standardized echography

JAN SCHUTTERMAN

Summary

A 75 years old man presented with a one year long history of successive visual deterioration he had noticed in his right eye. On examination it was found that v.a. was only CF in his right eye, and a slightly protruding whitish lesion was seen in the right macula. Patient serum was analyzed for *Toxocara canis* immunology and was found positive. The lesion was examined with standardized echography and fluorescein angiography. The results will be described.

A 75 years old Swedish gentleman was referred by a practising ophthalmologist to our department for fundus examination, echography and fluorescein angiography of a lesion she had found in the fundus of his right eye. She saw him in her office because he had noticed progressively deteriorating vision for the last year. In her office record full v.a. (1.0) was found a little more than 4 years earlier, when examined for itching and tearful eyes, and a bilateral blepharoconjunctivitis was described together with normal central fundi at that earlier visit. When now reexamined v.a. was only CF 1.5 metres in his right eye, but the left eye retained an acuity of 0.7 and some letters on the 0.8 and 0.9 lines. His reading ability was good (Jaeger 1 with a + 3 dptr add). IOP was normal. In the macula of the right eye she found a 3–4 discdiameters sized protruding white lesion and around the margins of the lesion the retina was slightly and locally detached. Retinal blood vessels seemed intact. The left eye did not show any of these macular findings, but a seemingly normal macula. Perimetry produced a central scotoma of the right eye; the left eye had normal Goldmann perimetry.

Arriving in our clinic the clinical findings were confirmed: v.a. was in the RE 'some' optotypes corresponding to 0.06 and the left eye had best corrected v.a. of 1.0. Examination with 60-diopter lens *biomicroscopy* seemed to show a whitish, dense membrane covering the foveal part of the

Dept. of Ophthalmology, Södersjukhuset Hospital, S- 100 64 Stockholm, Sweden

R. Sampaolesi (ed.), Ultrasonography in Ophthalmology 12, 261–265.

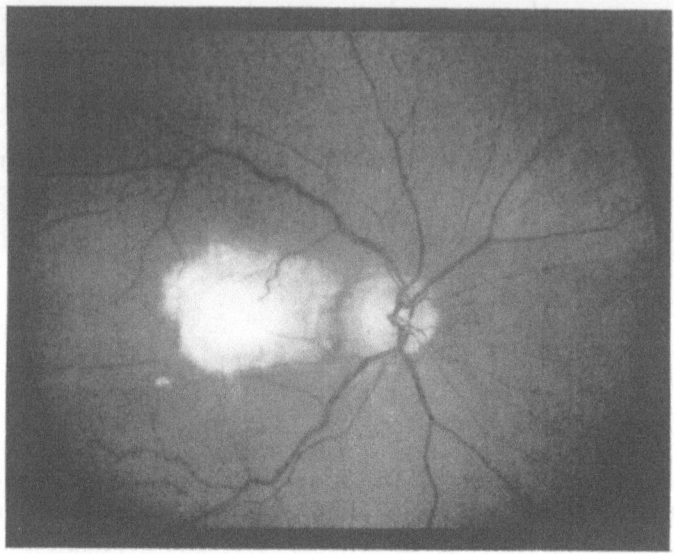

Fig. 1. Fundus appearance of the lesion. Note retinal vessels as they are entering the margins of the lesion.

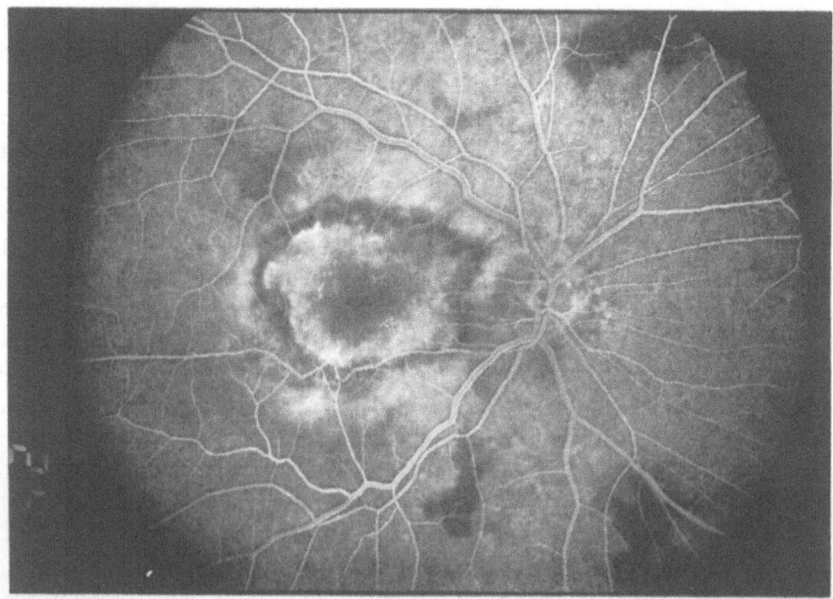

Fig. 2. Fluorescein angiogram of the granulamatous lesion showing diffuse hyperfluorescence except for the central parts as well as bizarre retinal vessel changes in the same area (late arterio-venous phase).

retina and from the lesion, traction folds were seen radiating in the internal limiting membrane for quite a distance and in all directions, reaching areas with slightly, seriously elevated retina surrounding the central parts of the lesion. The superficial retinal blood vessels were seen plunging under the opaque membrane sized approximately one disc area, as they approached it from the perifery of the lesion.

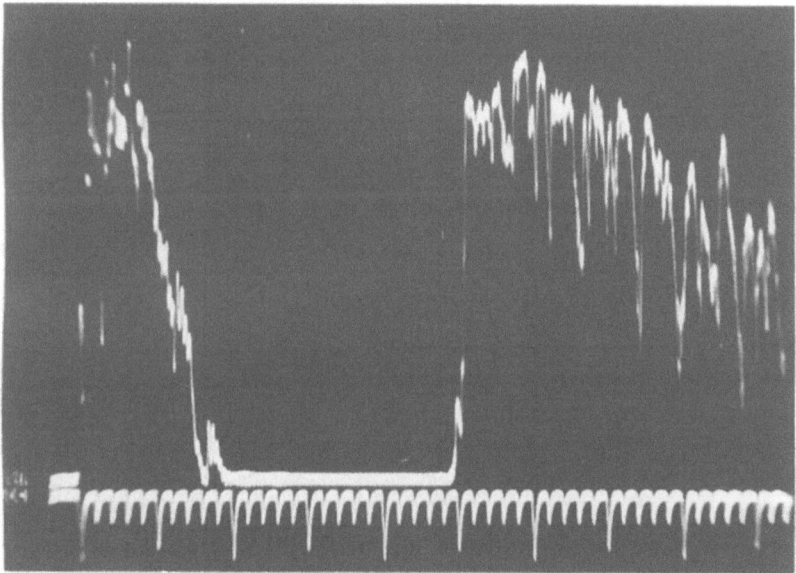

3(a)

3(b)

Fig. 3a & b. Legend, see next page.

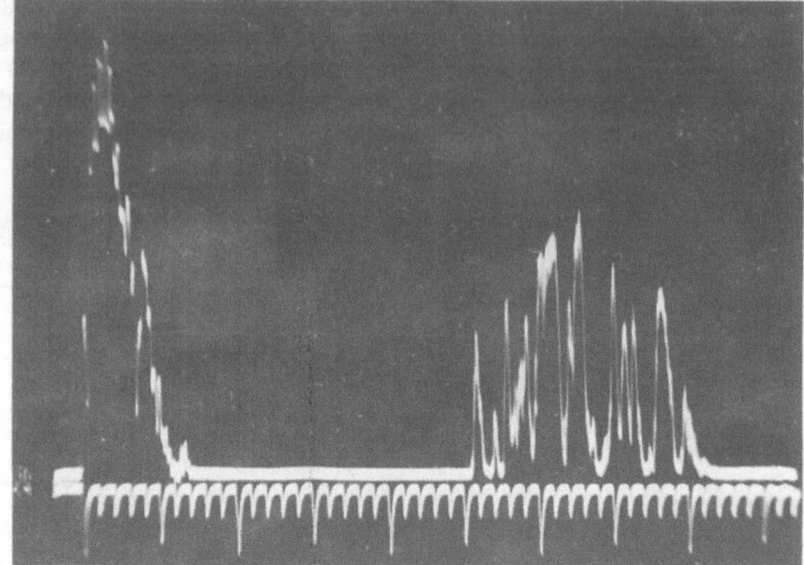

3(c)

3(d)

Fig. 3a–d. (a and b) standardized A-scan echogram (Kretztechnik 7200MA) with tissue sensitivity, showing the regular internal structure and high reflectivity of the lesion, (c) standardized A-scan with reduced sensitivity to show increased thickness of retino-choroidal layer, (d) B-scan (Sonometrics Ocuscan 400) showing the topography of the lesion.

Fluorescein angiography showed blocked choroidal fluorescense in the first stages, followed by an almost uniform fuzzy hyperfluorescense except for the very centre of the lesion, which remained hypofluorescent for some time. The retinal vessels were seen to hyperfluorescense in a bizarre pattern of small irregularities in the margins of the lesion. Up to this stage the lesion was surrounded by a dark rim in the angiogram. In the late stages there was an increasing staining of the lesion and the retinal vessels were by now seen to be dark and to contrast with the hyperfluorescent tissues as they plunged into them.

Standardized echography showed a central thickening of the tissues compared to normal retino-choroidal layer thickness. In this case the corresponding thickness was about 3 mm in the central part of the posterior pole as compared to normal thickness of up to 1.6 mm, as described by Ossoinig (1979). The internal structure was mostly regular with high reflectivity about 85–95% of the display height, but there were some smaller areas with a more membrane like structure. Because of the peculiar appearance of this macular lesion together with the normal findings of the macula of the contralateral eye, blood sera were sent for examination for *toxocara*. The results were positive with repeated examinations, although 'border line'. Titers were 62/87 and 72/87.

At follow-up examinations the disease state seemed stable and there was no obvious inflammatory response from the eye except for the granuloma formation itself.

As we found in literature (Smith and Nozikh, 1983), that it is recommended, that no therapeutic measure, as e.g. systemic or periocular steroid treatment or specific antihelminthics as e.g. thiabendazole are taken, unless there are complications such as retinal detachment or endophthalmitis, the gentleman was not treated but was only informed of the probable cause of the lesion. He has been followed for 8 months and the condition has been stable so far.

Végh and Danka described a 'cystic' lesion in a child examined with B-scan echography. The lesion described here seems to be more 'massive', possibly due to its 'coarser' granuloma kind of tissue with a higher reflectivity, yet with a regular internal structure.

References

Ossoinig K C. 1979. Standardized echography: basic principles, clinical applications, and results. In: International Ophthalmology Clinics 19, No. 4: Dallow R L (ed) Ophthalmic Ultrasonography: Comparative Techniques; Little, Brown and Company.

Smith RE, Nozik R M. 1983. Uveitis: a clinical approach to diagnosis and management. Williams & Wilkins.

Végh M, Danka J. 1987. Das Krankheitsbild und die Behandlung der Toxocara-canis-Uveitis im Kindesalter (Clinical picture and treatment of juvenile uveitis caused by toxocara Canis), Klin. Mbl Augenheilk 191: 395–396.

Intraocular tumours

35. Ultrasonography in intraocular tumours

MARY ABRAHAM, MYTHILI SRIRAM, S. M. OKE,
CHANDRAN ABRAHAM and S. S. BADRINATH

Summary

113 eyes of 103 patients had ultrasonography to confirm or rule out an intraocular tumour. The clinical diagnosis in 65 clear media eyes comprising 33 retinoblastomas, 21 malignant melanomas, 1 parasitic cyst and others could be confirmed in 93%. In 48 eyes with a doubtful diagnosis or opaque media, ultrasonography revealed malignancy in 52%, hamartomas in 12.5% and conditions other than tumours in 27%. Among the 33 enucleated eyes, histopathology confirmed the ultrasonographic diagnosis in 84.8%. Errors in diagnosis were evident in large tumours without specific characteristics and in tumours too small to be picked up.

Introduction

The role of ultrasonography as a non-invasive diagnostic aid in intraocular tumours in eyes with opaque or clear media is well established [2, 4, 9, 10]. The characteristic features of benign, primary and secondary tumour deposits in the eye have been described [1, 2, 3, 5, 6, 7, 8]. It has been however recognised that tumours less than 1 or 2 mm can not picked up by ultrasound [4, 5] and that large tumours filling the entire vitreous cavity and anteriorly placed tumours may lead to diagnostic errors [4]. Errors in diagnosis also include mistaking subretinal haemorrhage for a malignant melanoma [2]. Choroidal excavation, a characteristic sign of malignant melanoma has been occasionally observed in haemangiomas, naevi and metastatic tumours [5]. A negative co-relation between the acoustic profile of malignant melanomas and the cytological features have been reported [2]. the reported accuracy of ultrasonographic diagnosis when compared with the histopathological diagnosis following enucleation or post-mortem varies from 89–100% [2, 10].

Sankara Nethralaya, 18, College Road, Madras 600 006, India

R. Sampaolesi (ed.), Ultrasonography in Ophthalmology 12, 269–279.
© *1990. Kluwer Academic Publishers, Dordrecht*

We have described the ultrasonographic features in eyes with clear and opaque media that were referred to either confirm or rule out an intraocular tumour.

Material and methods

113 eyes of 103 patients diagnosed or suspected to have an intraocular tumour were evaluated by A- and B-scan ultrasonography at Sankara Nethralaya between January 1980 and May 1988. This comprised 42 eyes with retinoblastoma, 28 eyes with malignant melanoma and 43 eyes with hamartomas, haemangiomas or intraocular tumours suspected clinically. Of the 96 eyes with clear ocular media, a definite ophthalmoscopic diagnosis was available in 65 eyes and a doubtful diagnosis in 31. The media was opaque in 17 eyes. Serial ultrasonography was performed in 2 eyes with malignant melanoma and 5 eyes with retinoblastoma to pick up an initially small tumour, document growth or document regression after photocoagulation or irradiation. 33 eyes underwent enucleation and histopathological examination. The findings were analysed to co-relate the ultrasonographic diagnosis with the ophthalmoscopic and histopathological diagnosis.

Table 1. Histopathological co-relation with ultrasonographic features.

U/S features	Histopathology		
	Spindle A/B	Epithelioid	Mixed
Acoustic hollowing	4	3	1
Choroidal excavation	4	2	1

Results

Among the 42 eyes with retinoblastoma, an ophthalmoscopic diagnosis was available in 33 eyes where the media was clear. Ultrasonography substantiated the diagnosis of retinoblastoma in 32 out of 33 eyes (96.96%). In the remaining eye, the mass had the features of a vitreous haemorrhage with no specific tumour characteristics. All 8 eyes with opaque media showed ultrasonographic features of retinoblastoma. One eye with a doubtful diagnosis was found to have ultrasonographic features of retinoblastoma. Ultrasonographic documentation of regression of the mass was obtained in 3 photocoagulated eyes and 2 irradiated eyes (Figs. 1 and 2). Rapid increase in tumour size could be documented in 1 eye following irradiation and a prolonged follow-up. Ultrasonography helped to rule out an intraocular mass in 2 eyes with an ophthalmoscopic diagnosis of retinal detachment

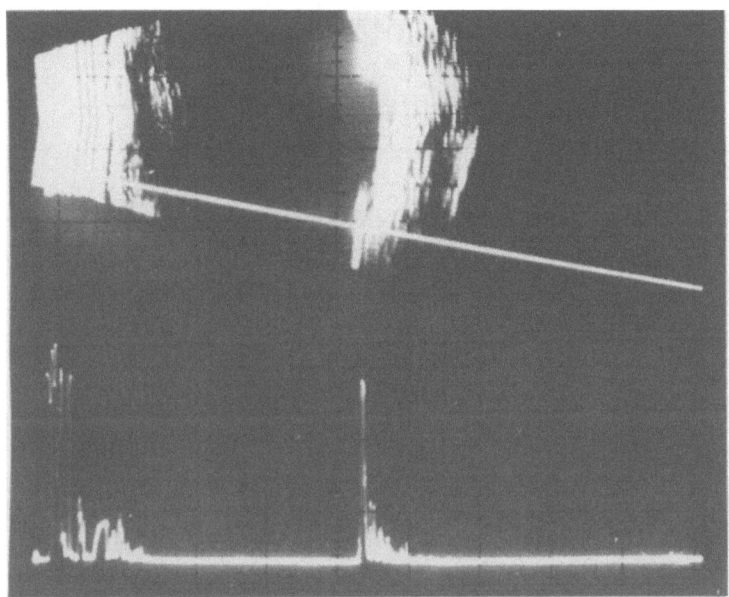

Fig. 1. Ultrasonogram showing small retinoblastoma in the periphery.

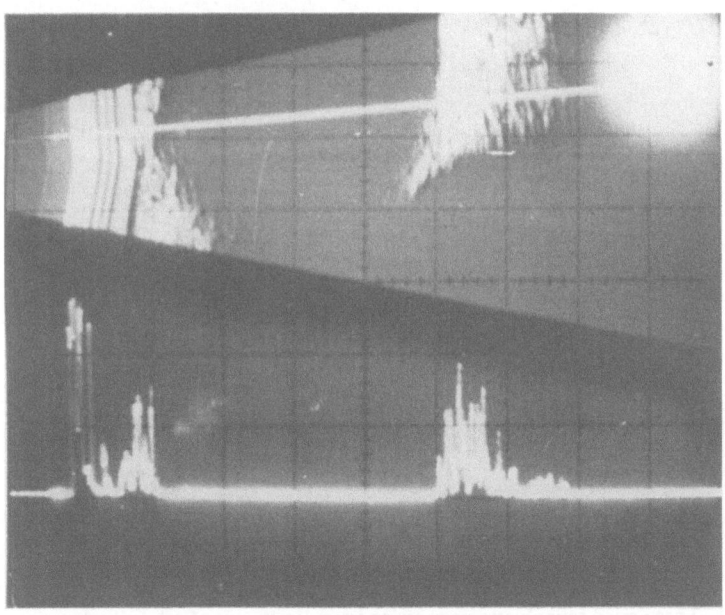

Fig. 2. Ultrasonogram showing regression of retinoblastoma after photocoagulation.

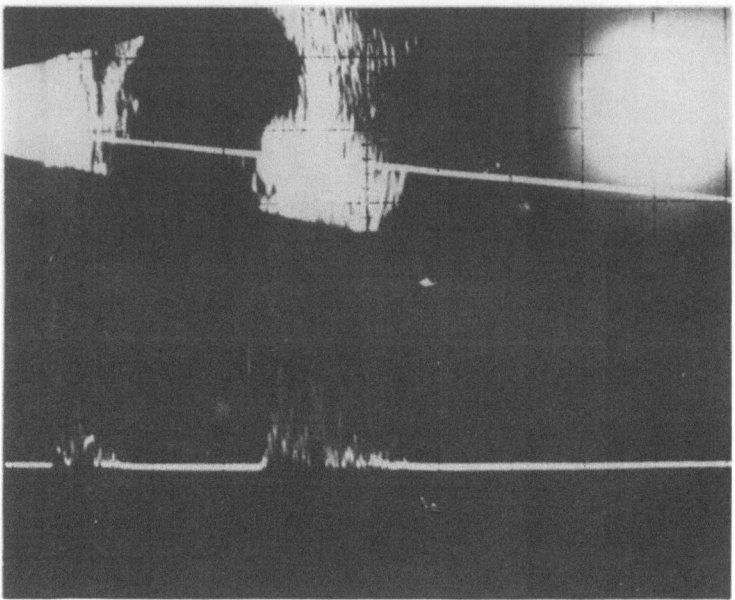

Fig. 3. Medium sized retinoblastoma showing compact tall amplitude internal echoes.

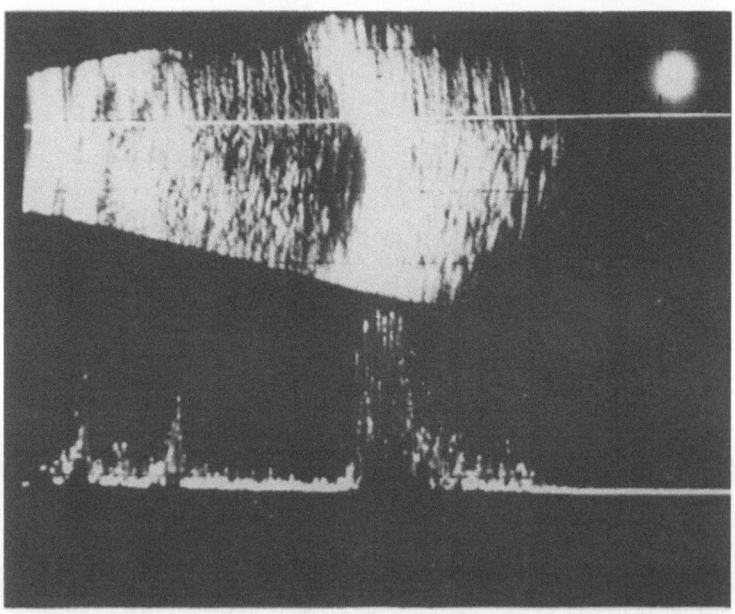

Fig. 4. Large sized retinoblastoma showing irregular clumps of echoes and cystic spaces.

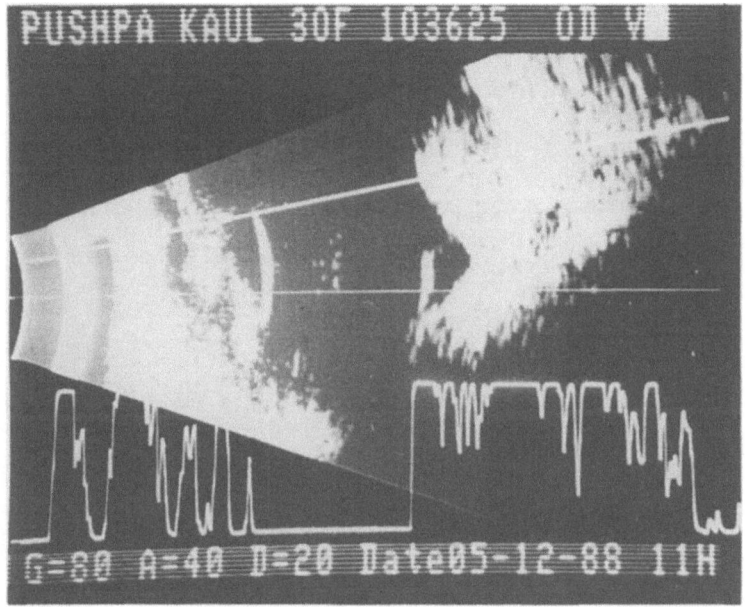

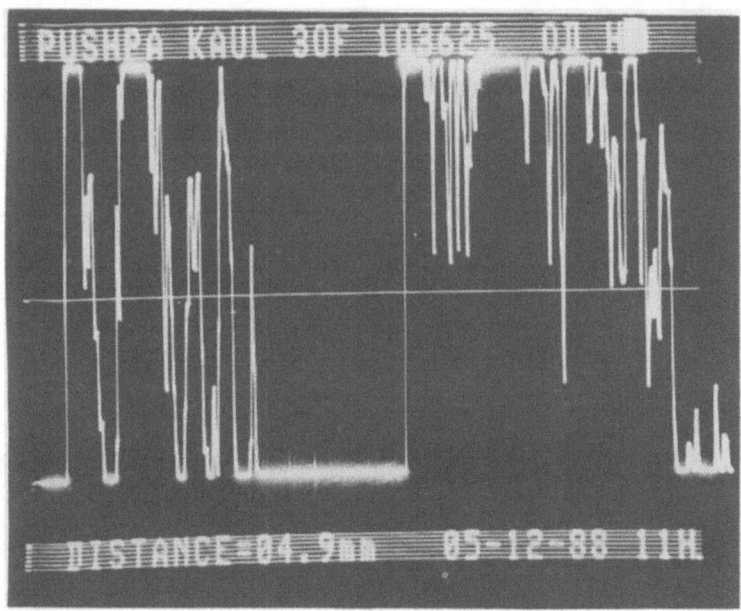

Fig. 5. Malignant melanoma prior to photocoagulation.

274

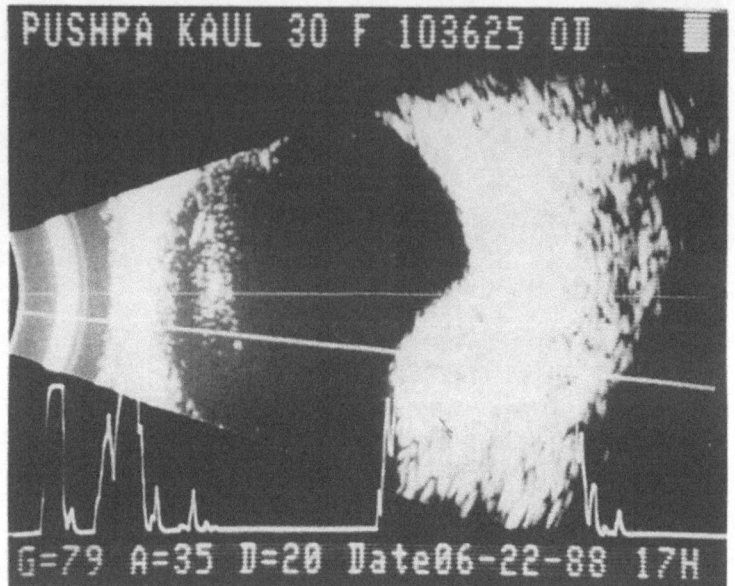

(a)

(b)

Fig. 6 (a + b). Reduction in tumour size after photocoagulation.

secondary to a retinoblastoma and in another with a suspected retino-blastoma like tumour. The most characteristic features were an initial tall amplitude echo followed by tall amplitude internal echoes. The internal echoes were compact in medium size tumours (Fig. 3). Irregular clumps of echoes alternating with cystic spaces were seen in large nectoric tumours (Fig. 4). Calcification was evident in 18 eyes. Orbital shadowing was seen in 12 eyes. Of the 14 enucleated eyes histopathology confirmed the diagnosis of retinoblastoma in 12 (85.7%). The histopathological diagnosis was Coat's disease in one and Retinal Dysplasia in another; both these eyes had an opaque media.

Among the 28 eyes with malignant melanoma an ophthalmoscopic diagnosis was available in 21 eyes where the media was clear. Ultrasonography substantiated the diagnosis of melanoma in 18 out of the 21 eyes (85.7%). In 2 eyes, an ophthalmoscopically visible tumours was too small to be picked up by ultrasound and the other showed features of a disciform macular degeneration. Of the 31 eyes where the clinical diagnosis was in doubt, malignant melanoma was suspected in 12 of these cases. Characteristic ultrasonographic features of melanoma were evident only in 7 out of the 12 eyes. In one eye in which the tumour was too small to be picked up was found to have malignant melanoma on histopathological examination. Ultra-

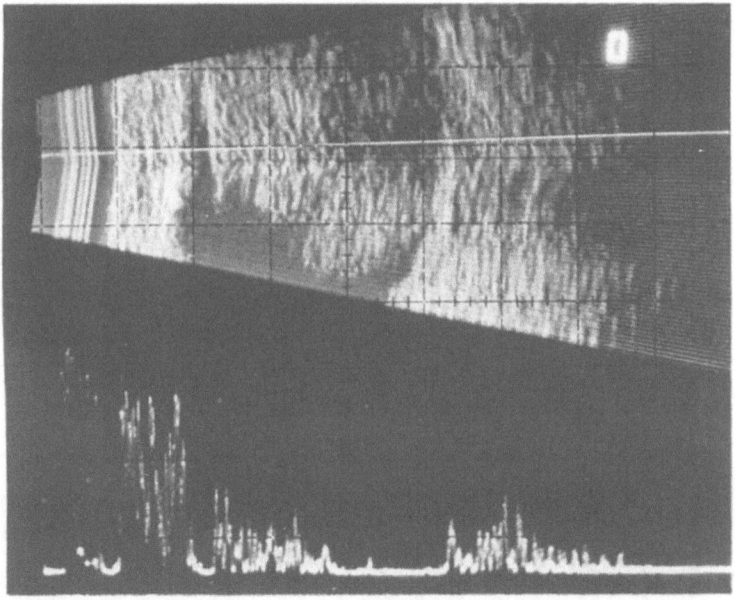

Fig. 7. Malignant melanoma showing acoustic hollowing, choroidal excavation and orbital shadowing.

sonography helped in the diagnosis of disciform macular degeneration in 2, choroidal haemangioma in 1, and choroidal haemorrhage in 1 in the remaining eyes that were suspected to have a melanoma. Reduction in tumour size could be documented in 1 eye following photocoagulation (Figs. 5 and 6). The characteristic features of an initial tall spike and orbital shadowing were evident in all the eyes that were diagnosed ultrasonographically (Fig. 7). Acoustic hollowing was evident in 18 eyes. The decay slope could be appreciated in 12 eyes and choroidal excavation in 11. Histopathological findings were available in 14 out of the 19 enucleated eyes and all 14 eyes were found to have malignant melanoma. There was no co-relation between the ultrasonographic features and the cell-type (Table 1).

In 43 eyes, the diagnosis comprised of hamartomas (10 eyes), retinal detachment with PVR (5 eyes), choroidal haemangioma (3 eyes), secondary deposits (2 eyes), paracytic cyst (2 eyes), posterior hyperplastic primary vitreous (1 eye), Coat's disease (1 eye) and choroidal haemorrhage (1 eye). In 8 eyes the diagnosis remains unknown and in 7 with either a clear media and a secondary retinal detachment or with an opaque media, no mass could be found.

Though only large angiomas could be picked out, ultrasonography was helpful in the diagnosis of this condition in 2 eyes where the ophthalmoscopic diagnosis was doubtful and in 1 eye with an opaque media (Fig. 8). Ultrasonography was helpful in the diagnosis of PHPV in an eye suspected to have retinoblastoma, helped to rule out retinoblastoma in 2 eyes with

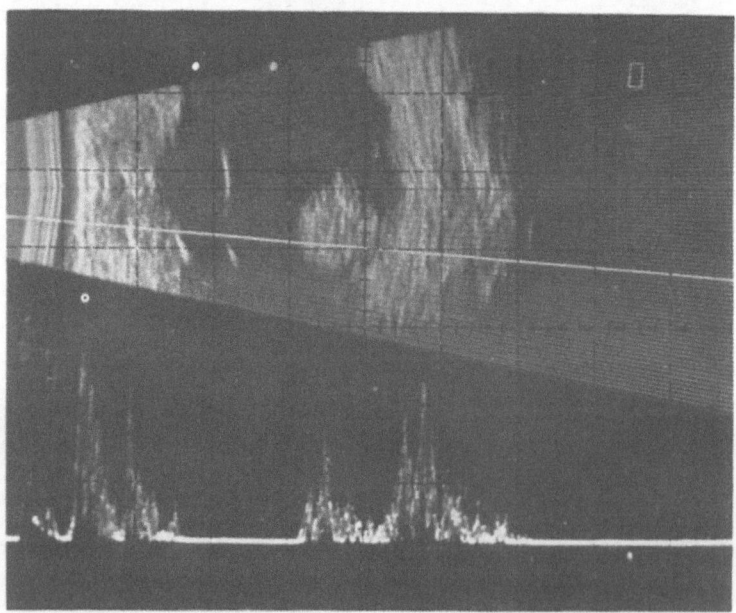

Fig. 8. Small angiomatous mass showing compact moderate amplitude internal echoes.

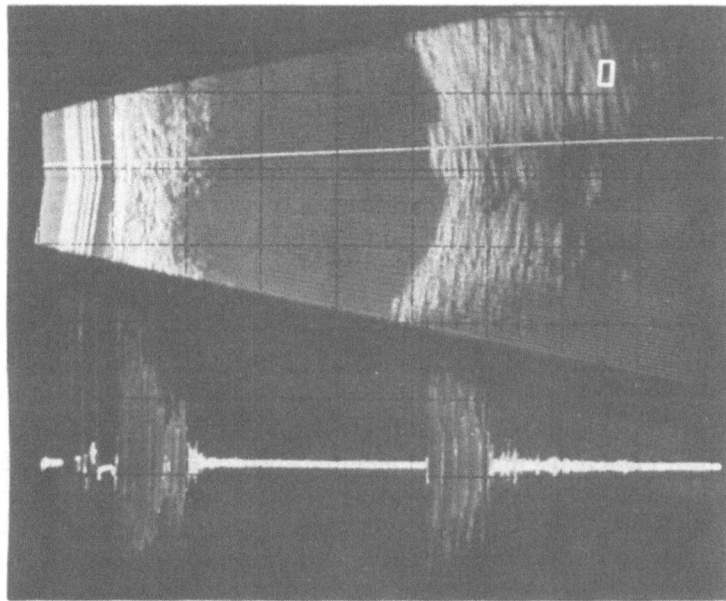

Fig. 9. Melanocytoma of optic nerve head showing compact low amplitude echoes.

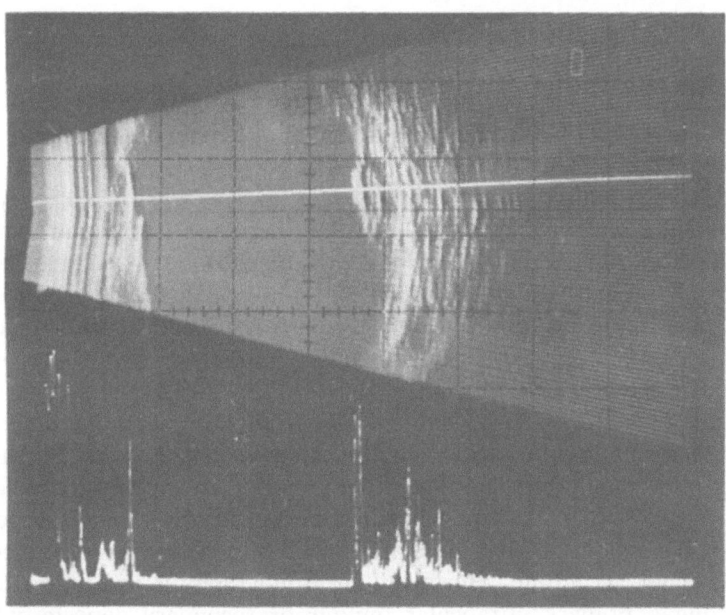

Fig. 10. Paracytic cyst with smooth anterior and posterior surfaces and absence of internal echoes.

retinal detachment with PVR. One of the 7 eyes where no mass was detected had an opaque media and was enucleated. Histopathology revealed a small malignant melanoma. The diagnosis in 8 eyes remains unknown as neither the ophthalmoscopic nor ultrasonographic features fit into a definite pattern. The 4 melanocytomas were characterised by the presence of a convex border with compact medium amplitude internal echoes (Fig. 9). The two paracytic cysts were characterised by smooth borders, well defined anterior and posterior walls and absence of internal echoes. The parasite though visible could not be picked up in either eye (Fig. 10).

If one considers all of the tumours as a whole, it was found that the ultrasonographic diagnosis co-related with the definitive ophthalmoscopic diagnosis in 59 out of 65 (90.76%) clear media eyes. In 48 eyes where the ophthalmoscopic diagnosis was doubtful or the media opaque, ultrasonography revealed a malignant tumour in 18 eyes (37.5%), hamartomas in 4 eyes (8.3%) and helps to rule out an intraocular tumour in 18 eyes (37.5%). In 8 eyes both clinical and ultrasonographic diagnosis remained in doubt (16.7%). Among the 33 enucleated eyes, histopathology confirmed ultrasonographic diagnosis in 28 (84.8%). The errors were evident when the tumours were large and without specific characteristics or when they were too small to be picked up.

Discussion

The reason for including eyes with conditions other than tumours such as retinal detachment, retinal dysplasia, PHPV, choroidal haemorrhage, choroidal haemangioma and Coat's disease is because these eyes had undergone ultrasonography to rule out an intraocular tumour. The inclusion of such eyes allows a better evaluation of ultrasonography as a diagnostic procedure. Though used mainly in eyes with opaque media, when used in eyes with clear media with intraocular tumour or suspected intraocular tumour, it augments or refutes the ophthalmoscopic diagnosis. It also facilitates a co-relation between the fundus and the ultrasonographic features, enhances the acumen of the clinician and can be of immense value when opaque media eyes are being examined. This has been evident in eyes with retinoblastoma, choroidal melanoma and hamartoma in this series. The fact that all 8 opaque media eyes suspected to have retinoblastoma did indeed have retinoblastoma on ultrasonography probably reflects the fact that this is the commonest condition in this age group. Conversely our results of not being able to detect a malignant melanoma in any of the 17 eyes suspected to harbour one indicates that there are several other reasons for opaque media in the older age group. However, ultrasonography is the only method of detecting a primary intraocular tumour or secondary deposits when the media is opaque.

The accuracy of ultrasonography in this series is similar to that of others

[2, 10]. The fact that very small tumours could not be picked up and that large tumours lacked specific characteristics [4, 5] is also borne out in this series. Though refinements in techniques to overcome these shortcomings can be suggested, it must be realised that small tumours can be followed up closely without much risk and the large ones enucleated and subjected to histopathology if the visual acuity is grossly affected. Large undiagnosed tumours with good visual acuity however pose a problem because enucleation is not necessarily the best manner of management. Despite some of these limitations the results of this study indicate that ultrasonography is an important diagnostic technique, useful in detecting, confirming or ruling out an intraocular tumour in clear and opaque media eyes.

References

[1] Baum G. 1967. Ultrasonographic characteristics of malignant melanoma. Arch Ophthalmol 78: 12–15.
[2] Char D H, Dudley Stone R, Irvin A R. 1977. The diagnosis of uveal malignant melanoma in eyes with opaque media. Am J Ophthalmol 83: 95–105.
[3] Coleman D J, Abrahamson D H, Jack R L, Frenzen L A. 1974. Ultrasonographic diagnosis of tumours of the choroid. Arch Ophthalmol 91: 344–354.
[4] Coleman D J 1977. Ultrasonography of the eye and orbit. Philadelphia, Lea and Febiger. 209–242.
[5] Fuller D G, Snyder W B, Huton W L, Vaiser A. 1979. Ultrasonographic features of choroidal malignant melanoma. Arch Ophthalmol 97: 1462–1472.
[6] Gitter K A, Meyer D, White R H, Ortolon, Sarin L K. 1968. Ultrasonic aid in evaluation of Leucocoria. Am J Ophthalmol 65: 190–195.
[7] Hodes B L, Chromokos E. 1977. Standardized A Scan Echographic Diagnosis of choroidal malignant melanomas. Arch Ophthalmol 95: 593–597.
[8] Jack R L, Coleman D J. 1972. Detection of retinal detachments secondary to choroidal melanoma with B Scan Ultrasound. Am J Ophthalmol 74: 1057–1065.
[9] Shammas H J. 1984. Atlas of Ophthalmic ultrasonography and biometry. St. Louis, C V Mosby Co. pp. 57–107.
[10] Shields J A, McDonald P R. 1977. The diagnosis of uveal malignant melanoma in eyes with opaque media. Am J Ophthalmol 83: 95–105.

36. Morphological parameters of intraocular tumours taking part in ecographical tracings

J. O. ZÁRATE[1] and R. SAMPAOLESI[2]

Introduction

It has been of great interest over the last years to construe ecographical tracings on histopathological bases in different intraocular tumour pathologies.

This is the way in which a direct correlation between mode A ecography and the morphological types of the lesions studied has been described in the different case reports of Prof. Sampaolesi's book: 'Ultrasonidos en Oftalmología' [1].

In said book when we refer to the factors that determine the small interphases we take into consideration the primary ones (cellular disposition, connective-vascular stroma) and the secondary ones (added substances such as calcium and melanin). Necrosis, bleedings, cystic areas, membranes and capsules).

The aim of this communication is to establish which are the morphological parameters belonging to intraocular tumours which take part in a great extent in the several ecographical tracings and as a result of this to support the hypothesis about the potential usefulness of ultrasonography in the preoperative diagnosis of the tumour morphological type.

In vivo studies

Ten case reports of intraocular tumours already analyzed by us have been studied, by making the histological analysis of each one of them with semiserial sections of the eyeball.

In each one of them all the primary and secondary factors referring to the small interphases mentioned in the introduction were determined.

In this paper we determinate in each case the cellular concentration per mm^3.

[1] Department Ophthalmic Pathology, University of Buenos Aires, Parana 123 g-la, Argentina
[2] Ophthalmology Department, Universidad del Salvador, Buenos Aires, Argentina

R. Sampaolesi (ed.), Ultrasonography in Ophthalmology 12, 281–292.

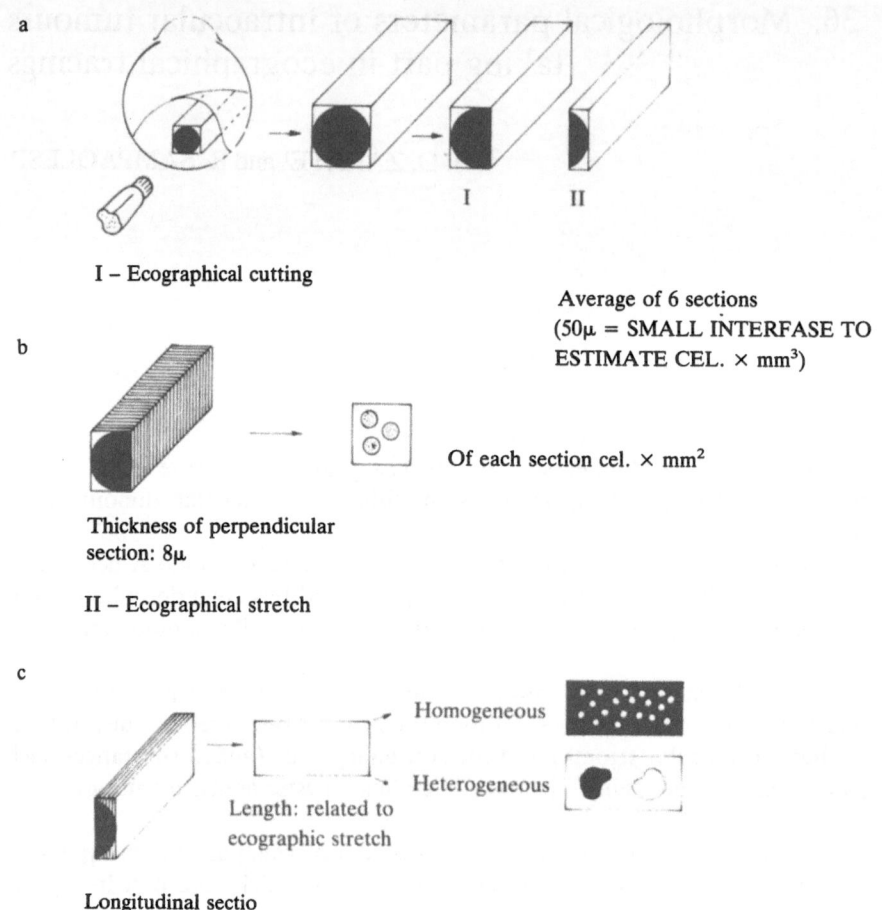

I – Ecographical cutting

Average of 6 sections
(50μ = SMALL INTERFASE TO
ESTIMATE CEL. × mm³)

Of each section cel. × mm²

Thickness of perpendicular
section: 8μ

II – Ecographical stretch

Homogeneous

Heterogeneous

Length: related to
ecographic stretch

Longitudinal sectio

Fig. 1. Pathological examination of the eye (histogram methodology).

Said measurement was taken by making an average of the cellular count of the different analyzed histological sections done by means of lenses of 4x; 10x; 20x; 40x and 100x in 20 different areas of each individual section.

Cellular concentration/mm³ was correlated to the ecographical reflectivity.

In vitro studies

Ten case reports of intraocular tumours differing from the ones studied in Part I have been studied. Block reserves from our laboratory, in general semisections were used. Ecographies were performed in vitro by means of a mode A Kretz-Technik 7200 MA ecographer. The piece was

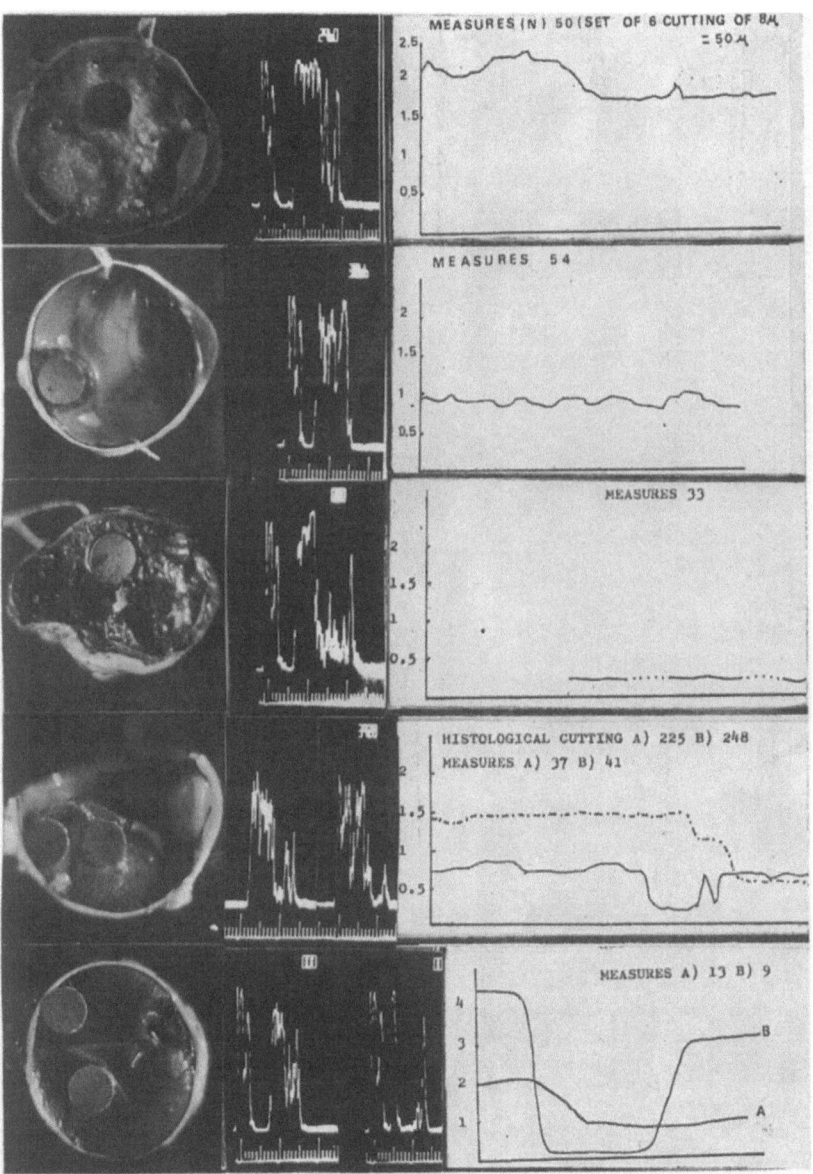

Fig. 2a.

284

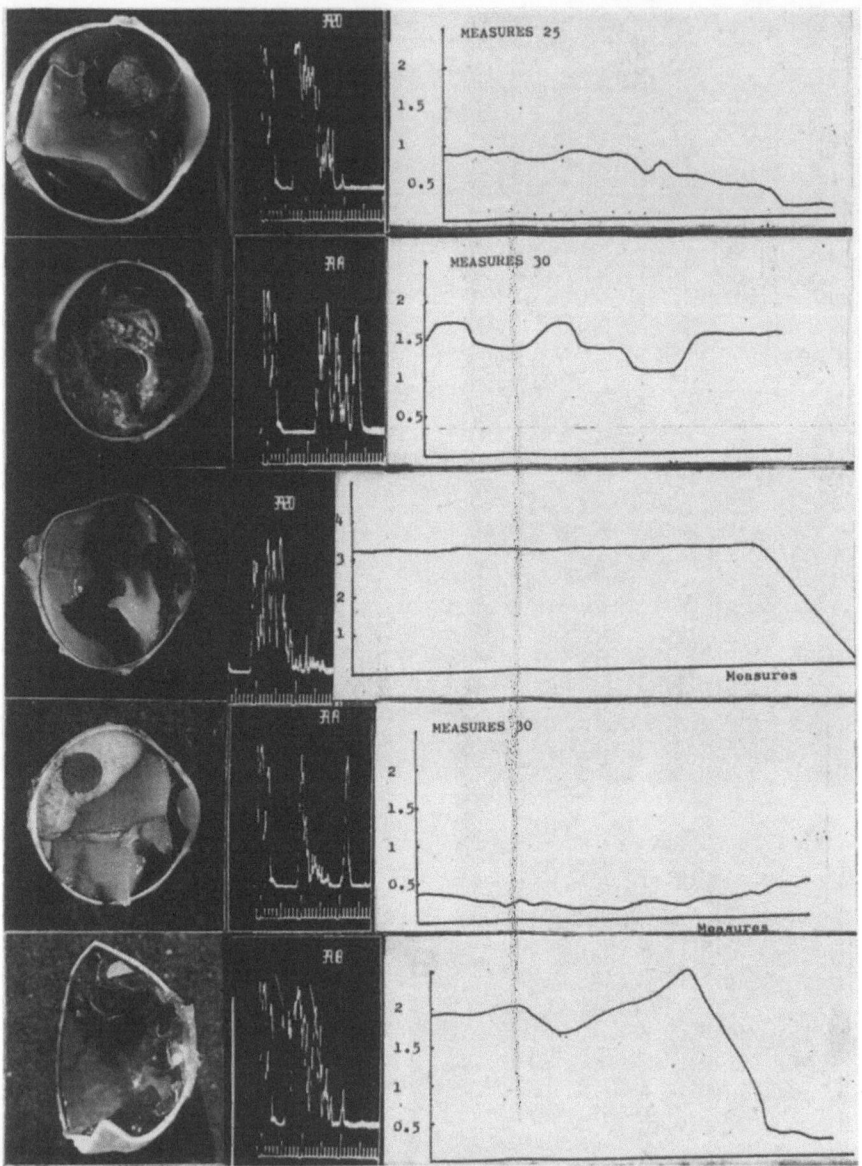

Fig. 2b

Fig. 2. Histogram summing up the data in each case.

placed in a vessel containing physiological salt solution. The probe was directed towards the areas marked with a circle (Fig. 1) in each case.

The specimen was divided into two. One part was from five to seven mm thick and the other part from two to three mm thick (Fig. 1a).

Afterwards one part was cut into perpendicular sections and the other one into longitudinal sections (Fig. 1b, c).

From the former we obtained between 50 and 300 cuttings (according to its size).

Preparations corresponding to the perpendicular section (Fig. 1b) of the tumour which represent the successive planes through which ultrasound runs have been called echographical cuttings. They are numbered from the surface to the interior individually. In each one of the cuttings 3 histological fields were taken at ramdom to calculate the number of cells per mm^2. In order to estimate the number of cells per mm^3 we took the average of 6 consecutive sections (50μ: small interface).

At the same time both in the 'echographical cutting' (Fig. 1b) preparation as well as in the 'echographical stretch' (Fig. 1c) vascularization, necrosis, pigment, calcium and septum were evaluated.

The data obtained was summed up in each case in a scheme called histogram (Figs. 2a and b).

Echograms were analyzed in the following manner: 1) Lesion size in miroseconds and its transformation into mm using the conversion table (from the Ophtalmology Department, University of Iowa, Iowa City USA) and relating it to the size in mm by direct macroscopic measure of the piece; 2) number of peaks of the tracing, dividing them into series of peaks by areas, according to their reflectivity.

As from these values the data obtained for their correlation to the corresponding histogram have been summed up in a table (Table 2).

Results

Table 1 shows the values obtained in the determination of the number of cells per mm^3 in the 10 case reports studied in part 1.

Table 3 shows the results obtained in the evaluation of the morphological parameters of each type of tumour, in relation to the reflectivity and the primary factors already numbered, establishing in every one of them the cellular concentration per mm^3.

In Fig. 3 the cellular concentration data and the kind of reflectivity found in the echographical tracing were compared. (Part 1 presurgical *in vivo* echography).

Table 1. Determination of the number of cells per mm^3 in ten intraocular tumours.

Case No.	A_I	A_{II}	A_{III}	A_{IV}	A_V	A_{VI}	A_{VII}	A_{VIII}	A_{IX}	A_X	Average	c/mm^2	c/mm^3
1 Spindle A	220	210	225	205	215	220	225	215	220	225	218	10.900	1133600
2 Spindle B	160	161	170	180	170	160	162	161	162	160	164	8.200	738000
3 Spindle B	180	170	168	166	170	160	170	170	130	160	164	8.200	738000
4 Epitelioid	50	55	60	60	62	60	50	46	70	60	57	2.850	151050
5 Mixed	100	92	95	110	100	90	90	95	100	102	97	4.850	339500
6 Necrotic	190	N.V.	150	N.V.	N.V.	175	N.V.	N.V.	N.V.	N.V.	171	8.550	786600
7 Necrotic	N.V.	N.V.	80	N.V.	200	N.V.	200	N.V.	N.V.	N.V.	160	8.000	712000
8 Hemangioma	530	530	540	550	540	520	530	540	510	610	540	27.000	428000
9 Retinobl.	360	370	360	378	390	310	320	385	240	290	340	17.000	2210000
10 Metast. Ca.	340	310	320	310	320	320	400	280	280	320	320	16.000	2016000

(Figures of average number to be observed 20/CMA (greatest increase field 100x) in surface, specified in ten different horizontal or vertical histological sections in relation with the tumour. Out of its total average we get cells/mm^2 and out of the latter the number of cells per mm^3).

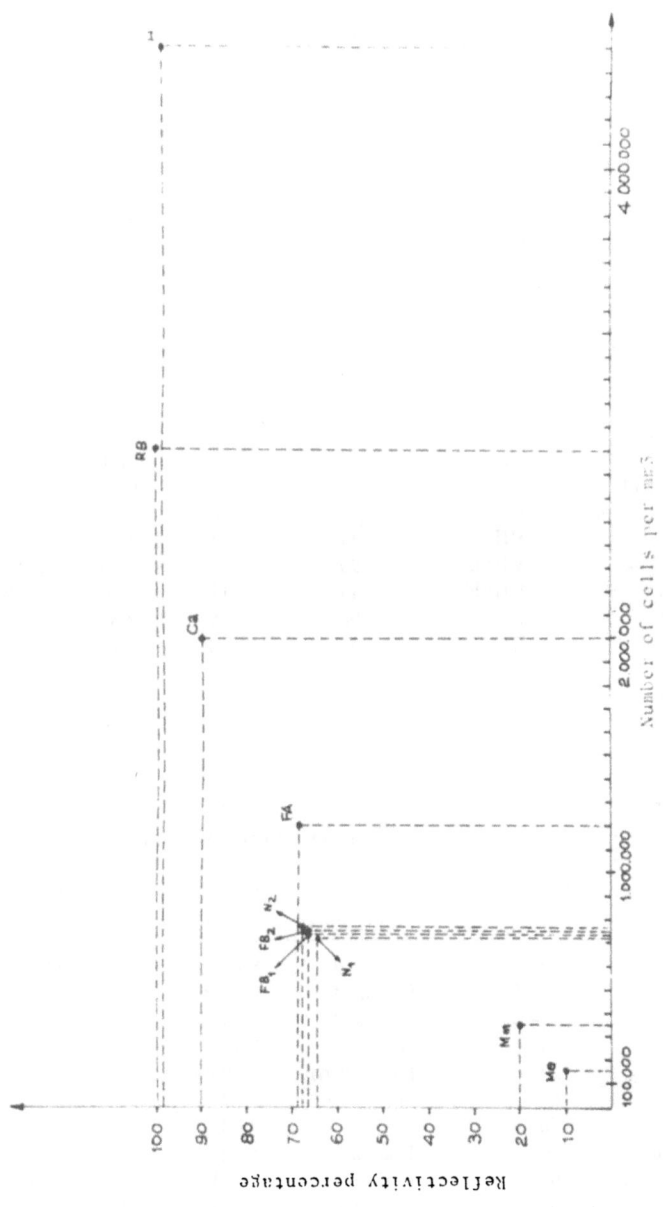

Fig. 3.

Table 2. Data obtained for correlation to the corresponding histogram.

Case	Pathologic diagnosis	Ecographical zone	Reflectivity	Number of echo	Stretch size	Cellularity (per mm^3)
I	Undifferentiated	I a	100	6	5,43	2.090.000
	Retinoblastoma	I b	80	3	4,65	1.730.000
II	Mixed melanoma	II	80–85	6	8,9	909.090
III	Necrotic	III a	100	5	4,65	No valorable Necrosis
	Melanoma	III b	40–60	8	8,9	214.800
IV	Mixed melanoma	IV Aa	80	9	5,04	783.300
		IV Ab	50	7	5,43	465.700
		IV Ba	85	7	6,98	1.434.347
		IV Bb	25	3	5,43	431.666
V	Spindle	V Aa	85	4	3,49	1.925.400
	Melanoma	V Ab	50	3	4,26	800.750
		V Ba	100	2	1,55	4.410.000
		V Bb	2	6	3,88	40.000
		V Bc	80	2	2,33	3.113.333
VI	Mixed	VI a	85	8	5,43	833.230
	Melanoma	VI b	40	5	2,71	600.500
		VI c	10	3	2,71	218.000
VII	Undifferentiated	VII a	75	9	6,20	1.650.000
	Retinoblastoma	VII b	40	3	1,55	1.140.000
		VII c	75	3	2,33	1.650.000
VIII	Lymphoma	VIII a	90	12	7,75	3.241.792
		VIII b	15	11	6,20	140.608
IX	Epithelioid	IX a	90	5	2,33	324.300
	Melanoma	IX b	20	6	6,20	197.388
		IX c	90	3	2,33	392.333
X	Suprachoroid	X a	90	19	8,53	1.980.250
	Hemorrhage	X b	25	1	3,10	303.500

Table 3. Evaluation of the morphological parameters of each type of tumour.

Case No.	Reflectivity (%)	Cell arrangement	Cell attachment	Cellularity (per mm^3)
1 Spindle A	70	Fascicled	Strong	1.200.000
2 Spindle B	65–70	Fascicled	Strong	738.000
3 Spindle B	65–70	Fascicled	Strong	738.000
4 Epithelioid	10	Alveolar	Weak	150.000
5 Mixed	20	Fas. and Alv.	Variable	339.500
6 Necrotic	65	—	Null	786.600
7 Necrotic	70	—	Null	712.000
8 Hemangioma	100	Lobular	Null	4.428.000
9 Retinoblastoma	100	Diffuse	Weak	2.210.000
10 Metastatic CA.	90	Alveolar	Weak	2.016.000

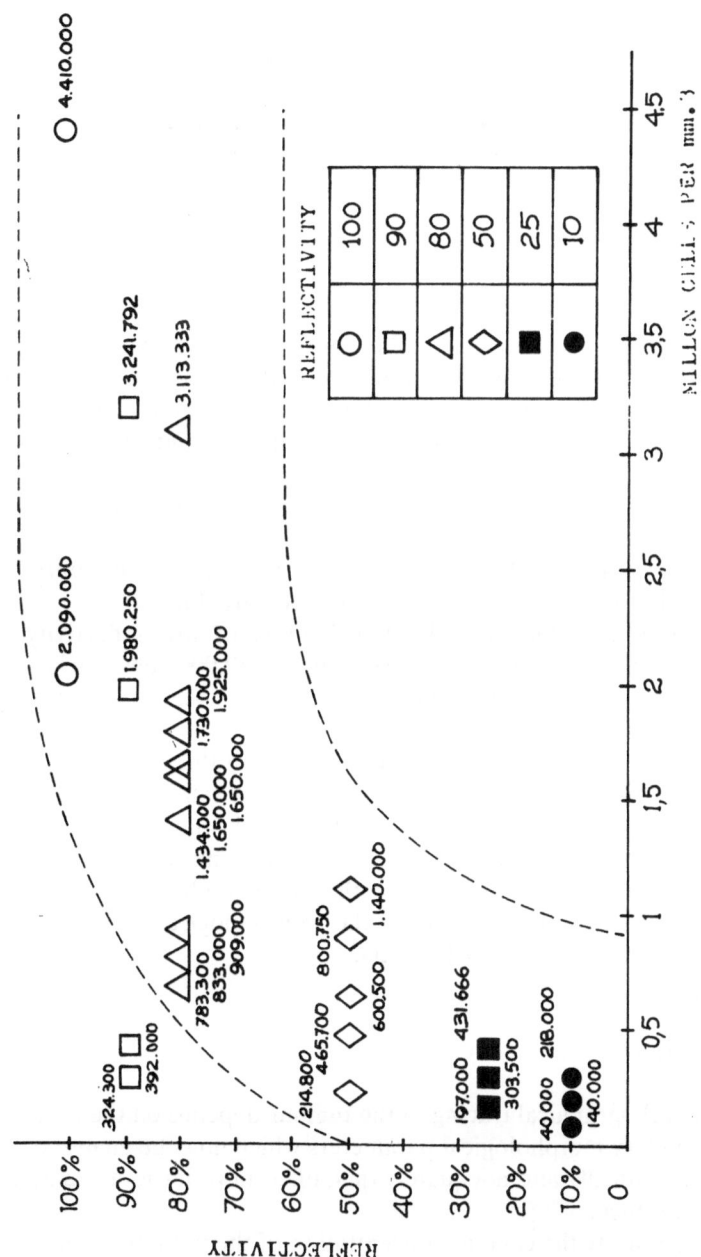

Fig. 4.

The results belonging to part II (12 in vitro echographical tracings in 10 intraocular tumours and the corresponding measures of the cellular concentration per mm³) have been summed up in Table 2 and in Fig. 2a and b the same are analyzed individually.

In Fig. 4 there is a summary of the information obtained so far: each histological type of tumour has a different cellular concentration. We left aside the histological type and only related the average cellularity with the same reflectivity which showed a positive lineal correlation between them (Fig. 5).

Discussion

Although the different histopathological types of a tumour must have some meaning in the echographical result of the same, in this study we have devoted ourselves with special interest to the relationship between the cellular concentration per mm³ of the tumours and the type of reflectivity found.

It is evident that the cellular concentration keeps a close relation with the cellular size and the neoplasia cellular attraction in question.

The existing cellular correspondence between the tumours studied and the kind of echographical reflectivity is remarkable.

It is so that the epithelioid melanoma of low reflectivity is in close relation to the low cellular concentration (150.000 cells/mm³ average) while the A and B fusocellulars melanoma are in close relation to high cellular concentration (800.000 cells/mm³ average).

We may add to the foresaid the fact that in the metastatic carcinoma and the retinoblastoma high reflectivity is in direct relationship with high cellular concentration (2.000.000 and 2.800.000 cells/mm³ respectively) as in the hemangioma with a 4.500.000 cells/mm³ concentration.

This paper is the first one in the bibliography which partly explains a numerical relationship between the morphological and the echographical aspects of the intraocular tumours.

Conclusions

- The echographical tracing of the tumour depends on the primary and secondary morphological parameters which must be analyzed systematically and adequately quantified in order to evaluate its real importance.
- In this study the cellular concentration of the tumour estimated in the cells quantity per mm³ appears as a determining factor of the echographical reflectivity. At low reflectivity low cellular concentration and the other way round.

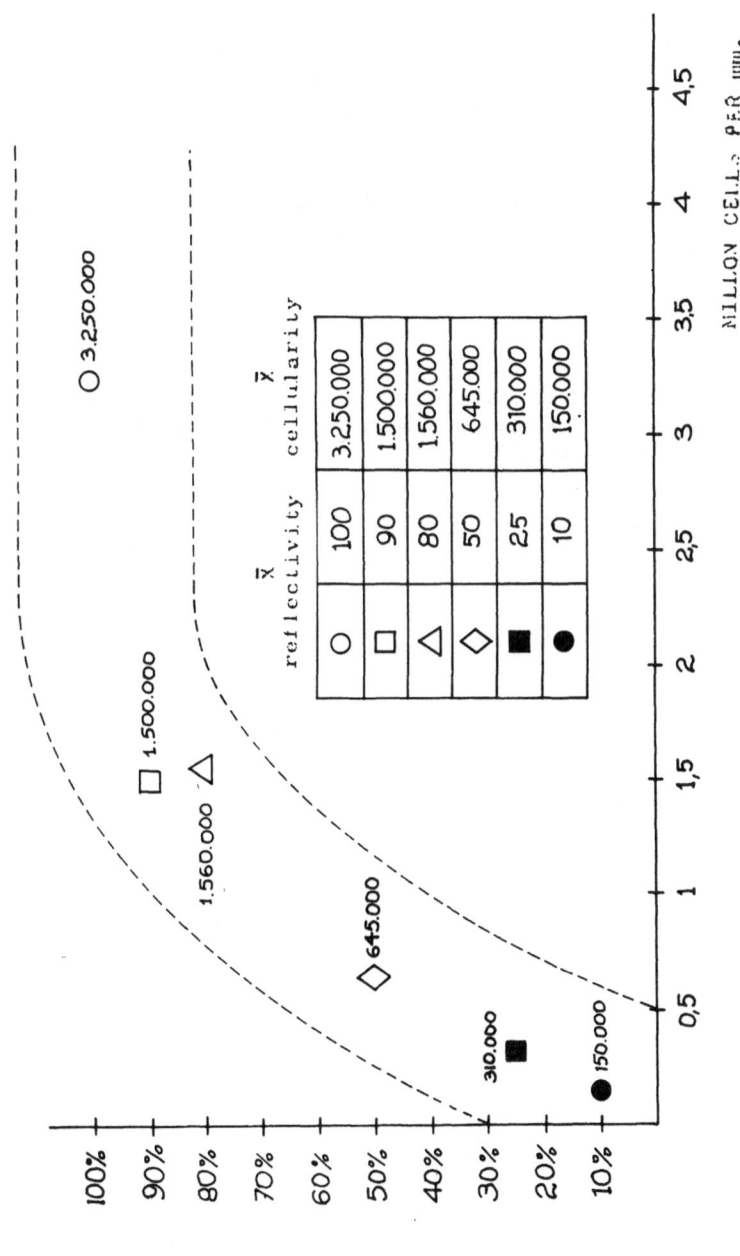

Fig. 5.

- This fact should not be surprising if we bear in mind Ossoinig's experience [2] in tissular patterns when analyzing eight sanguineous samples with different number of cells.
- Both vascularization and necrosis help modifying the number of cells per mm^3 and therefore, their relationship to reflectivity.
- Uveal melanoma shows differences in the cellular concentration in different areas.
- What has been observed supports the hypothesis on the potential utility of ultrasonography in the diagnosis of the morphological type of lesion, especially where referred to intraocular tumours.

References

[1] Sampaolesi R. 1984. Ultrasonidos en Oftalmología. Editorial Médica Panamericana.
[2] Ossoinig K C. 1974. Quantitative echography. The basis tissue differentiation. Journal of clinical ultrasound. II, 1: 33.

37. Tissue characterization by ultrasound

JOHAN M. THIJSSEN

Abstract

Two distinct approaches are outlined: the estimation of acoustic parameters of tissues and the analysis of echographic images by statistical methods. Two acoustic parameters are accessible: the attenuation coefficient and the backscattering coefficient. The latter anables the estimation of the effective size of the scattering sites within the tissue. The statistical analysis of images yields a quantification of the mean reflectivety level, the textural signal-to-noise ratio and the mean 'speckle' size. These parameters may be employed to estimate the volume density of the scatterers. Combining all these parameters in lineair discrimant analysis yields a powerful means to detect or even differentiate neoplasms.

Introduction

The diagnostic potentials of echography are presently well established in ophthalmology. The diagnosis is based on visual assessment of the A- and B-mode echograms. This assessment comprises quantitative features like reflectivity level, amplitude decrease and regularity of the pattern which are available at the A-mode traces, and anatomical and morphological features like shape and changes from the normal (e.g. choroidal excavation) at the B-mode. It should be mentioned that some way of standardization of equipment performance characteristics as well as careful calibration of the transducer-equipment combination are essential prerequisits to the quantitative employement of A-mode echograms. A fundamentally more powerful method for echographic diagnosis is the analysis of signals and images by a digital computer (c.f. Thijssen, 1987). The most sophisticated studies are enabled by digitizing the radiofrequency (rf) echographic signals. The spectral contents of these signals can be calculated and corrected for the

Biophysics Laboratory of the Institute of Ophthalmology, Academic Hospital and University, Nijmegen, the Netherlands

R. Sampaolesi (ed.), Ultrasonography in Ophthalmology 12, 293–304.
© *1990. Kluwer Academic Publishers, Dordrecht*

depth-dependence induced by the beam formation (diffraction and focussing) as was shown by the author (Cloostermans and Thijssen, 1983; Verhoef et al., 1985).

The corrected signals can be analysed in various ways to obtain acoustic tissue parameters, which are frequency dependent: the attenuation coefficient (Cloostermans, 1986) and the backscattering coefficient (Feleppa et al., 1986; Romijn et al., 1988). It will be obvious that these parameters can not be estimated by employing the normal 'video' echogram that is displayed at the A-mode image. Moreover, the above mentioned correction employs both the amplitude and the phase information of the rf-echograms, the latter of which is lost in the demodulation producing the video signal.

\The diffraction corrected spectra are furthermore corrected for the attenuation and transformed back to rf-lines and then the demodulation is performed by an algorithm, i.e. B-mode images are calculated by the computer (Oosterveld et al., 1985). In the following it is assumed that the A-mode and B-mode images have been corrected in this way before the analysis. This analysis comprises the first order statistics, i.e. the mean (reflectivity) level of the echogram and the so-called signal-to-noise ratio (SNR) which is the mean over the standard deviation of the video echogram ('gray level'). The second order statistics is a quantification of the mean size of the 'speckle' that governs the texture of B-mode echograms and the width of the peaks of an A-mode echogram. It should be mentioned that this analysis (Thijssen, 1987; Thijssen and Oosterveld, 1985, 1987; Thijssen et al., 1987, 1988; Oosterveld et al., 1985) is confined to the 'tissue' echograms, which incorparates the scattering from soft tissues and excludes the specular reflections from large anatomical interfaces.

Physics of ultrasound

Transmission and beam formation

The pulse-echo principle implies that the tranducer is activated by a very short electrical impulse. The surface of the transducer transmits a short duration longitudinal wave which is essentially coherent. The frequency of the acoustic pulse is determined by the dimensional and acousto-electrical properties of the employed piezoelectric material (a ceramic, mostly PZT). The time waveform of this pulse can be assessed by registering the echo from a plane interface (Fig. 1 left). The transducer frequency is to be seen from the periodicity of this waveform. The right side of Fig. 1 displays the (logarithmic) spectrum corresponding to the echo. The central frequency of the spectrum corresponds to the transmission frequency. The width of the spectrum is *inversely* related to the width of the sound pulse: the shorter this pulse, the wider the spectrum will be.

The sound field produced by a focussed transducer when operating in the

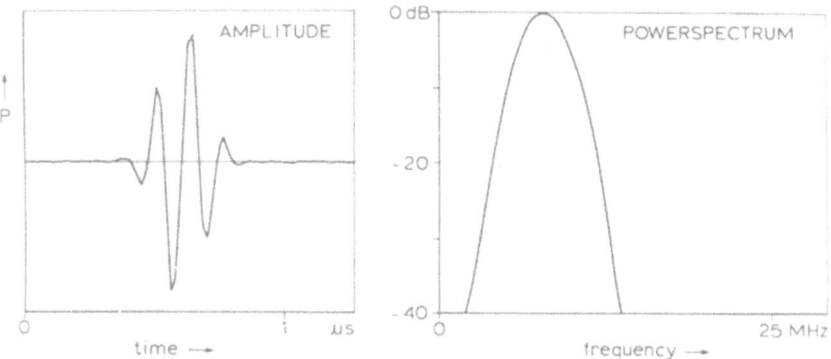

Fig. 1. Left: Waveform of transmitted ultrasound pulse.
Right: Corresponding amplitude spectrum (Logarithmic ordinate)

continuous wave (CW) mode is shown in Fig. 2 (top). This operation of the transducer yields in addition to coherence also monochromaticity. Therefore, the beamformation is identical to the one of an optical laser. The interference and the side lobes in front of the focus are called diffraction effects which are due to the finite size of the employed transducer. When the transducer is operated in the pulsed mode (Fig. 2, bottom) most of the interference in the near field has disappeared, although the field is still not homogeneous. It has to be concluded that the distribution of acoustic

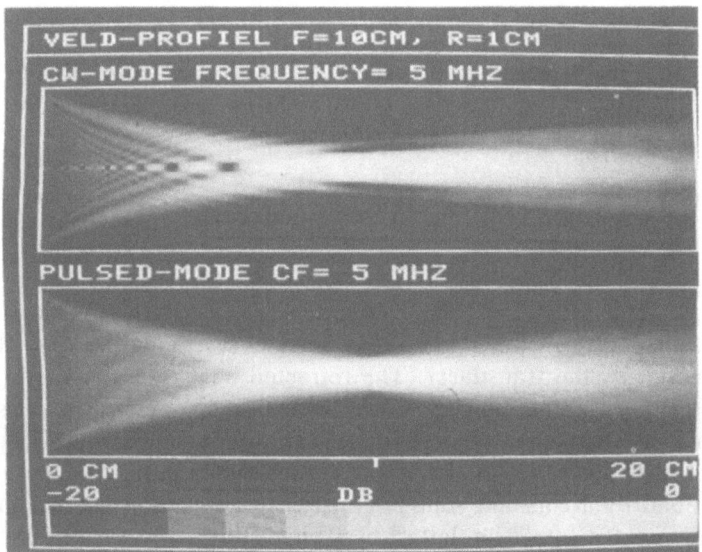

Fig. 2. (Top) Cross section of the ultrasound field produced by a continuously transmitting transducer, frequency 3 MHz, focus at 10 cm. (Bottom) Same as above for pulsed mode of transmission (Verhoef, et al., 1984).

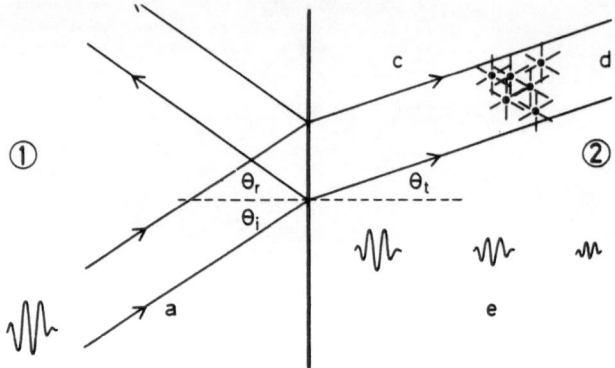

Fig. 3. Mechanisms of interaction of ultrasound with tissue. (a) Beam incident at interface between media 1 and 2; (b) reflected fraction of beam; (c) refracted fraction of beam; (d) scattering by small inhomogeneities; (e) decrease of amplitude due to attenuation.

energy is depth dependent due to diffraction and focussing, so that any parameter, either acoustic or from the image, will be dependent on the localization of the 'region of interest' with respect to the transducer, i.e. depth dependent. For that reason it is essential to correct for these effects prior to any analysis of the echograms.

Interaction mechanisms and tissue model

The sound beam, modelled by a cylindrical shape (a) in Fig. 3, is partly reflected (b) on the interface between two media according to the first of Snell's laws, i.e.:

$$O_i = O_r$$

and partly refracted (c) into medium 2 according to the second law:

$$\frac{\text{Sin } O_i}{c_1} = \frac{\text{Sin } O_t}{c_2}$$

The reflected fraction, at perpendicular incidence, yields the echo that can be registered by the transducer. The refracted beam is attenuated (d) and scattered (e) within medium 2, which mechanisms are characteristics of the medium and when quantified yield 'acoustic' parameters of this medium. The appropriate acoustic model of a tissue, as shown in Fig. 4, can therefore be described by a constant sound velocity, an absorption coefficient and a scattering coefficient. The latter two yield both a contribution to the (frequency dependent) attenuation coefficient. As is shown in Fig. 4 the attenuation coefficient as well as the backscattering coefficient can be estimated. It should be remarked that the attenuation within the medium

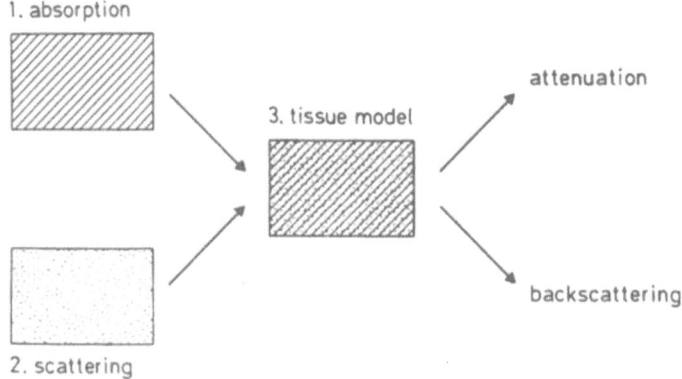

Fig. 4. Acoustic tissue model: medium with a constant velocity containing absorption and scattering (homogeneous and isotropic respectively). Attenuation and scattering can be estimated.

has to be compensated for prior to the estimation of the backscattering coefficient.

Estimation of the attenuation coefficient

An example of a rf-signal backscattered by solid tissues is shown in Fig. 5 (top). As will be discussed furtheron the reception of the backscattered echoes yields interference and therefore the echogram is quite irregular. It may be appreciated still that the amplitude of the rf-signal decreases with depth. When the spectra corresponding to the time windows 1 and 2 are calculated (Fig. 5, middle), the attenuation becomes visible by a lowering of the spectrum at the largest depth (2). In addition to this lowering the latter spectrum appears to be shifted to lower frequencies. This is due to the fact that the higher the frequency the stronger is the attenuation. When the logarithm is taken of the ratio of the spectra a striking characteristic becomes evident (Fig. 5, bottom): the attenuation increases *linearly* with frequency, hence, a single parameter corresponding to the slope of this straight line characterizes the attenuation. This parameter is called the attenuation coefficient linear slope, or just attenuation coefficient and it is expressed in dB/cm. MHz.

The irregularity of the rf-signals is transferred to the corresponding spectra and therefore the attenuation coefficient can not be reliably estimated from a few time windows. In general many spectra obtained at equal depth have to be averaged before the division is carried out; in other words the rf-lines corresponding to the whole region of interest (e.g. a tumour) are taken.

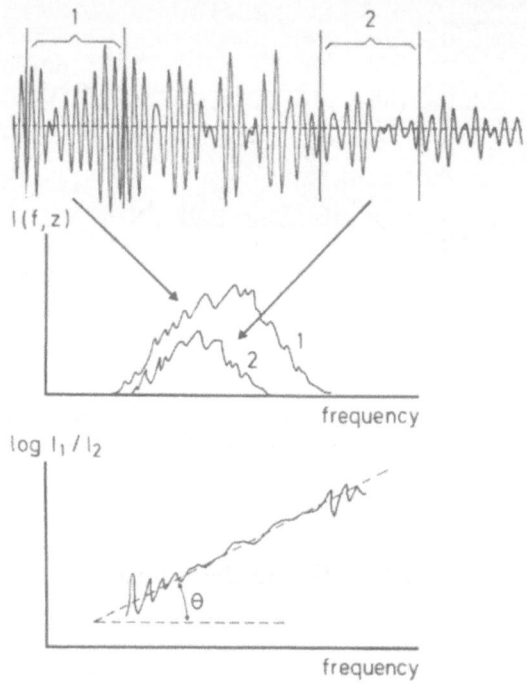

Fig. 5. Attenuation; (top) RF signal obtained from scattering in attenuating medium, time windows at depth 1 and 2; centre: amplitude spectra corresponding to RF signal in time windows, (bottom) logarithm of ratio of spectra 1 and 2, note linear increase of attenuation with frequency.

Estimation of the effective scatterer size

The scattering in biological tissues can be modelled as a random distribution of small (with respect to the wavelength) spherical inhomogeneties in the 'acoustic impedance'. The scattering by collagen rich microstructures (microvasculature) will dominate, but it cannot be excluded that also cell conglomerates and small liquid filled vacuoles contribute to the scattering. Small spheres scatter in all directions equally and the amplitude (strength) of the scattering is frequency dependent. This latter property can be calculated for various sizes, as is shown in Fig. 6 for the range from 20 μm to 500 μm. It can be seen that these curves, displaying the backscattering coefficient vs. frequency, can be fairly well approximated by straight lines in the diagnostic frequency range from 5–10 MHz.

Therefore, the slope of these lines is uniquely related to the size of the scatterer. In practice a tissue may contain a range of scatterer dimensions. The analysis will produce a 'mean effective' scatterer size, which neverthe-

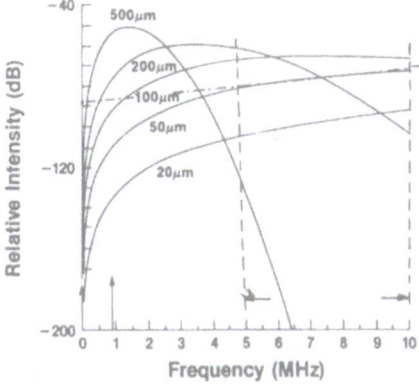

Fig. 6. Backscattered intensity vs. frequency for various sizes of the scatterer. Within the diagnostic frequency range (5–10 MHz) linear approximation. Slope of these lines uniquely related to the size.

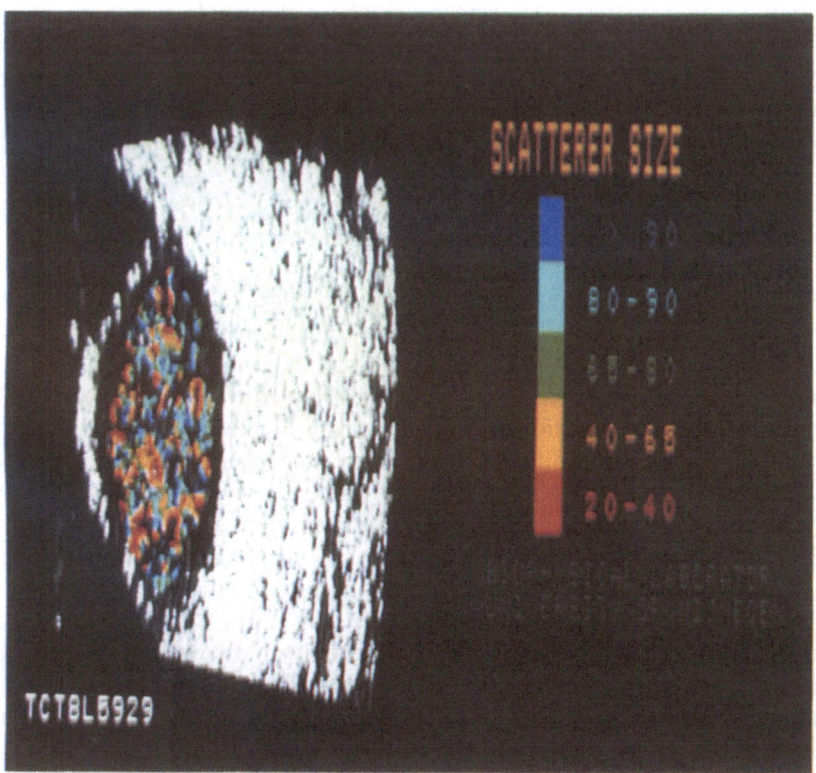

Fig. 7. B-mode image of posterior part of an eye (in vivo registration) calculated from RF-data by computer. The local size of scatterers within tumour is colour coded.

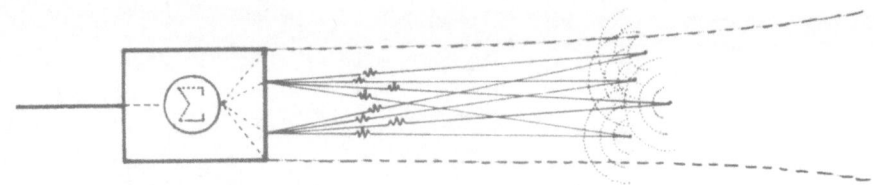

Fig. 8. Principle of generation of echogram from scattering in solid tissues. Rayleigh scattering yields spherical wave fronts arriving on transducer at slightly different moments.

less is a very promising parameter as was shown by correlation studies with histological data obtained from intraocular tumours after enucleation (Coleman et al., 1985; Romijn et al., 1989). The procedure to estimate the backscattering coefficient, i.e. the amplitude of the spectrum vs. frequency, is to calculate the diffraction corrected spectra from the region of interest and to estimate and correct for the attenuation. This procedure results in a series of (linear) spectra at various depths, which can either be averaged to obtain a single scatterer size (mean value) for the whole region of interest, or alternatively, the local scatterer size can be estimated. This is of course a relatively inaccurate estimate, but it is possible to create a 2-D image now of the scatterer size! By overlaying these values in colour over the original B-mode image a very informative *new* kind of image is obtained (Fig. 7).

Construction of B-mode images and statistical analysis

The basic principle of the texture in B-mode images of scattering media, like solid tissues, is illustrated by Fig. 8. The transducer insonates a medium in which a large number of small scatterers is randomly positioned (cf. Fig. 8). Four of the scatterers are depicted. According to the Rayleigh theory the scattering is omnidirectional, i.e. spherical. Since, the distances of the scatterers to the transducer are different, the four waves arrive at the transducer surface at slightly different moments. The resulting echoes are additively registered, hence, the electrical wavelets are linearly summated (Fig. 9). Because the wavelets are replicas of the transmission pulse, which are similarly changed by attenuation, strong interference occurs.

In other words because the differences in depth are smaller than the resolution limit the resulting rf-signal is actually an interference pattern with no direct relation to the individual scatterers. Because of the quasi-monochromaticity this interference pattern (after demodulation) is similar to the 'speckle' occuring when viewing a reflection of laserlight. During the scanning of the B-mode transducer this speckle is depicted on the image as a texture of white 'blobs' which is the familiar aspect of any echogram obtained from a solid tissue.

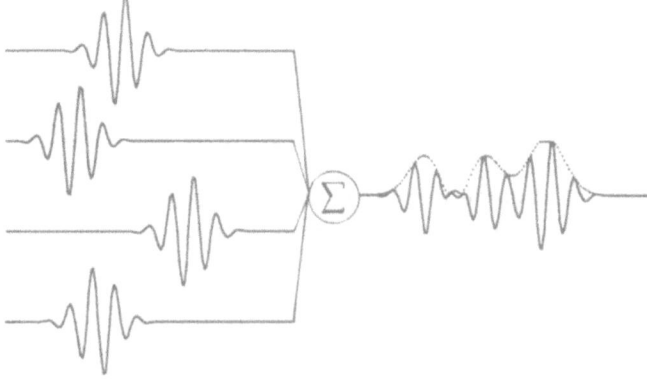

Fig. 9. Principle of generation of echogram from scattering in solid tissues. Linear summation of echo waveforms received by transducer within resolution limit and yielding interference pattern instead of true image of scattering structures (Fig. 8). Dotted line video signal after demodulation, peaks are similar to 'speckle'.

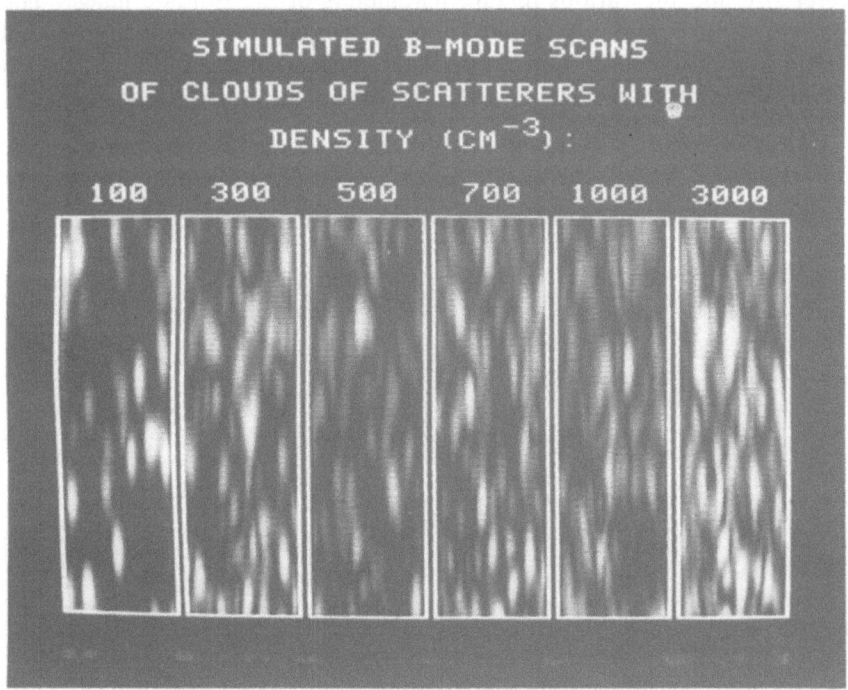

Fig. 10. Simulated B-mode images of media containing scatterers with an increasing volume density (from left to right) (Oosterveld et al., 1985).

The size (and also the density) of the speckles is completely governed by the frequency, the bandwidth, the diameter and the focal distance of the transducer, when the volume density of the scatterers is relatively large. However, at lower densities the size of speckles increases and thereby reveals the histological structure of the tissue (Fig. 10). The mean echolevel is proportional to the square root of the volume density. These characteristics of the texture of B-mode echograms can be assessed by proper statistical analysis, after the depth depence has been removed as before, by correcting the rf-signals prior to image construction.

Techniques

At the author's laboratory a data acquisition and processing system has been developed (Fig. 11) which can be readily connected to a commercial B-mode scanner (Triscan, Biophysic Medical). It digitizes the rf-lines at a 40 MHz rate and stores 128 Kb corresponding to a region of interest of one quarter of the B-mode image, in a single sweep. The data to correct for the beam diffraction are stored in the computer memory and are employed before the analysis starts. The analysis comprises the attenuation coefficient, the scatterer size and the various texture parameters of the B-mode image. These parameters are presently employed in a retrospective study, where data are taken from intraocular tumours prior to enucleation and pre- and posttreatment by radiotherapy.

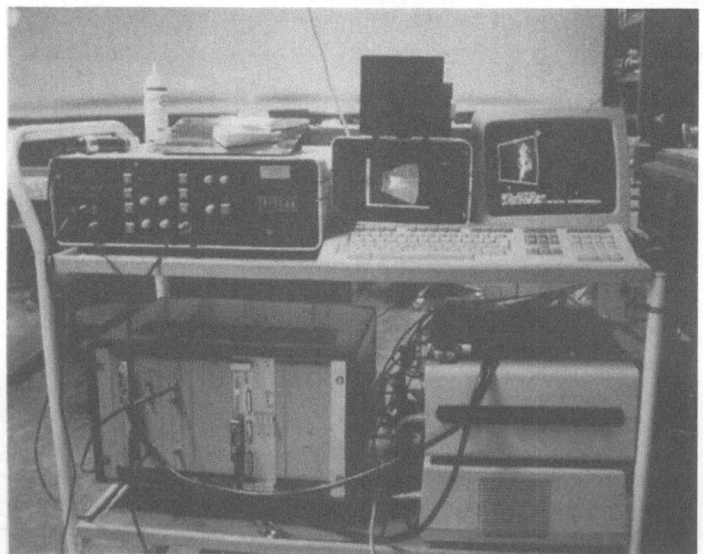

Fig. 11. Data-acquisition and processing system developed at the author's laboratory (Kruimer et al., 1985).

The preliminary results are confirming those obtained by Coleman et al. (1985), showing that it is not only possible to differentiate various kind of tumours, but also the different types of melanomas. The latter result is rather important when prospectively employed in the planning of the treatment of these tumours.

Acknowledgements

This work is supported by grants from the Netherland's Cancer Foundation-Koningin Wilhelmina Fonds and the Foundation for Technological Research of the National Science Foundation. It was carried out within framework of the Concerted Action Programme on Ultrasonic Tissue Characterization and Echographic Imaging of the European Community (Project leader: J M Thijssen).

References

Cloostermans M J T M, Thijssen J M. 1983. A beam corrected estimation of the frequency dependent attenuation of biological tissue from back-scattered ultrasound. Ultrasonic Imag 5: 136–147.

Cloostermans M J T M, Mol H J, Verhoef W A, Thijssen J M, Kubat K. 1986. In-vitro estimation of acoustic parameters of the liver and correlation with histology. Ultrasound Med Biol 12: 39–51.

Coleman D J, Lizzi F L, Silverman R H. et al. 1985. A model for acoustic characterization of intraocular tumours. Invest Ophthalmol Vis Sci 26: 545–550.

Feleppa E J, Lizzi F L, Coleman D J, Yaremko M M. 1986. Diagnostic spectrum analysis in ophthalmology: a physical perspective. Ultrasound Med Biol 12: 623–631.

Kruimer W H, Lammers J H E, Thijssen J M. 1985. Ultrasonic Biopsy apparatus. In: Berkhout, A J et al. (eds) Acoustical Imaging, vol. 14, Plenum, New York. pp. 481–486.

Oosterveld B J, Thijssen J M, Verhoef W A. 1985. Texture of B-mode echograms: 3-D simulations and experiments of the effects of diffraction and scatterer density. Ultrasonic Imag 7: 142–160.

Romijn R L, Thijssen J M, Van Delft J L et al. 1989. In-vivo ultrasound backscattering estimation for tumour diagnosis: an animal study. Ultrasound Med Biology 15: 471–479

Thijssen J M, Oosterveld B J. 1985. Texture in B-mode echograms. In: Berkhout A J et al. (eds) Acoustical Imaging, Vol. 14, Plenum, New York, pp. 481–486.

Thijssen J M. 1987. Ultrasonic tissue characterization and echographic imaging Med Progr Technol 13: 29–46.

Thijssen J M, Oosterveld B J. 1987. Performance of echographic equipment and potentials for tissue characterization. In: Viergever M A, Todd-Prokopek A (eds) Proceedings NATO-ASI on Mathematics and Computer Science in Medical Imaging, Springer, Berlin, pp. 455–468.

Thijssen J M, Oosterveld B J, Romijn R L. 1987. Texture in amplitude modulated and phase derivative echograms. In: Ferrari L A et al. (eds) Proceedings Intl. Symp. Pattern Recognition and Acoustical Imaging, SPIE, Bellingham, pp. 162–167.

Thijssen J M, Oosterveld B J. 1988. Texture of echographic B-mode images. In: Thijssen J M et al. (eds) Ultrasonography in Ophthalmology 11, Doc. Ophthal. Proc. Series, Vol. 51, Kluwer Acad. Publ., Dordrecht, Boston, London, pp. 77–83.

304

Verhoef W A, Cloostermans M J T M, Thijssen J M. 1984. The impulse response of a focused source with an arbitrary axisymmetric surface velocity distribution. J Acoust Soc Am 75: 1716–1721.

Verhoef W A. Cloostermans M J T M, Thijssen J M. 1985. Diffraction and dispersion effects on the estimation of ultrasound attenuation and velocity in biological tissue. IEEE Trans Biomed Eng BME-32: pp. 521–529.

38. Retinoblastoma conservative treatment: ultrasonographic follow-up

GUILHERME MARTINELLI NETO*, HÉLIO FERNANDO HEITMANN DE ABREU** and JOÃO ALBERTO HOLANDA DE FREITAS

Introduction

Retinoblastoma conservative treatment was first attempted in 1903 by H L Hilgartner with radiotherapy [1]. Since then many authors reported their experience with this method and with radioative isotopes, chemotherapy, photocoagulation, LASER and cryotherapy [1].

Since 1982 we have treated selected cases of retinoblastoma with cryotherapy and radiotherapy, with the intent of preserve some useful vision in these patients. In twelve cases, we had the opportunity to document the progressive flattening of the tumor with A and B ultrasonography.

Methods

First examination

The child with leucocoria was first examined in the office without general anesthesia. An indirect binocular ophthalmoscopy and A and B ultrasonography with a contact transducer of the ophthascan-B (Biofisic Medical) were performed.

The Clinical [4] and ultrasonographic [2, 3] diagnosis of retinoblastoma are well established. In positive cases the B image was frozen when the tumor presented its maximum elevation. Afterwards a biometry with A-mode was made. (Fig. 1)

Clinical and laboratorial study

In the following days all patients with diagnosis of retinoblastoma were submitted to clinical and laboratorial procedures to exclude the possibility of

* Centro Oftalmológico Campinas, R. Souza Compos 515, Campinas, 13025 Sao Paulo, Brazil
** From Centro Infantil de Investigação Dr. Domingos Boldrini (Hematologia/Oncologia Infantil — UNICAMP)

R. Sampaolesi (ed.), Ultrasonography in Ophthalmology 12, 305–311.

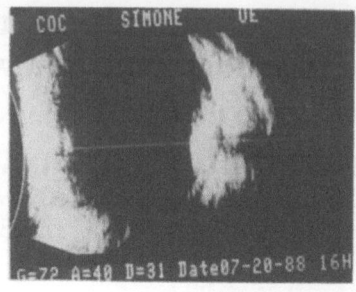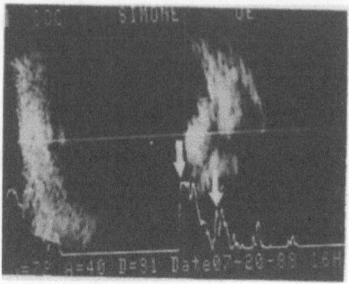

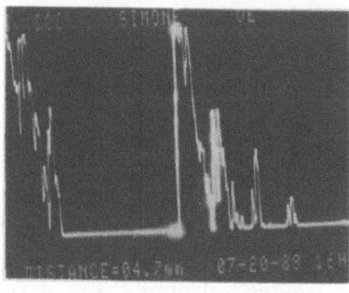

Fig. 1. (Top left) Maximum tumor elevation in frozen B image. (Top right) B image, cross vector and A image simultaneously. Arrows indicates the spikes choosen for biometry (Bottom) biometry between the spikes choosen.

metastasis. They included: spinal fluid examination, bone marrow evaluation, liver function, long-bone X-rays, liver and bone radioisotope study and skull and orbit CT scan.

After all of these procedures, the appropriate treatment was decided upon

The eyes choosen for conservative treatment were those which have a flat retina, with tumor involving less than half retina and had no evidences of metastasis [4]. Otherwise they were enucleated.

Second examination

Second examination was performed under general anesthesia in the Hospital. Both eyes were better examined with indirect binocular ophthalmoscopy with escleral depression. The treatment indicated was made: enucleation, cryotherapy or both.

Treatment

1. Cryotherapy: Was indicated for peripheral retinoblastomas, alone in small tumors and accompanied by irradiation in larger tumors.

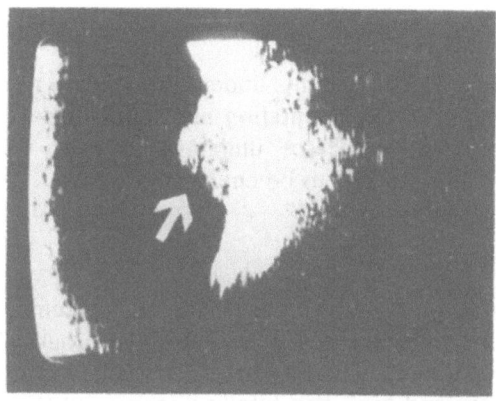

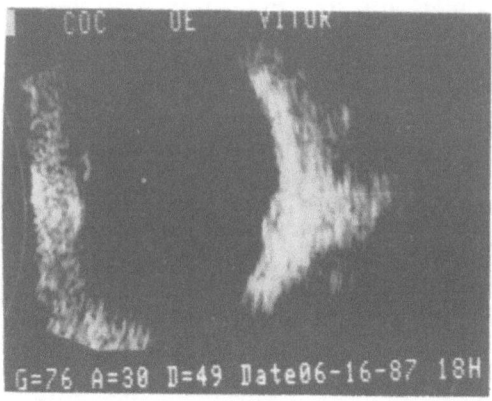

Fig. 2. (Top) B image of tumor before treatment. (Bottom) B image of tumor two years after treatment (radiotherapy). Notice the diminution of tumor volume.

2. External irradiation: Was indicated in large and multiple tumors, vitreous seddings and small tumors near the macula or optic disk. The total dose used was 3.500 rads divided in 9 sessions during three weeks.
3. Chemotherapy: Was indicated when the other eye was enucleated or when metastasis appeared in the follow-up. The drugs used were: Cyclophosphamide, Vincristine, Adriamycin and methrotexate.

Follow-up

After the initial treatment, the child was examined every 30 to 90 days under general anesthesia with indirect binocular ophthalmoscopy, when another session of cryotherapy was done if indicated. The ultrasonography was made in the office one day before or after this procedure.

308

Results

Since 1982, we have had 62 patients under conservative treatment, but only 12 with ultrasonographic documentation and follow-ups Ten of these cases had bilateral tumors and two cases, unilateral. In every bilateral case, one eye had a large tumor and had to be enucleated.

Ultrasonography

Treated cases showed a progressive flattening of the tumor (Fig. 2). The B image became more reflective while the tumor was progressively calcificated (Fig. 3). The acoustic shadow became more dense and in some instances the image of the esclera and orbit had totally disappeared (Fig. 4). In one case with three years of follow-up, the image was the same, showing a calcificated elevation near the optic disk (Fig. 5).

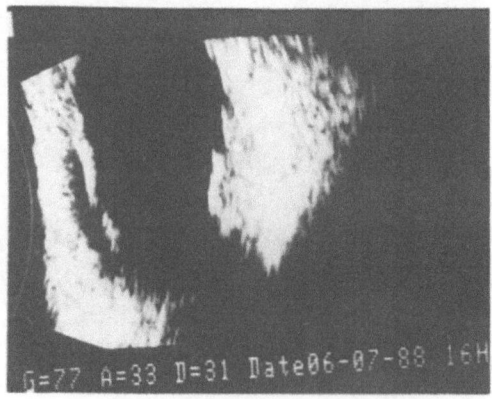

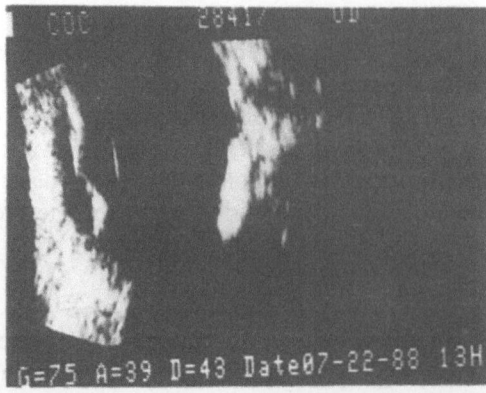

Fig. 3. (Top) B image of tumor before treatment. (Bottom) B image of tumor after cryo-theraphy and radiotherapy. Notice the great reflectivity of the tumor.

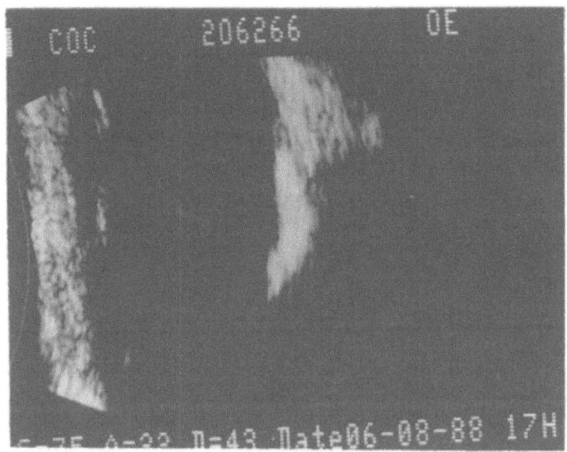

Fig. 4. Dense acoustic shadow in calcificated tumor after treatment.

Indirect binocular ophthalmoscopy

Treated cases present a shrunken white mass, sometimes surrounded by scar tissue and pigmentary alterations [4]. In some instances it was very difficult to predict that the tumor was inactive.

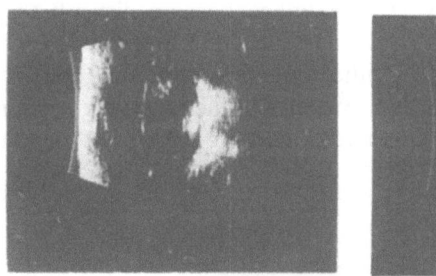 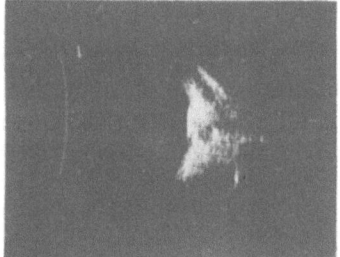

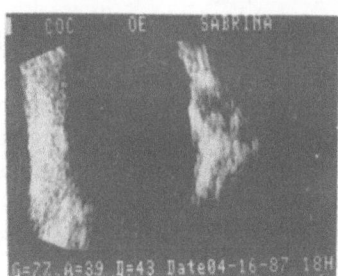

Fig. 5. (Top left) B image of tumor before treatment. (Top right) B image tumor 3 months after radiotherapy. (Bottom) B image of tumor three years after treatment.

310

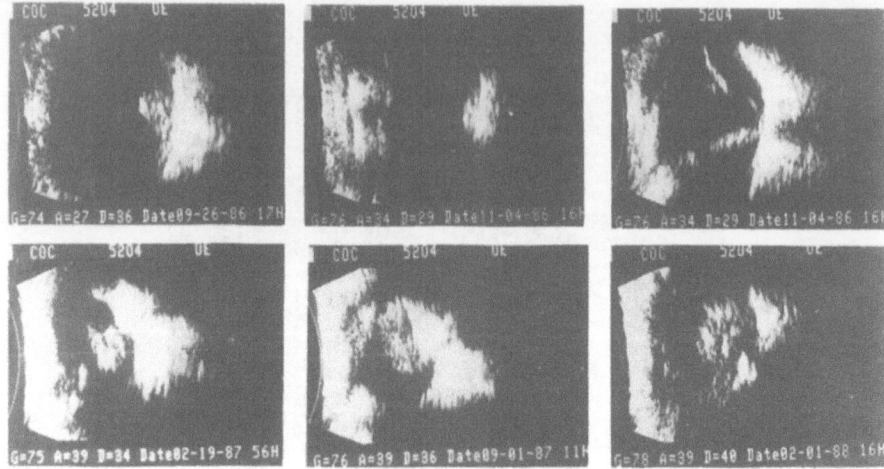

Fig. 6. (Top left) B image of tumor before treatment. (Top center) B image of tumor after cryotherapy and radiotherapy. (Top right) On the same day total retinal detachment (was noted). (Bottom) B images showing shrunken retina over the tumor mass.

Follow-up

During the follow-up two eyes had to be enucleated. One had total retinal detachment with dialisis and shrunken retina over the tumor mass, after cryotherapy and radiotherapy. The B image became difficult to be inter-pretated and enucleation was indicated (Fig. 6). The pathological examin-ation showed tumor activity. The other one presented a vitreous hemorrage and the eye became atrophic. No evidence of activity was encountered in patological examination. The other ten cases are doing well and still under periodic examination. (Fig. 7).

Discussion

Ultrasonography seems to be a good method of follow-up these cases. It is easy to compare the volume of the tumor in pictures of the B image before and after treatment. We can also compare with biometry their elevation. The exam is a non invasive method that can be made without general anesthesia and is less expensive then other methods.

There are however, some restrictions:

1. Impossibility to show far periferic tumors because of using a contact tranducer.
2. During the follow-up, after treatment, when the tumor becames a calci-ficated mass with dense acoustic shadow, it may be impossible to take biometry of the elevation.

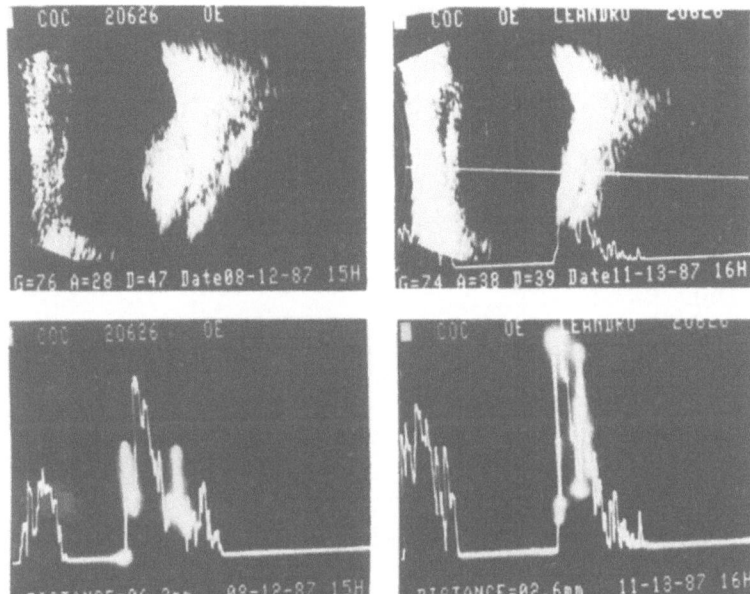

Fig. 7. (Right) Images of tumor before treatment. (Left) Images of tumor after cryotherapy and radiotherapy.

Conclusion

Ultrasonography is a good method for diagnosis, documentation and follow-up eyes with retinoblastoma not at far periphery, treated by cryotherapy, radiotherapy or both.

References

[1] Albert D M. 1987. Historic Review of Retinoblastoma Ophthalmology 94: 654–662.
[2] Ossoinig K C. 1972. Clinical echo-ophthalmology. In: F C Blodi (ed) Current Concepts in Ophthalmology Mosby, Saint-Louis.
[3] Poujol J. 1981. Echographie en ophtalmologie. Monografie, Masson, Paris.
[4] Shields J A, Augsburger J J. 1981. Current approaches to the diagnosis and management of retinoblastoma. Survey of ophthalmology 25: 347–372.

39. Ultrasonographic findings in selected cases of masquerading syndrome

A. LOMBARDI, L. A. IRARRAZAVAL, J. O. CROXATTO,
R. HULSBUS, R. FERNÁNDEZ MEIJIDE and E. S. MALBRÁN

Summary

Two patients, 9 and 12-years-old, were examined because of marked uni-lateral intraocular inflammatory signs. Vitreous opacity precluded visualiz-ation of the ocular fundus.

Ultrasonography revealed in both cases a slight thickening of the chorio-retinal layers. Evaluation of lactate dehydrogenase disclosed a high aqueous to plasma ratio in both cases.

Histopathologic examination after enucleation gave the diagnosis of mycobacterial endophtalmitis in one case, and a diffuse infiltrating retino-blastoma in the other. The echographic findings in these two cases will be discussed.

Introduction

Masquerade syndromes include conditions that are not primarily inflamma-tory, but may resemble acute or chronic uveitis. In this paper we present two cases previously reported [2, 5]. One of them was a diffuse infiltrating retinoblastoma that initially looked like a chronic uveitis with marked intraocular inflammation, an externally quiet eye and media opacity. The other case was a mycobacterium endophthalmitis that began in a very similar way. Although the latter isn't really a masquerade syndrome, we report them together to show how similar the clinical, laboratory and echographic findings may be.

Centro Oftalmológico Malbran and Fundación Oftalmológico Argentina 'Jorge Malbran,' Parera 162, Buenos Aires, Argentina

R. Sampaolesi (ed.), Ultrasonography in Ophthalmology 12, 313–319.

314

Case reports

Case 1 A 9-year-old girl [2] was examined in February 1980 for progressive hypopyon in the right eye with 6 months of evolution and resistant to medical therapy. Previous studies made elsewhere included normal ultrasonography, CT scan with an inferior solid area probably related to condensed exudates, negative aqueous culture and aqueous citology informed as purulent exudate.

Family history was negative for ocular and systemic deseases. Visual acuity was light perception in the right eye; the IOP was 45 mmHg. Ophthalmologic examination showed an external non inflamed painless, quiet eye. The anterior chamber was partially filled with chalky-white flocculent material that floated like talcum-powder with movement. Vitreous opacity precluded fundus visualization. The left eye was normal. A diagnosis of retinoblastoma was considered, but it was not supported by previous studies.

A and B scan ultrasonography performed with an Ocuscan 400 showed a few point-like, mobile low reflective spikes in the vitreous cavity. There was no evidence of an intraocular mass or calcification.

A vitrectomy was performed and an iris biopsy was obtained at the same time. Fundus examination during vitrectomy showed multiple white lesions on the retinal surface. Histopathologic study of the biopsy specimen was reported as consistent with granulomatous iritis.

Examination in March 1980 disclosed keratic precipitates, increased hypopyon and whitish nodules on the anterior surface of the iris. The IOP was 15 mmHg. Ophthalmoscopic examination revealed exudates covering the pars plana and a few white plaques which were interpreted as foci of retinochoroiditis.

Another vitrectomy, with lensectomy and iris biopsy, was performed. Cytological study of the vitreous was nondiagnostic. Fundus lesions remained unchanged.

The results of clinical and laboratory test for sarcoidosis, lymphoma and nematode endophthalmitis were negative. Because of the increased hypopion, vitreous haze and strong suspicion of a malignant process, the eye was irradiated in July 1980. The patient did well for some months. In November 1980 the condition worsened. Visual acuity was "no light perception" and the IOP rose to 42 mmHg. Ultrasonography showed multiple mobile point-like echogenic opacities that filled diffusely and uniformly the vitreous cavity, and a double linear image consistent with a flat thickening of the chorioretina in the suprapapillary region (Figs. 1–2). Because a diffuse variant of RTB could not be ruled out, a new paracentesis was performed. The cytological study revealed neoplastic cells consistent with retinoblastoma, and an aqueous to plasma lactate dehydrogenase (LDH) ratio of 9. Enucleation was performed in April 1981. No additional therapy was given and the patient is alive, without evidence of local recurrence or systemic disease 7 years after enucleation.

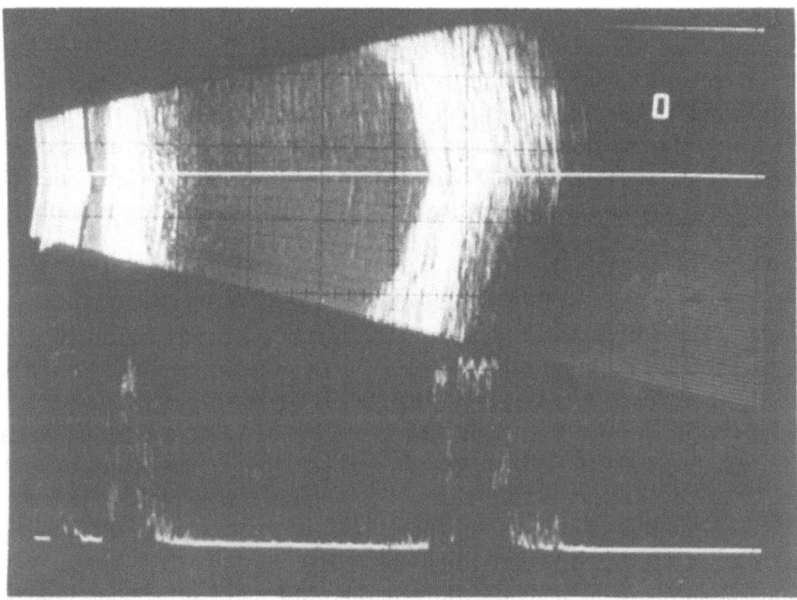

Fig. 1. Case 1: B-scan showing scattered echoes in the vitreous cavity and a thickened chorioretina.

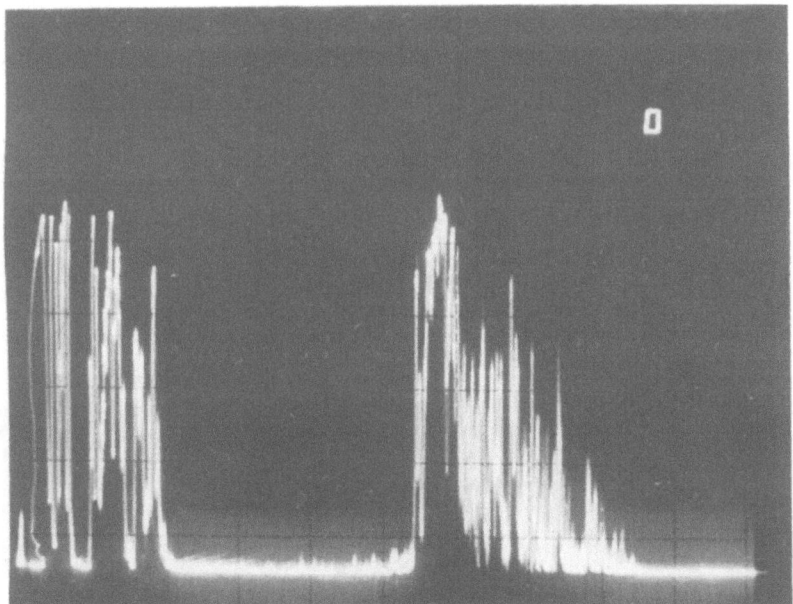

Fig. 2. Case 1: A-scan of retinoblastoma. The vitreous cavity is full of very low-reflective echoes.

316

On gross examination the anterior chamber was filled with a whitish exudate. The iris was thickened and deformed. The ciliary body and the retina were covered by patches of flocculent white material. Microscopically there were small tumor cells all over the inner aspect of the globe. The retina was slightly thickened and diffusely infiltrated by neoplastic cells with ocasional rosette formation. There were no foci of calcification. The choroid and sclera were normal. The diagnosis of diffuse infiltrating retinoblastoma was made.

Case 2   A 12-year-old boy [5] was seen in February 1986 with a two months history of granulomatous uveitis in the left eye resistant to medical treatment. Clinical, radiological and serological studies were negative for tuberculosis, toxoplasmosis or systemic disease. Visual acuity was light perception. Examination revealed a slight ciliary injection with an otherwise quiet external eye, corneal edema, keratic precipitates, chalky-white exudates in the anterior chamber, whitish nodules on the iris and lens opacity that precluded fundus visualization. The other eye was normal. Ultrasonography revealed a few point-like lesions within the vitreous, a posterior vitreous detachment with distinct aftermovements and a double linear image considered a diffuse thickening of the chorioretinal layers (Figs. 3–4). There was no mass and we could not detect any calcification. An anterior chamber paracentesis revealed atypical mononuclear cells without unequivocal evidence of neoplasia. The LDH aqueous to plasma ratio was 6.13. A vitrectomy was performed and an iris biopsy was obtained that showed granulo-

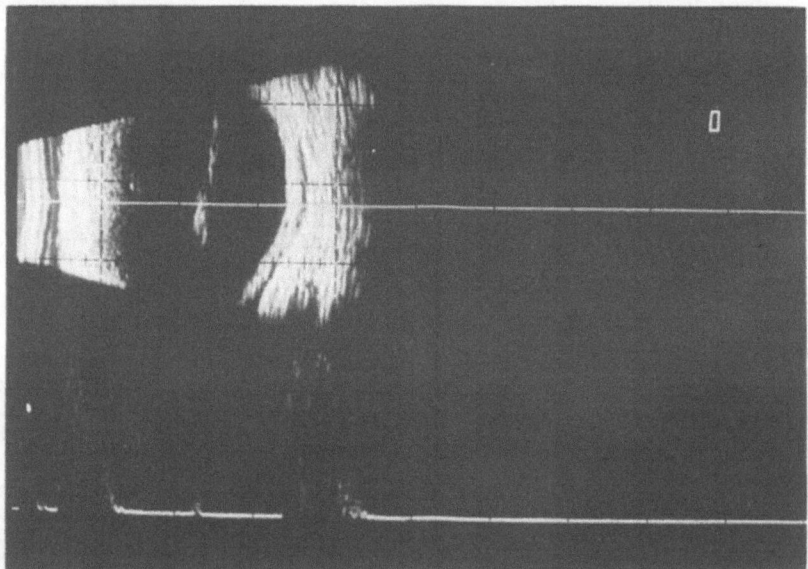

Fig. 3.   Case 2: Contact B-scan showing posterior vitreous detachment, condensation of the vitreous and chorioretinal thickening.

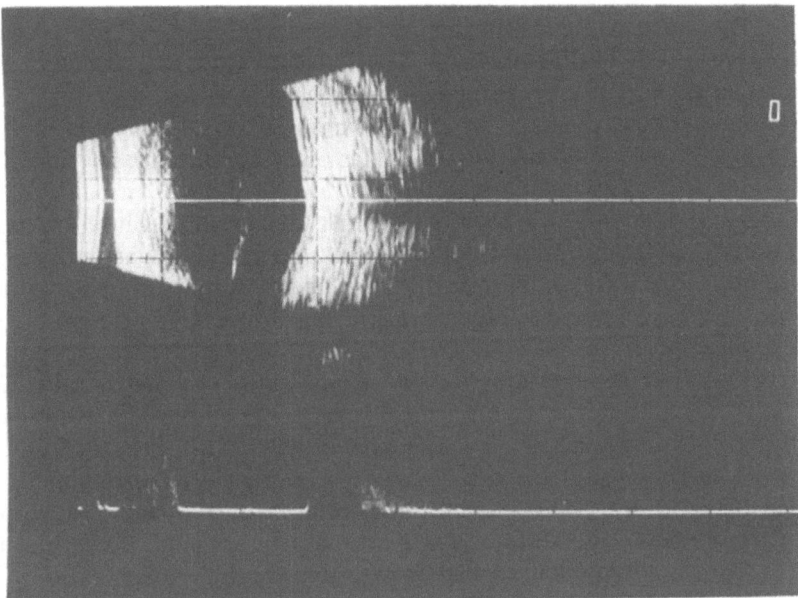

Fig. 4. Case 2: B-scan with posterior vitreous detachment not conected to the optic nerve and chorioretinal thickening.

matous infiltration. Fundus visualization during surgery revealed papillary edema with multiple yellow-white nodules on the retina.

During the postoperative period the ocular condition worsened and neovascular glaucoma developed. The decision to enucleate the blind painful eye was made and subsequently performed in March 1986. Pathologic findings: The anterior chamber and vitreous cavity were partially filled by exudates with fibrinous strands. Microscopically the retina was thickened with granulomatous inflammation and caseous necrosis. The choroid was of normal thickness and showed patchy infiltration and granulomas at the periphery. Ziehl-Neelsen stain revealed acid-fast bacilli in the vitreous adjacent to areas of caseous necrosis consistent with the diagnosis of mycobacterium endophthalmitis.

Discussion

A significant number of retinoblastoma patients are initially misdiagnosed as having primary ocular inflammation [13] as seen in case 1. The opposite situation is seen in case two where in a chronic granulomatous uveitis, the possibility of diffuse infiltrating retinoblastoma is considered. Cytologic evaluation of intraocular fluids, an LDH level assay in aqueous and a matching serum sample [9] may be helpful in making the diagnosis prior to enucleation but we must be aware of the possibility of some lack of specificity as seen in these cases.

Classic echographic evaluation of retinoblastoma [8, 14] is based on a description of the presence of a tumor mass with calcifications in it. In patients with diffuse infiltrating retinoblastoma, ultrasonography is of little help and may show only some mobile low amplitude vitreous echoes, corresponding to cellular seeding, retinal thickening because of diffuse infiltration, sometimes a localized retinal detachment [7, 10] and the absence of an intraocular mass or calcification. In our cases we use the term chorioretinal thickening because echographically we could not distinguish the retina from the choroid.

The term diffuse infiltrating retinoblastoma has been widely used [1, 2, 6, 7, 10, 11, 12, 13] and describes a tumor that grows and infiltrates the retina with vitreous and anterior chamber seeding [12]. This gives rise to great difficulty in diagnosis, often masquerading as intraocular inflammation.

Echographically, some authors have coined the misleading descriptive term of diffuse retinoblastoma for a postnecrotic retinoblastoma that produces low amplitude echoes that invade the vitreous cavity diffusely and uniformly with an absence of mass or vacuolated spaces. This tumor has a very poor prognosis but, on the other hand, diffuse infiltrating RTB has a good prognosis [6], with only one reported case of extraocular invasion.

We do think that in the presence of unilateral uveitis in older children with a quiet eye, even without a demonstrable intraocular mass or calcification, we must rule out the possibility of a diffuse infiltrating retinoblastoma.

This can only be accomplished by the close collaboration of ophthalmologists, echographists, pathologists and experienced cytologists when analyzing the different tests and procedures.

References

[1] Ashton N. 1958. Cited by Schofield [10].
[2] Croxatto J O, Fernandez Meijide R, Malbran E S. 1983. Retinoblastoma masquerading as ocular inflammation. Ophthalmologica 186: 48–53.
[3] Fernandez Vigo J, Cuevas Alvarez J. 1983. Formes echographiques typiques et atypiques des retinoblastoma. J Fr Ophthalmol 6/1: 43–49.
[4] Galli G, Perri P, Mazzeo V. 1984. Retinoblastoma of the diffuse type on the A and B scan. Ophthalmic Echography Proceedings of the 10th SIDUO Congress 419–423.
[5] Hulsbus R, Lombardi A, Croxatto J O. 1989. Unsuspected mycobacterial endophthalmitis with increased aqueous lactate dehydrogenase levels in a child. 21: 233–237 (Ann of Ophthalmol).
[6] Morgan G. 1971. Diffuse infiltrating retinoblastoma. Brit J Ophthal 55: 600–606.
[7] Nicholson D H, Norton E W D. 1980. Diffuse infiltrating retinoblastoma. Tr Am Ophth Soc 78: 265–289.
[8] Ossoinig K C, Cennamo G, Green R L, Weyer N L. 1981. Echographic results in the diagnosis of retinoblastoma. Docum Ophthal Junk Proc. Series. 29: 103–107.
[9] Piro P A, Abramson D H, Ellsworth R M, Kitchin D. 1978. Aqueous humor lactate

dehydrogenase in retinoblastoma patients: Clinicopathologic correlations. Arch Ophthalmol 96: 1823–1825.

[10] Schofield P B. 1960. Diffuse infiltrating retinoblastoma. Br J Ophthal 44: 35–41.

[11] Soll D B, Turtz A I. 1960. Retinoblastoma diagnosed as granulomatous uveitis. Arch Ophthalmol 63: 687–691.

[12] Spencer W H. 1985. Ophthalmic Pathology. W B Saunders (eds.) Philadelphia.

[13] Stafford W R, Yanoff M, Parnell B L. 1969. Retinoblastomas initially misdiagnosed as primary ocular inflammations. Arch Ophthal 82: 771–773.

[14] Sterns G K, Coleman D J, Ellsworth R M. 1974. The ultrasonographic characteristics of retinoblastoma. Am J Ophthalmol 78: 606–611.

40. Choroidal melanomas—correlations between A- and B-scan ultrasonography, nuclear magnetic resonance imaging and histopathology

R. GUTHOFF, J. MAAS, A. MOLINARI, R. W. BERGER
and D. VON DOMARUS

Summary

NMR-imaging and ultrasonography has been performed in 2 different groups of patients.

1. Prior to enucleation followed by histopathological examination.
2. Before and after Ruthenium-plaque therapy.
   In Ruthenium-treated patients we found a significant rise in spikeheight and internal reflectivity, but no change in NMR-signal-intensities.
   An unusually report is given of a patient were necrotic tumor areas could be well identified ultrasonography as well as in NMR-imaging techniques.

Introduction

In the management of patients with choroidal melanomas where we are dealing with the life threatening conditions diagnosis has to be made as safe as possible. All non-invasive diagnostic techniques should be applied in questionable cases to justify vision threatening therapy such as local irradiation or even enucleation.

Ultrasonography provided great help in diagnosis and planning conservative treatment such as ruthenium-irradiation (Guthoff et al., 1986). In general we found a raised internal reflectivity after irradiation but of course this cannot be regarded as an absolutely safe parameter for total necrosis, so recently we started to examine large melanomas with NMR-imaging techniques. The idea behind this quite costly and time-consuming procedure was not principally to establish the diagnosis but to gather basic information on signal behaviour of untreated tumors (Wollensak and Seiler, 1983).

Department Ophthalmology, University Hospital Eppendorff, Martinistrasse 52, D-2000, Hamburg, FRG

R. Sampaolesi (ed.), Ultrasonography in Ophthalmology 12, 321–326.

The next step should be to look for changes inside the tumor after beta irradiation.

To our knowledge what happens inside a large irradiated tumor in case of missing or unsatisfactory volume reduction is still a vexed question. We thought it might be of help in cases where unnecessary enucleation sometimes had been performed in the past (Guthoff et al., 1906).

Material and methods

Since the beginning of 1986 we have been able to examine 15 patients with malignant melanomas including 3 after Ruthenium plaque treatment. The examinations were performed with a Siemens Magnetom using a 0.35 and lateron 0.5 Tesla superconducting magnet. More recently a Phillips Gyroscan which allows one to perform mixed sequences for calculations of relaxation times was used. Ultrasonographical examinations have been performed with the Cooper vision instrument Digital B and additionally the Kretz 7200 MA unit.

Results

All but 2 tumors were defined by NMR as of homogeneous high signal intensity in the T1-weighted image and of low signal intensity also homo-

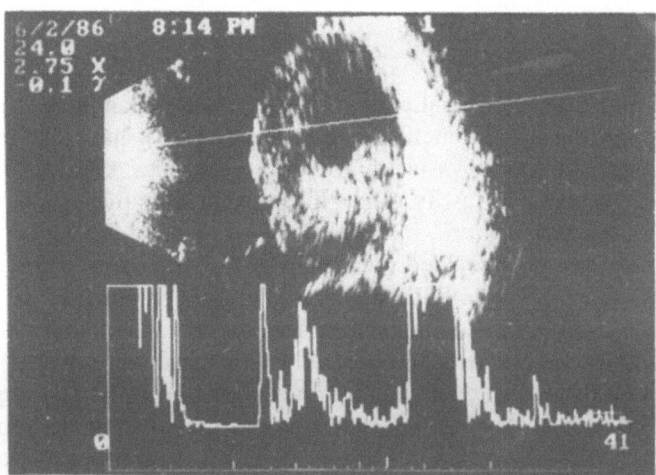

Fig. 1. Frontal section through a large choroidal melanoma, prominence 12.0 mm, tumor volume 1.900 cm. The superior part of the tumor showed low amplitude signals, the inferior part mainly consists in tissue with higher reflectivity. (Aus. Guthoff R. et al. 1967. Versuch einer praeoperativen Differenzierung des malignen Melanoms der Aderhaut. Klin Mbl Augenheilk 191: 45).

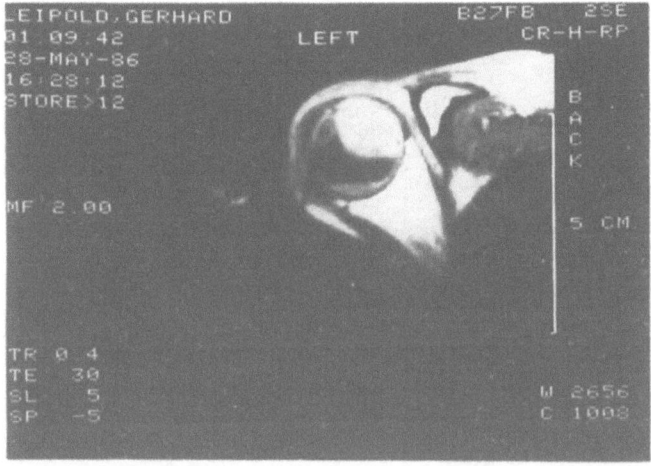

Fig. 2. T1-weighted NMR-image reveales a compound structure of the tumor with a central area of slightly reduced signal intensity.

geneously spread over the tumor in the T2-weighted images. All but 1 tumor showed medium to low reflectivity using standardized techniques in the Kretz unit as well as in the image regenerated by the B-scan pictures stored in the Digital B.

Those phenomena are already well known and described in literature (Gomorry et al., 1986). To demonstrate the possible influence of histo-pathology on NMR-imaging and ultrasonography one exception from this general rule should be presented in detail.

In a melanoma of 12 mm in prominence with a tumor volume of 1900 cm (Guthoff, 1980) ultrasonography demonstrated (Fig. 1). An inhomogenity of the internal structures. In the frontal section the superior part of the tumor showed low amplitude signals, the inferior part mainly consists of tissue with high reflectivity.

In the T1-weighted NMR-images (Fig. 2) a compound structure of the tumor might be suggested by a central area of reduced signal intensity surrounded by tissues of extremely high signal intensity. The fluid collection in the subretinal space was clearly to distinguish from the vitreous structure. Relations from tumor to lens were well outlined. In T2-weighted images (Fig. 3) the questionable central tumor area flashes up with high signal intensity surrounded by tumor tissue of low intensity. Signal behaviour of vitreous was comparable with that of the tumor center, subretinal fluid with that of the tumor periphery.

Conservative treatment of the melanoma seemed not to be advocated in a patient of 45 years of age with an intact 2nd eye. Therefore, enucleation was performed.

324

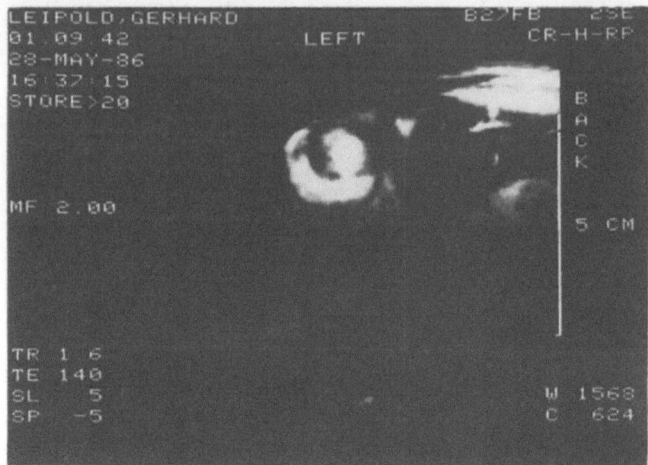

Fig. 3. In the T2-weighted image the questionable central tumor area flashes up with high signal intensity surrounded by tumor tissue of low intensity. (Aus Guthoff R. et al. 1967. Versuch einer praeoperativen Differenzierung des malignen Melanoms der Aderhaut. Klin Mbl Augenheilk 191: 45).

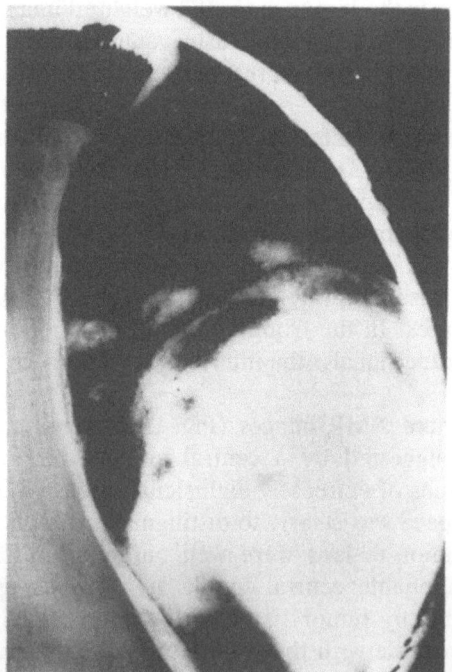

Fig. 4. Low magnification histopathology reveales a large melanocytic tumor which includes an area of unpigmented tissue. This corresponds anatomically with the region of low reflection ultrasound as well as high signal intensity in T2-weighted NMR-sequences. (Aus Guthoff R. et al. 1967. Versuch einer praeoperativen Differenzierung des malignen Melanoms der Aderhaut. Klin Mbl Augenheilk 191: 45).

Histopathology

Low magnification histopathology (Fig. 4) reveales a large melanocytic tumor which includes an area of unpigmented tissue. This corresponds anatomically with the region of low reflexion ultrasound as well as high signal intensity in the T2-weighted NMR-sequences.

High magnification identifies dark tumor areas as densely packed melanin loaded spindel shaped cells. In the unpigmented area were groups of partly necrotic tumor cells separated by large regions of extravascular blood and its remains.

Discussion

How to interprete the ultrasound pattern: The small amount of sound reflecting tissue interfaces in the unpigmented areas separated by homogeneous blood remains should be considered as responsible for the low reflective regions in A- and B-scan ultrasound images. This had been already found in a study we made 7 years ago, which showed that connective tissue was more likely to be present in tumors with high reflectivity.

Interpretation of NMR-pattern

At the present state of knowledge the higher amount of water seemed to be the reason for the atypical signal behaviour of the central tumor area. The signals of the peripheral parts correspond with the typical melanoma pattern reported in literature (Wollensak et al., 1983; Sobel et al., 1985; Sassani et al., 1984). This is probably due to the high concentration of melanin as a paramagnetic substance.

This signal behaviour was found in the pigmented areas of the enucleated tumors as well as in 2 melanomas after Ruthenium-treatment.

Using NMR-imaging technique no difference could be found in our 2 patients comparing pigmented tumors prior to treatment. In ultrasonography using a setting comparable with the standardized conditions described by Ossoinig a raise of internal reflectivity as previously described occurred also in those 2 patients.

Only recently applying mixed sequence techniques we were able to measure relaxation times in special areas of interest.

At the moment according to our experience and to the reports in literature there seems to be no answer in NMR-imaging techniques to the major question: What is going on in an irradiated choroidal melanoma. Most basic information is gathered in an article of Gomorry and co-workers (1986) who were able to correlate melanin-content of melanomas with exact measurement of relaxation times. May be those measurements including phosphor metabolism will prove to be of some help in the future.

Reference

Guthoff R. 1980. Modellmessungen zur Volumenbestimmung des malignen Aderhautmelanoms. Albr v Graefe's Arch klin exp. Opthalmol. 214: 139–146.

Guthoff R, von Domarus D, Steinhorst U, Hallermann D. 1986. 10 Jahre Erfahrung mit der Ruthenium-106/Rhodium-Behandlung des malignen Melanoms der Aderhaut. Bericht über 264 bestrahlte Tumoren. Klin Mbl Augenheilk 188: 576–583.

Gomorry J M, Grossmann R I, Shields J A, Augsburger J G, Joseph P M, Desimeone D. 1986. Choroidal Melanomas: Correlation of NMR Spectroscopy and MR Imaging. Radiology 158: 443–445.

Sassani J W, Osbakken M D. 1984. Anatomic features of the eye disclosed with nuclear magnetic resonance imaging. Arch Ophthalmol 102: 541–546.

Sobel D F, Kelly W, Kjus B O, Char D, Brant-Zawadzki M, Norman D. 1985. MR-Imaging of Orbital and Ocular Disease. AJNR 6: 259–264.

Wollensak J, Seiler T. 1983. Kernspintomographie am menschlichen Auge. Albr v Graefe's Arch klin exp Ophthal 220: 71–73.

41. Doppler ultrasonography in the follow-up of malignant melanoma of the choroid

R. W. BERGER, R. GUTHOFF, K. HELMKE* and P. WINKLER*

Summary

The sensitivity of modern pulsed duplex-scanners has been experimentally proven to be sufficient for measurements of flow velocity in the central retinal vessels. Clinical examinations were performed in 158 eyes with various diseases, including 27 malignant melanomas of the choroid. In vascular disturbancies the findings did not show significant deviations from the normal values.

In almost all malignant choroidal melanomas Doppler signals could be detected within the tumour. In the ultrasonographic follow-up conservatively treated melanomas Doppler examinations provided valuable additional information, when the findings before, directly after and four to six months after beta-irradiation were compared.

Introduction and objectives

Ultrasonographic imaging techniques have reached a high standard, due to the basic work of authors like Buschmann (1972), Coleman (1979), Ossoinig (1979), and others. Many attempts have been made to add information to the conventional grayscale picture like colour coding or frequency analysis, as worked out by Coleman and Lizzy (1979) and the group of Trier (1979).

Only recently, mainly due to sophisticated digitized equipment, it was possible to include Doppler signal analysis in high resolution B-scan devices. At present, an instrument specially designed for ophthalmic use is not available. But, influenced by the most interesting results in the field of cardiology and pediatrics, we tried to adapt their equipment to ophthalmological use and are going to present our first results we obtained during the last year.

Department of Ophthalmology,* Pediatric Department, University of Hamburg, Martinistr. 52, D-2000 Hamburg 20, FRG

R. Sampaolesi (ed.), Ultrasonography in Ophthalmology 12, 327–331.

Material and methods

The instrument used in our experiments and examinations was the ATL-Ultramark-8. In this apparatus B-scanning is performed with a nominal frequency of 7.5 MHz and Doppler signal analysis with 5.0 MHz.

In a pilot study in 12 healthy volunteers flow velocities of the central retinal artery and central retinal vein were measured. As a second step, the examinations were repeated after artificial elevation of the intraocular pressure up to a maximum of about 80 mm Hg by a suction cup dynamometer (Boucke-Oculo-Oscillodynamograph after Ulrich (1985)).

The clinical examinations comprised 72 eyes with normal findings, 27 eyes with choroidal melanoma, 8 eyes with central artery and 9 with central vein occlusion, 5 eyes with carotid cavernous fistula, sixteen with glaucomatous or vascular atrophy of the optic nerve, 4 eyes with hemangiomas, 8 eyes with inflammatory diseases and 9 others with various diagnoses. Altogether we can report the findings of 158 examinations.

Results

In normal eyes the mean systolic flow velocities were 9.5 cm/sec ($\pm$ 3.1) in the central retinal artery, 5.7 cm/sec ($\pm$ 1.5) in the central retinal vein, and 31.6 cm/sec ($\pm$ 9.0) in the ophthalmic artery.

There was a close correlation between time-averaged maximum flow velocity in the central retinal artery and the intraocular pressure as indicated in the diagram (Fig. 1). In all cases at intraocular pressures of more than

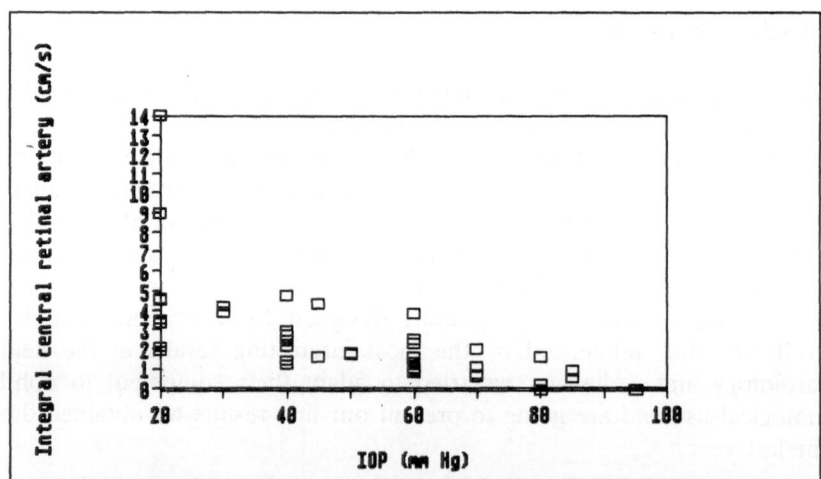

Fig. 1. When Doppler examinations were performed during artificial elevation of the intraocular pressure (IOP), there was a strong correlation between time-averaged maximum flow velocity in the central retinal artery (= integral, ordinate) and IOP (abscissa).

80 mm Hg the central retinal circulation was no longer detectable according to our measurements, with a sudden onset after pressure release.

For general evaluation of our results we analyzed various parameters, such as the age of the patient, systolic blood pressure, uninfluenced intra-ocular pressure and the different flow parameters of the central retinal vessels as well as the ophthalmic artery. The only correlation we could find to be statistically relevant was the decrease of ophthalmic artery flow velocity with increasing age (coefficient $r = -0.36$; $p < 0.01$).

Intraocular tumours

In all but two out of 24 intraocular melanomas examined before enucleation or irradiation there was a Doppler signal inside the tumor tissue (Fig. 2). Directly after Ruthenium treatment (two days up to one week, nine patients), average flow velocities were unchanged. In general, after four to six months after treatment (those examinations were performed in seven out of nine patients after irradiation) a decrease of flow velocity was recorded in two patients, a total lack of Doppler signals was found in three patients.

In three patients with cavernous haemangiomas of the choroid there had been Doppler signals comparable with those of melanomas.

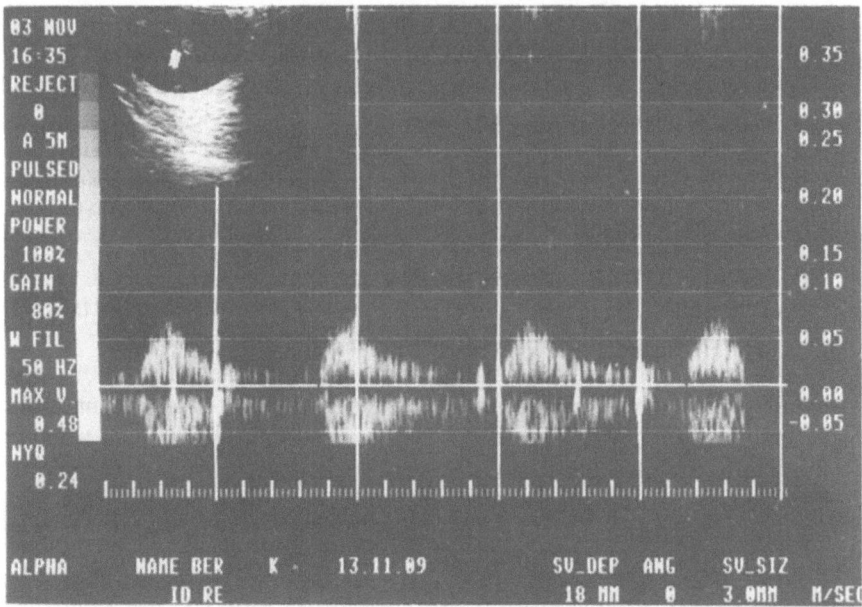

Fig. 2. In all but two out of 24 malignant melanomas Doppler signals were detected within the tumour. The flow velocities were comparable with those reached in the central retinal artery. Upper left: B-mode picture of malignant melanoma of the choroid, with white rectangle indicating the sampling volume for Doppler measurement.

Discussion

Measurements of flow velocity of orbital and ocular vessels have drawn attention already in the past. It was Niesel in 1962, who in calorimetric measurements of uveal blood-flow rates in rabbits was able to show an adequate response of intraocular blood-flow to changes produced by carotid ligation or jugular compression. Recently, laser Doppler examinations of retinal vessels have been reported by Riva and coworkers (1983).

The combination of soft tissue imaging and simultaneous Doppler measurement in ophthalmology is to our knowledge in a very early phase of development. Sufficient sensitivity of commercially available equipment has been proven in our first experiment, where intraocular pressure was strictly correlated with blood-flow velocity in the central retinal vein and artery.

We had been confronted with quite astonishing results, when after clinically proven central retinal vein and artery occlusion already two to five days after the first symptoms we were no longer able to detect changes in the retinal circulation. This obviously can only be explained by the fact that nerve fibre necrosis has taken place in the very first hours so that the restored retinal blood flow, as proven in our measurements, came too late to regain visual function.

Our results concerning Doppler signals received out of choroidal tumours are obviously nothing but the reconfirmation of the fast, continuous flickering vertical motion of tumour spikes in A-scan ultrasonography as reported by Ossoinig (1979) in more than 90% of choroidal melanomas.

In one example of an extensive extrascleral growth of a huge intraocular melanoma, which had already caused secondary angle closure glaucoma (IOP 45 mm Hg) the correlation between intraocular pressure and flow dynamics could be demonstrated. The maximal flow velocities obtained inside the eye reached only 40% of the maximal flow velocity in the orbital part of the tumor.

Follow-ups in conservatively treated melanomas have shown that in a very early phase changes in the vascular structure of the tumour take place even before volume reduction can be recorded.

To summarize, we think that systematic studies and evaluation of Doppler signals using high resolution duplex scanners will offer us meaningful additional information at least in the area of tumour diagnosis and treatment. The role in the evaluation of circulatory disturbances of eye and orbit, after our first experiences, remains still uncertain.

References

Buschmann W. 1972. Ophthalmologische Ultraschalldiagnostik. In: Velhagen K (ed) Der Augenarzt, Vol II. VEB Thieme, Leipzig, pp. 391–464.
Coleman D J, Lizzi F L. 1979. In vivo choroidal thickness measurement. Am J Ophthalmol 88: 369–375.

Niesel P. 1962. Messungen von experimentell erzeugten Änderungen der Aderhautdurchblutung bei Kaninchen. Basel, 1962. Quoted in: Duke-Elder (ed) System of Ophthalmology, Vol IV. Kimpton, London (1968).

Ossoinig K C. 1979. Standardized Echography: Basic principles, clinical applications, and results. In: International Ophthalmology Clinics, Vol 19, No. 4. Little, Brown & Co, Boston, Massachusetts, p. 144.

Riva C E, Grunwald J E, Petrig B L. 1983. Reactivity of the human retinal circulation to darkness: A laser Doppler velocimetry study. Invest Ophthalmol Vis Sci 24: 737–740.

Trier H G, Lepper R D, Reuter R. 1979. Das Projekt 'Rechnergestützte Gewebsdifferenzierung' der Arbeitsgemeinschaft Bonn/Stuttgart, I und II. In: Gernet H (ed) Diagnostica ultrasonica in ophthalmologia. Proceedings of SIDUO VII meeting. Remy, Münster, pp. 35–39, 40–43.

Ulrich W-D, Ulrich C. 1985. Okulooszillodynamographie, ein neues Verfahren zur Bestimmung des Ophthalmikablutdruckes und zur okulären Pulskurvenanalyse. Klin Mbl Augenheilkd 186: 385–388.

42. Possibilities and limitations of ultrasonographical localisation of ruthenium-106-radioactive plaques during treatment

R. GUTHOFF and K. LAURITZEN

Introduction

Treatment with Ruthenium-106-radioactive plaques has proven to be an effective method achieving local tumor control of choroidal melanomas. (Lommatzsch and Vollmar, 1966; Lommatzschn, 1983; Förster et al., 1983; Förster et al., 1984) Success rates are dependent on a proper localization of the plaque as well as the exact measurements of tumor dimensions to calculate the irradiation dose required. Both parameters are highly dependent on ultrasonographical examinations. (Guthoff et al, 1983)

Fried et al. (1982) and Hasenfratz (1983) were the first who applied ultrasonography to identify fluid filled fissures between sclera and ruthenium plaques. It was our intention to find out the possibilities and the limitations of in situ localization in order to optimize the results of brachy therapy.

Material and method

In order to obtain ideal ultrasonograms of the ruthenium-plaque an inactive model with a diameter of 19 mm was examined in waterbath techniques. Simulation of in vivo condition was tried to achieve by using pig-eyes, liver tissue and various types of fat tissue whose ultrasonographical characteristics were comparable with those of the human orbit. For sound attenuation rubber gum material of 10 mm in thickness had proven to be most effective.

Fifteen patients with various types of the applicators in situ were examined between the first and eleventh day after fixation of the plaque and 12 of them also in the early postoperative period after the removal of the plaque.

The ultrasonograms were performed with the Cooper Vision Ultrascan 2 and Digital B Type 4 using a 10 MHz transducer.

Department of Ophthalmology, University of Hamburg, Montimistrasse 52, D 2000 Hamburg FRG

R. Sampaolesi (ed.), Ultrasonography in Ophthalmology 12, 333–337.
© *1990. Kluwer Academic Publishers, Dordrecht*

334

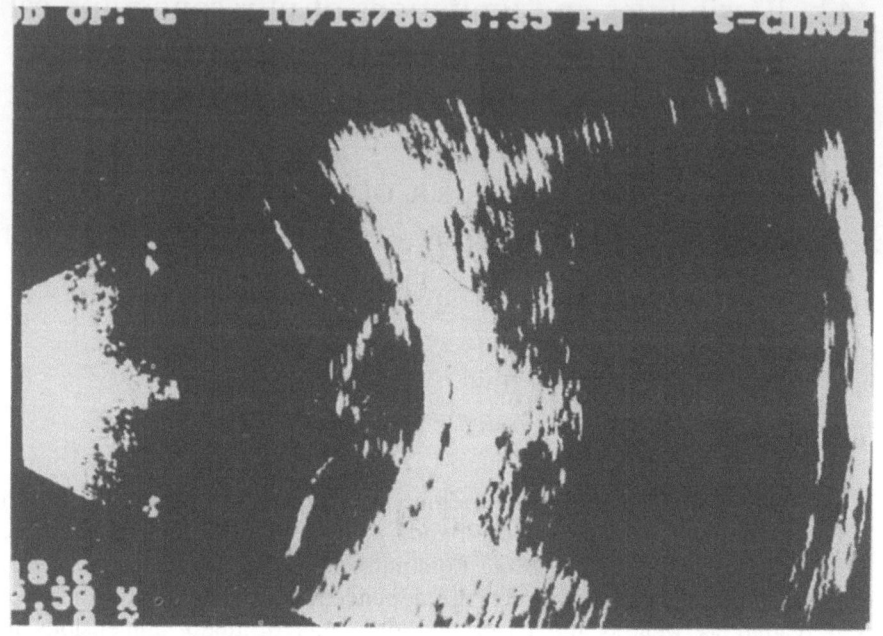

(a)

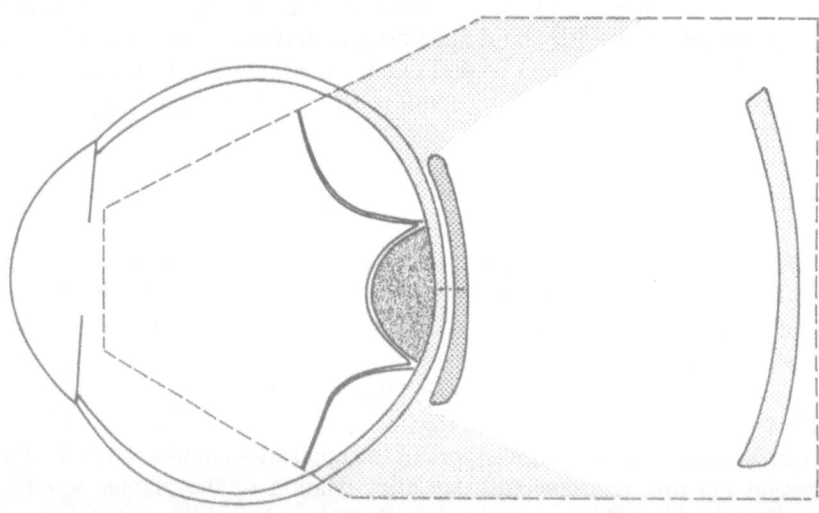

(b)

Fig. 1. (a) Ultrasonogram with Ruthenium-Beta applicator in place. The fluid filled fissure between applicator surface and posterior scleral surface was measured with 0.5 mm (see Calippers). The lateral extension of the plaque seems to be outlined by reduplication signals (aus R. Guthoff: Ultraschall in der Ophthalmologischen Diagnostik, Enke-Verlag Stuttgart (1988)). (b) Schematic drawing

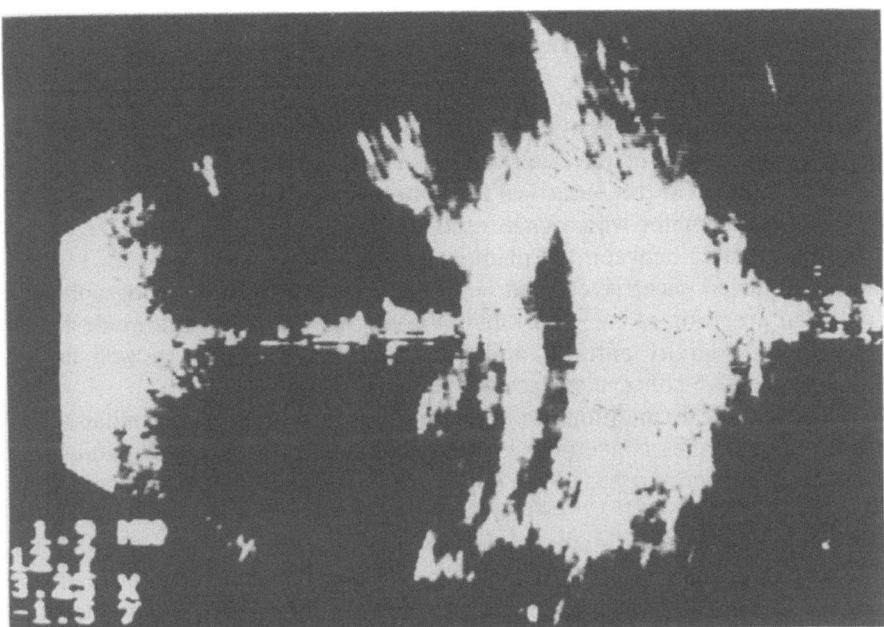

(a)

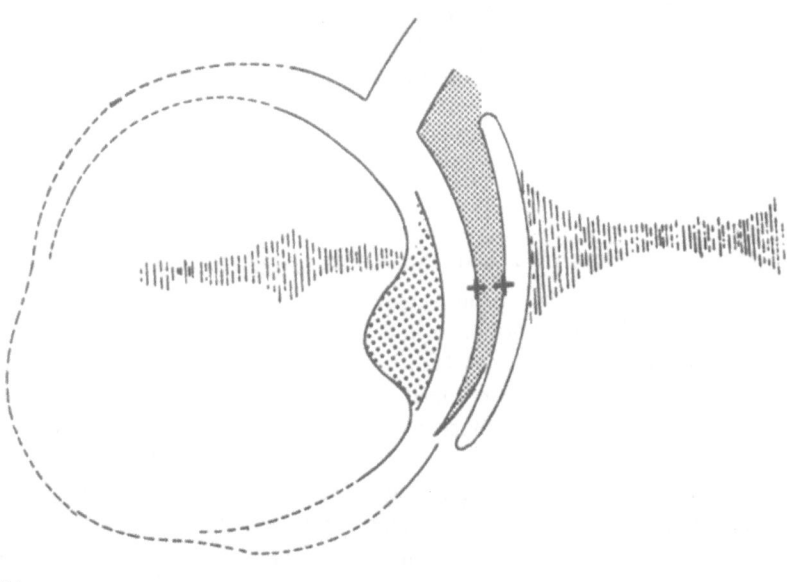

(b)

Fig. 2. (a) Ruthenium-Beta applicator in place with considerable formation of the fluid filled fissure between applicator and scleral surface. (Aus: R. Guthoff: Ultraschall in der Ophthalmologischen Diagnostik, Enke-Verlag Stuttgart (1988). (b) Schematic drawing

Results

Ultrasonograms obtained in vitro are characterized by well outlined image of the applicator-surface with reduplication echos of three major areas: The geometrical centre of the shell and both edges of the margin. Taking the sector geometry of the acoustical field into account we were able to measure the overall diameter which gave results 1–2 mm below the true size of the plaque. Fissures between the plaque and the overlying sclera of the pig-eye were produced successively and could be documented ultrasonographically with the precision of +/− 0.25 mm. Varying the amplification mode it was possible to identify anterior and posterior scleral surface as well as the highly reflective concave surface of the metal plate.

Under clinical conditions we obtained B-scan images quite similar to the experimental ones concerning the identification of fluid filled fissures and the major reflective areas of the applicator: centre and the two margins (Fig. 1).

Under low amplification conditions the highly reflected surface of the ruthenium plaque is well outlined where the soft tissues images are fading away. In one of the 15 patients examined a considerable fissure between posterior scleral surface and applicator was found (Fig. 2). With a 2 mm fissure we decided to leave the radioactive plaque in place for 18 hours longer to treat the most distant parts of the tumor with the precalculated radiation dose. One day after removal of the plaque an oedematous zone in Tenon's space was still clearly outlined. Recognition of lateral borders of the applicator easy to perform under in vitro conditions was not at all reliable in clinical examinations.

Discussion

Förster et al. mentioned 1983 problems in the localization of the applicator clinically. According to the results achieved experimentally the measurement of fluid filled fissures supposed into the Tenon's space should be easy to perform in clinical routine work (Guthoff, 1984). This could be confirmed in all of 15 patients. In one example it has proven to be very important to prolong the irradiation time, otherwise insufficient tumor regression would have been expected.

Localization of the plaque margins easy to perform experimentally seems not to be reliable in clinical work. This might be due to the following physical and ultrasonographical phenomena: The cross section of the ruthenium plaque is characterized by concentric surfaces forming the body which ends in semi-circular edges. If we take into account that the angle of the ultrasound sector of the B-scan probe is not identical with the radius of the curvature of the plaque, three major areas are defined as places where ultrasound hits metal surfaces perpendiculary. These areas are represented by the centre of the plaque and by well defined sectors in the curvature of the plaque margin. Only in these regions is it possible to obtain reduplication echoes. These are absolutely necessary for the identification and localization of the ruthenium plaque. (Haigis, 1988; Thijssen, 1988) Taking into account that the orbital margins do not allow to link the transducer probe freely to the globe, ideal measuring conditions are only achieved under exceptional situations where the applicator is sutured close to the posterior pole of the eye.

To summarize: According to our experience it is possible and necessary to perform ultrasonographical examinations while the applicator is in place. Finding a not full regression of the tumor in follow-ups of the patient this might be due to a fluid filled fissure not recognized early enough to prolong treatment time to the irradiation dose required. Any fissure that exceeds 1.0 mm should be considered to be unusual and recalculations concerning irradiation dose should be performed. Edges of the applicator are theoretically easy to identify but under clinical conditions no reliable measurements are possible. For daily work we still have to make all major efforts to place the applicator as exact as possible via microsurgical operation techniques and high power diaphanoscopy.

References

Buschmann W. 1972. Ophthalmologische Ultraschalldiagnostik. In: Velhagen, K. (Hrsg) Der Augenarzt, Bd. II. VEB Thieme, Leipzig; S. 391–464.

Foerster M H, Bornfeld N, Wessing A, Schulz U, Schmitt G, Meyer-Schwickerath G. 1984. Die Behandlung von malignen Melanomen der Uvea mit 106-Ruthenium-Applikatoren. Klin Mbl Augenhlk 185: 490–494.

Foerster M H, Fried M, Wessing A, Meyer-Schwickerath G. 1983. Tumor regression and functional results in sequential ruthenium therapy and photocoagulation for choroidal melanoma. In: Lommatzsch P K, Blodi F C. (Hrsg.) Int. Symposium of intraocular tumors, 17–20 May 1981. Akademie Verlag, Berlin, pp. 316–340.

Fried M, Foerster M H, Wessing A, Meyer-Schwickerath G. 1982. Echographische Größen-bestimmung von Tumor und Lageüberprüfung des Applikators in der Ruthenium-Therapie beim Aderhautmelanom. Fortschr Ophthalmol 79: 193–198.

Guthoff R. 1984. Die differentialdiagnostische Bedeutung des Tenonschen Raumes. Fortschr Ophthalmol 81: 388–390.

Guthoff R, Hallermann D. 1983 Ruthenium irradiation of choroidal melanomas—methods of planning and controlling therapy. In: Lommatzsch P K, Blodi F C (Hrsg.) Int. Symposium of intraocular tumors, 17–20 May 1981, Akademie Verlag, Berlin, p. 312–306.

Haigis W. 1988. Personal communications, Department of Ophthalmology, University of Würzburg, West-Germany.

Hasenfratz G. 1985. Echographische Befunde bei Aderhaut-Melanoblastomen nach Ruthenium-Therapie. Fortschr. Ophthalmol 82: 453–456.

Lommatzsch P K. 1983. β-Irradiation of Choroidal Melanoma With 106 Ru/106 Rh Applicators — 16 Year's Experience. Arch. Ophthalmol 101: 713–717.

Lommatzsch P, Vollmar R. 1966. Ein neuer Weg zur konservativen Therapie intraokulärer Tumoren mit Betastrahlen (Ruthenium 106) unter Erhaltung der Sehfähigkeit. Klin Mbl Augenheilk 148: 682–699.

Thijssen J M. 1988. Physikalische Grundlagen der ophthalmologischen Ultraschalldiagnostik. In: Guthoff R (Hrsg) Ultraschall in der ophthalmologischen Diagnostik. Enke, Stuttgart. Bücherei des Augenarztes Bd. 116 S.19ff.

43. Tumor volume calculations by ultrasonographical data in the evaluation of regression patterns in ruthenium-treated melanomas

R. GUTHOFF, D. VON DOMARUS, J. DRAEGER and A. BIEN

Summary

After 12 years experiences with Ruthenium-106-treatment a clinical impression that good local tumor control means high risk concerning tumor related mortality was evaluated by statistical methods. B-scan ultrasonography was used to calculate tumor volume regression speed. In patients who died from metastasies the average time to half the tumor volume was 4.4 months, in a matched group of survivors it tooks 6.6 months. This difference was proven to be statistically significant.

Introduction

Since 1975 we have collaborated with Lommatzch who introduced Ruthenium-plaque therapy in 1968. Since then more than 300 patients had been treated in Hamburg and a local tumor control could be achieved in about 85% of cases. We regard tumors as suitable for routine application of Ruthenium-plaques up to a prominence of 6 mm and a maximal diameter of 18 mm. Exceptions are made.

The irradiation time is planned to reach the apical part of the tumor with at least 15.000 rad.

To reach this aim a careful planning of therapy mainly guided by ultrasonographical measurements of tumor prominence is mandatory. About 6 mm away from the ruthenium surface only about 20% of the energy is present which is indicated in a very narrow isodose distribution. So far little is known about tumor mortality following conservative treatment of intraocular melanomas. First comparative studies gave rise to the suggestion that there is no difference compared with groups of patients whose tumors were treated by enucleation.

Department Ophthalmology, University Hospital Eppendorff, Martinistrasse 52, D-2000, Hamburg, FRG

R. Sampaolesi (ed.), Ultrasonography in Ophthalmology 12, 339–343.

Our working hypothesis that there might be a correlation between tumor related mortality and regression speed after irradiation treatment, was based on 3 suggestions:

Rapidly growing tumors are more likely to consist out of epithelioid cells (Augsburger et al., 1984). Secondly, tumors with high proliferation rates are more sensitive to irradiation compared with those of low proliferation rates (Hellmann, 1985), thirdly, in a statistical analysis published in 1986 we were unable to find any correlation between irradiation parameters and the speed of tumor regression.

Material and methods

We would like to give a first report on our analysis concerning factors influencing tumor related mortality in ruthenium treated patients. As a parameter to measure the reduction speed of the treated tumor we have chosen the time it takes to half the initial tumor volume.

Volume calculations are made on the basis of ultrasonographical measurements. To estimate the tumor volume we have to accept some simplifications: The melanomas suitable for radiotherapy should be considered as biconvexed shape which geometrically can be defined by its prominence and its smallest and largest diameter (Guthoff, 1980). For everyday use the computer print-out is available.

Two hundred forty-six patients were treated up to June, 1986. There were 17 missing data. We know of 12 patients who died from melanoma metastases, 3 from non tumor related reasons, 2 were alive with known metastasies and 212 were known to be alive and free from secondary effects?

In Table 1 patients who died from melanoma metastasies are outlined. It was obvious that in 6 out of 12 patients there was finally no tumor in the eye at all and in the others a considerable reduction of volume had taken place. Comparing the regression speed of the tumors between the group of patients who died and the ones alive and free from secondary effects we looked for a matched group with similar age and similar initial tumor volume. This group of patients finally consisted of 27 individuals.

Two different statistical methods were applied to aluticate tumor related mortality.
1. Cox regression analysis to evaluate the influence of pretreatment tumor volume
2. Covariance regression analysis to look for the correlation of tumor regression speed, initial tumor volume and tumor related mortality.

Results

According to Cox analysis there was only one factor that influenced tumor mortality significantly: Initial tumor volume was correlated on a level of P =

Table 1. Data of patients who died after a Ruthenium treatment of a chozoial melanoma. 6/75–6/87

	Alter, Ge-schlecht	Tumor volumen (mm^3)	V $\overline{2}$ (Mon.)	Überlebenszeit (Mon.)	Tumor-restvolumen
1	42, m	145 4×8×9	1	57.3	0
2	67, w	66 3×7×7	2	50.5	0
3	73, m	170 5×8×8	5.5	65.1	0
4	56, m	400 5×11×14	2.5	41.7	0
5	50, w	400 4×8×14	2.5	45	0
6	58, m	75 3×6×7	1.2	39	0
7	62, m	300 5×12×12	14.9	32	110
8	47, m	170 5×6×10	5	41.6	20
9	53, w	300 5×12×12	3.3	19	120
10	68, m	560 6×15×15	4.2	21.3	120
11	67, m	590 7×13×13	7.6	32.9	30
12	42, w	270 3×12×13	3.2	46.6	60

0.028. Concerning the regression speed a difference was obvious in both groups (Fig. 1). In patients who died from metastases the average time to half the volume was 4.4 months, in the matched group of survivors it took 6.6 months. According to Covariance selection this was significant on a level of P = 0.0058.

In this analysis there was a slight evidence of the influence of the initial tumor volume on regression speed after treatment.

To summarize our results there was strong evidence for a correlation between tumor related death and initial tumor volume as well as the regression speed after radiotherapy. To a minor extend the time to half the volume was influenced by the initial volume itself. How can this be interpreted?

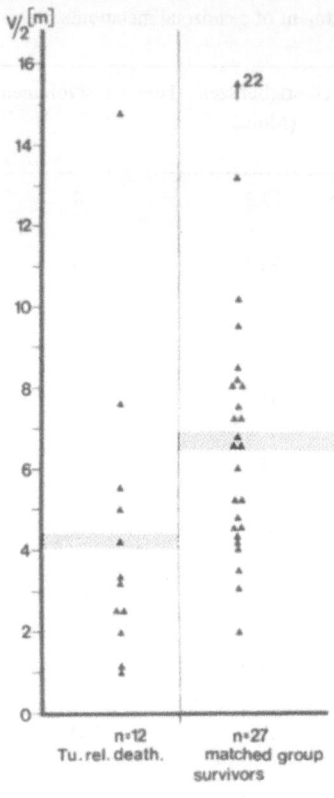

Fig. 1. Time to half the tumor volume in 12 patients known to have died from melanoma related metastasies compared with 27 patients known to be alive and free from secondary effects.

Discussion

It is generally accepted and proven by many authors that tumor size influences tumor mortality. So it was no surprise that this could be confirmed in a group of selected patients whose initial tumor size was suitable for plaque radiotherapy. Concerning the tumor regression speed as an indicator for malignancy we could not find some direct confirmation in literature. There was some evidence in a publication of Augsburger, where they analysed the response of Kobalt plaque therapy in correlation with pretreatment tumor growth. They found that rapid growth tumors responded better to radiotherapy than the ones with minimal proliferation activity prior to treatment. We do not have reliable pretreatment follow ups but taking Augsburgers' results into account we could conclude that a good local tumor control — a short time to half the tumor volume — gives evidence for the suggestion that we are dealing with a tumor with high proliferation rates prior to treatment. This means those patients suffered propbably from epitheloid type melanomas. We are well aware of the fact that these conclusions are still suggestive and need confirmation with larger number of patients.

In conclusion there seems to be evidence for a prognostic factor in Ruthenium treated patients which had not be paid attention to a larger extent in the past.

It is the postirradiation regression speed which can be measured as the time to half the tumor volume. In our group of patients it has shown to be of about the same significance than the pretherapeutic tumor volume itself.

References

Augsburger J, Gonder J R, Amsel J. 1984. Growth rates and doubling time of posterior uveal melanomas. Ophthalmology 91: 1709–1715.

Guthoff R. 1980. Modellmessungen zur Volumenbestimmung des malignen Melanoms. Albr v Graefe's Arch 214: 139–146.

Guthoff R, von Domarus D, Steinhorst U, Hallermann D. 1986. 10 Jahre Erfahrungen mit der Ruthenium-106/Rhodium-106-Behandlung des malignen Melanoms der Aderhaut. Klin Mbl Augenheilk 108: 576–583.

Hellman S. 1985. Principles of radiation therapy. In: DeVita VT Jr, Hellman S, Rosenberg S A (eds) Cancer Principles and Practice of Oncology. 2nd ed. Philadelphia: JB Lippincott Co., pp. 227–47.

Lommatzsch P. 1983. Betairradiation of Choroidal Melanoma-106-Ruthenium/106-Rhodium-Applicators. Arch Ophthalmol 101: 713–717.

44. Echographic patterns simulating extrascleral extension of malignant melanoma following plaque removal

GAIL L. DAUBERT and JAMES E. PUKLIN

Summary

Quantitative A-scan and contact B-scan patterns for extrascleral extension of choroidal malignant melanomas have been documented. We report a pattern that simulates these patterns. A-scan echography performed after the removal of iodine-125 plaques demonstrated a sharp decrease in reflectivity of the orbital spikes after the scleral spike. On B-scan echography there was an echolucent area posterior to the sclera behind the choroidal melanoma. These patterns simulate extrascleral extension of uveal melanomas and must not be confused with extrascleral extension.

Introduction

Six patients with posterior choroidal melanomas were evaluated and treated with iodine-125 plaques. Pre-operatively all patients had echographic examinations to assist in the diagnosis of melanoma [1]. A and B-scan echographic examinations were typical for melanoma. A-scans demonstrated vascularity, low to medium reflectivity, and regular acoustic structure. B-scans demonstrated a choroidal mass with some shadowing [4]. The tumor height ranged from 2.5 to 6.6 mm. Post-operatively all patients were examined echographically to determine the outcome of treatment. Once tumors are treated with radioactive plaques they demonstrate different patterns echographically. One post-operative pattern simulates extrascleral extension of the choroidal melanoma. This report describes these post-operative echographic changes in six cases treated with iodine-125 plaques.

Kresge Eye Institute, Wayne State University, 4717 St. Antoine, Detroit, Michigan, 48201–1423, USA

R. Sampaolesi (ed.), Ultrasonography in Ophthalmology 12, 345–349.

Material and methods

Six eyes with choroidal malignant melanomas were examined pre-operatively with either the Kretztechnik 7200 MA and/or the Ophthascan. A-scans were performed at tissue sensitivity and measuring sensitivity for quantitative and kinetic information. B-scans were performed for topographic information. Measurements of the tumor height and diameter were made and iodine-125 plaques constructed accordingly [3]. The plaques were sewn into place over the tumor and they remained in place until the apex of the tumor was treated with 10,000 rads. The plaques were removed and post-operative echograms performed at one month, three months, and six months.

Results

After radioactive plaque therapy characteristic changes begin to develop on both A-scan and B-scan echograms. These changes may be echographically visible as early as one month after plaque removal and they may continue to develop for years as the tumor responds to the radiation.

On B-scan echography the treated melanomas developed greater echogenicity. This differs from pre-operative echograms where there are areas of shadowing and echolucency. The areas of echolucency in the tumors decreased. Three of the six eyes developed a new area of echolucency behind

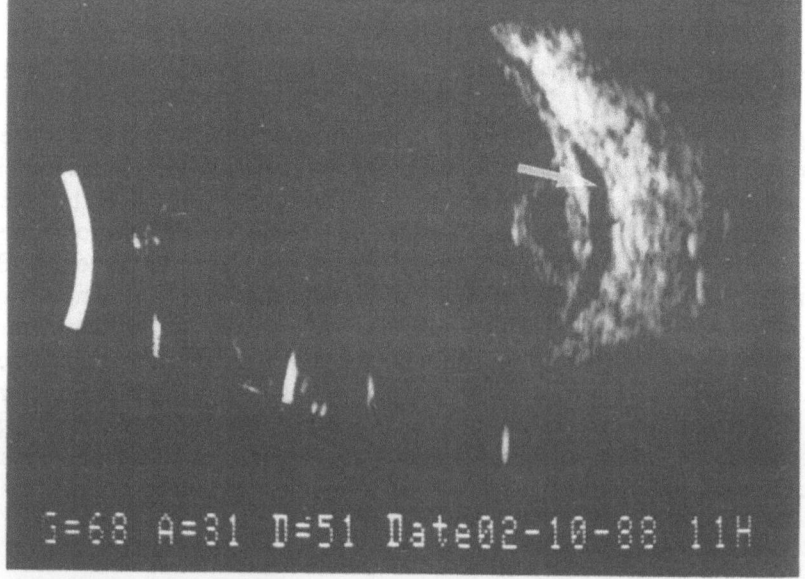

Fig. 1. Transverse contact B-scan echogram one month after plaque removal. Note the area of echolucency (arrow) behind tumor and sclera.

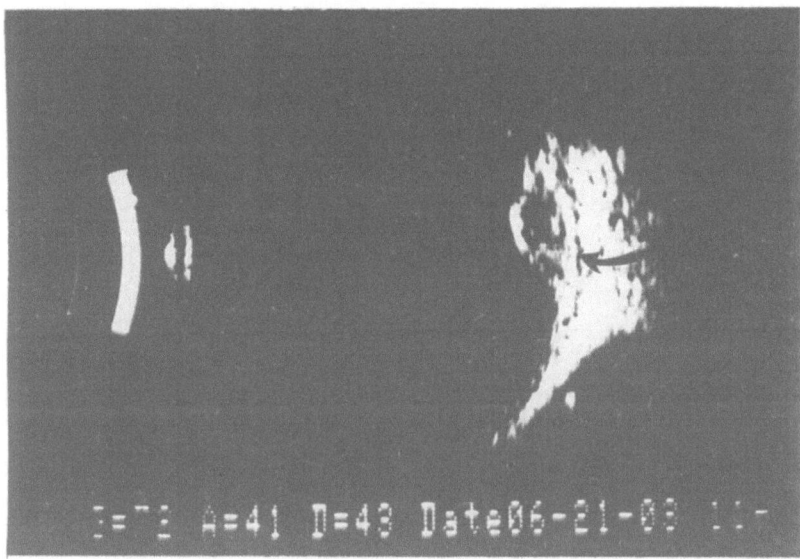

Fig. 2. Transverse contact B-scan echogram six months after plaque removal. Same tumor as Fig. 1. Note the area of echolucency (arrow) behind sclera and tumor. Echolucency is markedly diminished compared to Fig. 1.

the sclera that simulated extrascleral extension (Fig. 1). In one case, which demonstrated the most significant area of echolucency at one month post-operatively, when examined again at the six month post-operative visit the area of echolucency was markedly diminished but still present (Fig. 2). The two other cases exhibit areas of echolucency at both the one month and three month folow-up examinations.

These areas of echolucency were also demonstrated using A-scan echography at tissue sensitivity and measuring sensitivity (Fig. 3). After the scleral spike the orbital echoes sharply decreased in reflectivity and widened. Other changes observable on A-scan echography include a decrease in tumor height and changes in the internal reflectivity. The internal reflectivity of the tumors increased and their acoustical structures became irregular. These echographic findings are consistent with changes normally found in tumors treated with radiotherapy [5].

Discussion

The use of radioactive plaques as a treatment option in patients with medium-sized ocular melanomas is growing. A collaborative study is being conducted to determine whether enucleation or plaquing is the treatment of choice [2]. These results are not yet available. Echographic examinations are

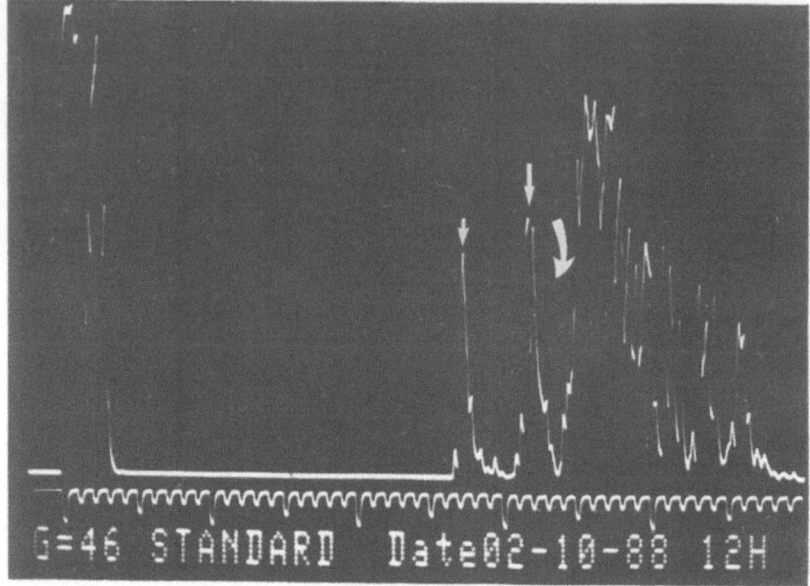

Fig. 3. A-scan taken at measuring sensitivity of tumor in Fig. 1 and 2. This is one month after plaque removal at the same time as Fig. 1. Note the retinal (small arrow) and scleral (large arrow) spikes are followed by a sharp decrease in reflectivity (curved arrow) behind the globe.

important in determining the effectiveness of radioactive plaque therapy. B-scan echography after plaque therapy should demonstrate a gradual decrease in size and shape of the tumor. A-scan echography should show regression in tumor height. Additionally, on A-scan echography the internal reflectivity of the tumor should increase as fibrosis and necrosis of the cells in the tumor occur [5].

Shammas and associates were apparently the first to describe areas of echolucency posterior to the sclera and patients treated with plaques [5]. They found such patterns in two of four patients with posterior melanomas treated with cobalt-60 plaques. These areas of echolucency persisted for up to one year subsequent to plaque removal in the two patients in whom they were found. Shammas did not comment on whether or not the areas of echolucency they observed diminished.

We have described this pattern of echolucency in three of six eyes treated with iodine-125 plaques. This pattern simulates extrascleral extension [6] and is an inconstant finding. The area of echolucency behind the sclera is probably a temporary condition resulting from inflammatory responses and serious fluid accumulation within the orbital tissue. These areas of echolucency decrease with time. They should not be confused with extraocular extension of the tumor. Periodic echography is necessary to evaluate tumor responses.

References

[1] Diamond J G, Ossonig K C. 1977. Contact A-scan and B-scan ultrasonography in the diagnosis of intraocular lesions. In: Intraocular Tumors. Peyman G A, Apple D J, Sanders D R. New York: Appleton Century Crofts. pp. 35–49.

[2] Fine S L. 1986. Do I take the eye out or leave it in? Arch Ophthalmol 104: 653–654.

[3] Packer S, Rotman M. 1980. Radiotherapy of choroidal melanoma with I-125. International Ophthalmology Clinics 20 Boston: Little, Brown and Company. pp. 135–141.

[4] Shields J A. 1983. Diagnosis and management of intraocular tumors. St. Louis: The CV Mosby Co., 46–52.

[5] Shammas H J, Boyer D S, Miller J B. 1987. Ultrasound characteristics of posterior uveal melanomas treated with cobalt plaque radiotherapy. Ophthalmic Echography. Proceedings of the 10th SIDUO Congress. K C Ossoinig (ed) Documenta Ophthalmolgica Proceedings Series 48. Dordrecht. Nijhoff/Junk. pp. 379–383.

[6] Verbeek A M. 1987. Uveal melanomas before and after ruthenium application therapy. Ophthalmic Echography. Proceedings of the 10th SIDUO Congress. K C Ossoinig (ed) Documenta Ophthalmolgica Proceedings Series 48. Dordrecht. Nijhoff/Junk. pp. 385–389.

45. Intraoperative use of ultrasound to document proper plaque placement in treating choroidal melanoma

GAIL L. DAUBERT and JAMES E. PUKLIN

Summary

Echography has been used to document proper radioactive plaque placement in the treatment of ocular melanomas. We have used echography to help diagnose and compute dimensions of intraocular tumors. In addition to accurate height measurement, we have used contact B-scan echography to help establish or confirm the basal diameter of tumors. We will discuss our methods of using intraoperative contact B-scan echography to ensure proper placement of iodine-125 plaques.

Introduction

We have used radioactive plaque therapy as the treatment of choice for six patients with choroidal malignant melanomas. The usual clinical and echographic measurements were obtained to help determine tumor size and plaque dimensions. After plaque placement, intraoperative contact B-scan echography was performed to assess the accuracy of plaque placement. This report describes the technique of intraoperative echography and its value in modifying and verifying radioactive plaque placement.

Methods

The Biophysic combined A- and B-scan contact ultrasound machine was used in the operating room. The B-scan probe was draped using a sterile, clear plastic steridrape with 2.5% methycellulose first applied to the probe tip. The methycellulose is, therefore, inside the tight-fitting steridrape. The probe is then placed directly on the eye opposite the tumor.

Kresge Eye Institute, Wayne State University, 4717 St. Antoine Ave, Detroit, Michigan 48201-1423, USA

R. Sampaolesi (ed.), Ultrasonography in Ophthalmology 12, 351–355.

The echography was performed in various meridians. The echograms were photographed and measurements were taken from them. By this method it is possible to verify and ensure that the plaque has been placed accurately and that there is an appropriate 2 mm tumor-free margin around the tumor.

Results

A posterior melanoma was clinically estimated to have a basal diameter of 9 mm by 9 mm. Evaluation of the fluorescein angiogram and color photographs suggested the tumor measured 10 mm by 10 mm. Measurements of the basal diameters from the echograms were 11 mm by 13 mm. These measurements all contain elements of error caused by the optics involved. The tumor borders were determined by transillumination in the operating room. Transillumination verified the accuracy of the echographic measurements.

The dummy plaque was positioned and the suture eyelets marked. Sutures were placed and the dummy plaque secured. Transillumination was performed and the plaque was thought to be in proper position in relation to the tumor. The gold-shielded iodine-125 plaque was sewn into place and the sutures tied. The plaque was thought to be in proper location. Transillumination was performed by the technique of Snyder. [1] It was thought that

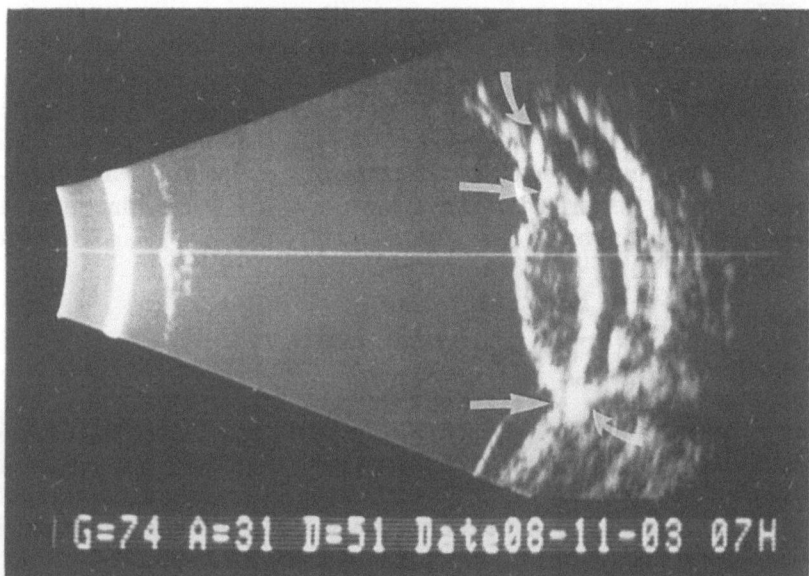

Fig. 1. Transverse intraoperative contact B-scan echogram. Straight arrows demonstrate the tumor margins. Curved arrows demonstrate plaque edges. Note the posterior edge of the plaque does not overlap the tumor margin.

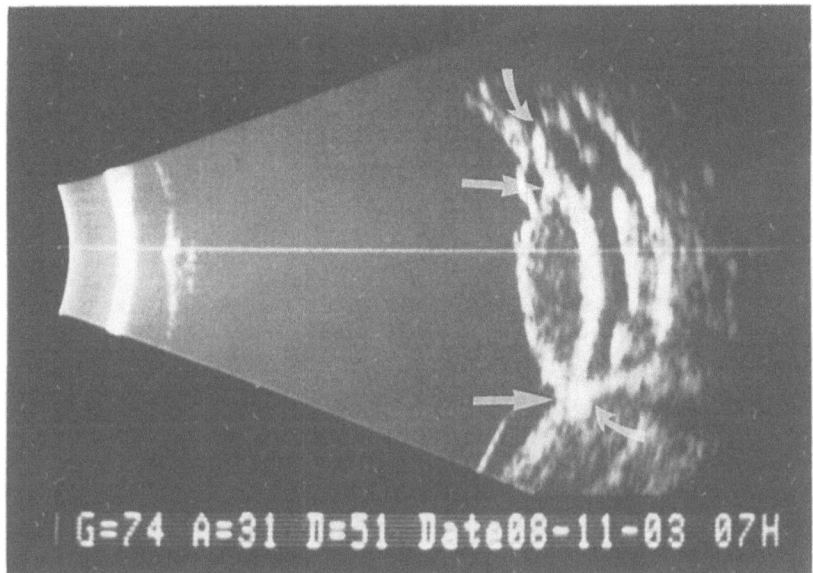

Fig. 2. Transverse intraoperative contact B-scan echogram of same patient as in Fig. 1 demonstrating the proper plaque placement after repositioning.

the posterior edge of the plaque did not provide enough tumor-free margin. Intraoperative contact B-scan echography was performed and verified improper plaque placement (Fig. 1). The plaque was repositioned and additional intra-operative B-scan echography performed both transversely and longitudinally to verify proper plaque placement (Fig. 2).

Echographically the gold shield of the radioactive plaque can be visualized and its relationship to the tumor determined. The silastic seed carrier in which the seeds are placed is not visible on echography. The radioactive iodine-125 seeds are echographically visible and produce various shadows. They may be seen in cross-section where they appear as dots. They may be seen tangentially or longitudinally where they are visible as echogenic lines (Fig. 3).

This technique of echographically visualizing the plaque and its relationship to the tumor has been used in five additional patients to verify proper plaque placement.

Discussion

The use of echography in the operating room to document proper plaque placement is valuable. It is an efficient, accurate method of assessing proper plaque placement and has not been utilized to its fullest capacity. Ophthalmic ultrasound machines are portable and may be moved to the operating room to aid in documenting proper plaque placement.

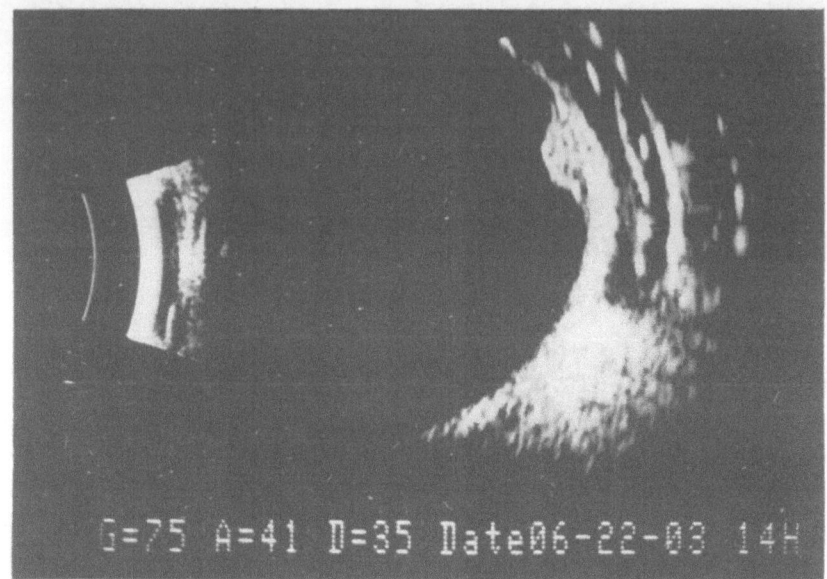

Fig. 3. Longitudinal intraoperative contact B-scan echogram demonstrating proper plaque placement. Note the iodine-125 seeds in the echolucent silastic carrier. They are seen in cross-section as dots and as various line segments when scanned tangentially.

Other methods for verifying proper plaque placement are not suitable. X-rays will demonstrate the plaque but not image the tumor. Magnetic resonance imaging and computerized tomography are feasible but cannot be done in the operating room. Therefore, if the plaque is not placed properly, results documented by these tests result in the patient undergoing another surgery. Transillumination can be done after the plaque is in place, but it is difficult to illuminate very posterior borders and it is not possible to measure the exact amount of tumor-free margin.

Intraoperative contact B-scan echography has been reported once before to our knowledge [2]. Pavlin and associates describe contact B-scan echography to verify proper placement of iridium-192 plaques. We have used this technique successfully to document proper plaque placement in five cases of malignant melanomas treated with iodine-125 plaques. In one case this technique permitted an intraoperative change in position of the plaque when the posterior border was not adequately covered.

Radioactive iodine-125 plaques are custom designed to each individual tumor to assure adequate treatment. Proper plaque placement is essential to proper tumor treatment. Intraoperative echography is a simple, effective method of achieving this goal. Tumor margins and plaque margins can be measured from the echograms to ensure a 2 mm tumor-free margin. Adjustments in plaque placement may be made if necessary. We feel echography is the best method available for verifying and ensuring proper plaque placement.

References

[1] Pavlin CJ, Japp B, Payne DG, Drysdale AM, Gallie BL. 1987. Intraoperative use of ultrasound in the management of choroidal melanomas. Ophthalmic Echography. Proceedings of the 10th SIDUO Congress. KC Ossoinig (ed). Documenta Ophthalmologica Proceedings Series 48. Dordrecht. Nijhoff/Junk. pp. 391–399.
[2] Snyder WB, Fuller DG, Fish GE. 1988. An inexpensive fiberoptic light pipe to aid in placement of episcleral radioactive plaques. Ophthalmic Surg 19: 62–63.

46. Acoustospectrography and histology of intraocular Greene's melanoma

J. M. THIJSSEN, R. L. ROMIJN, J. L. VAN DELFT*, D. DE WOLFF-ROUENDAAL*, J. A. VAN BEST*, and J. A. OOSTERHUIS*

Summary

This study has been performed to investigate the potentials of acoustospectrographic analysis for the characterization of biological tissues in general and of intraocular tumours in particular. The animal model employed was an amelanotic melanoma (Greene) implanted in the anterior chamber of Dutch rabbit. The eyes containing a tumour were scanned in vivo and after enucleation for a second time in vitro. The scanning was performed with a commercial B-scanner that was interfaced to a data-acquisition and processing system. The attenuation and backscattering parameters were estimated from the spectra calculated from the radiofrequency echograms.

The dimensions of histologically identified structures corresponded closely to the acoustically estimated backscattering dimensions.

Introduction

The differentation of intraocular tumours has been a major field of interest in Echo-ophthalmography for many years. Important progress was made by systematically employing a calibrated A-mode equipment (c.f. Ossoinig, 1974; Poujol, 1974; Verbeek, 1985). The differentiation of haemangioma, carcinoma and melanoma was stated to be possible with an accuracy of over 90%. This clinical success is impressive and deserves to be supported by scientific studies. Moreover, the question should be addressed as to whether this clinical experience can even be extended to further differentiation and at least to objective and quantitative figures of merit. A clear indication of the potentials of sophisticated signal analysis methods can be found in recent publications by the group of Coleman and Lizzi (Coleman et al. 1985;

Biophysics Laboratory of the Institute of Ophthalmology, University of Nijmegen,
* Department of Ophthalmology, University of Leiden, The Netherlands.
P.O. Box 9101, 6500 HB Nijmegen, The Netherlands.

R. Sampaolesi (ed.), Ultrasonography in Ophthalmology 12, 357–363.

Feleppa et al., 1986) who, from a retrospective correlation with histology, found a clear discriminability between mixed-epitheloid and spindle B-type melanomas in patients. Also the use of the developed methods of back-scattering analysis for the follow-up of radio-therapy of melanomas was shown to be feasible (Silverman, 1985).

In this contribution the accuracy and the precision of the method to estimate the dimension of backscattering structures are assessed by employing a tumour (Greene's melanoma) with a characteristic histology. Furthermore, some preliminary results of a simulation study will be presented.

Methods

Equipment

The experiments were performed with a Triscan (Biophysique Medical, Inc.) A- and B-mode equipment. The 8 MHz B-mode transducer was interfaced to a transient recorder (Bakker Electronics Inc.) which digitized the RF-signals in 8 bits at a 40 MHz sampling rate. During a single scanning sweep 128 lines of 1024 samples were stored, which correspond to the central half of the B-mode image and a 1.9 cm depth range. After transfer of the data to the microcomputer (Professional 380, Digital Equipment Corp.) the RF data were demodulated by software and redisplayed. By using the 'mouse' of the computer a region-of-interest (ROI) was selected and the encircling line drawn on the screen. This ROI was stored in RF-mode to be processed either on-line, or off-line (for further details see Romijn, 1990).

The effects of beam diffraction and focussing on the echograms (Cloostermans and Thijssen, 1983; Verhoef et al., 1985) was assessed by careful reference measurements using a plate reflector and a tissue mimicking phantom (Romijn et al., 1988). This procedure resulted in a look-up table containing a set of correction spectra at different depths. So, before any analysis was carried out the spectral information obtained from tumour echograms (RF) was corrected.

Animal model

Dutch rabbits were used in this study. The technique of implanting the tumour (Greene's amelanotic melanoma) has been described elsewhere (Franken et al., 1985). The tumour is growing very fast and 8 to 10 days after implantation the acoustic measurements were made. The dimensions of the disc-shaped tumour at that time were of the order of 8–10 mm diameter and 2–4 mm maximum thickness. After enucleation the eyes were measured in vitro and then stored in formaldehyde (10%). The next step was dehydration, embedding in celloidin, followed by slicing and finally staining by hematoxylin-eosin.

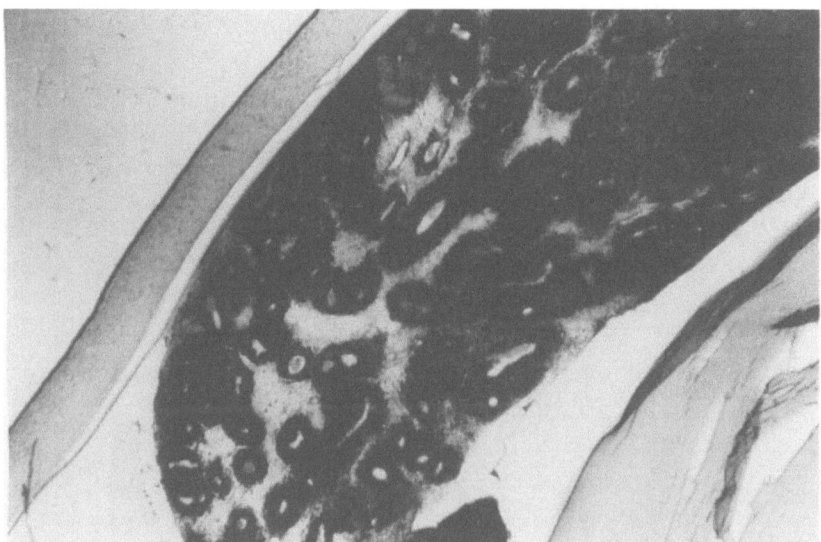

Fig. 1. Section through melanoma in anterior chamber Hematoxylin-eosin staining, magnification 400x.

An example of the histology of the Greene's melanoma is shown in Fig. 1. The proximal (corneal) part of the tumour shows a typical characteristic: small blood vessels which are surrounded by 4–6 layers of tumour cells, forming circular or elliptical 'islets' in the section plane. The interstitial space contains some necrotic debris and loose tumour cells. The distal part in some tumours consisted of more or less densely packed tumour cells. The short axis of the generally elliptical cross sections of the mentioned islets within the tumours was measured with an optical microscope in several sections of each tumour.

Theory

The backscattering in biological tissues can be modelled as an inhomogeneous continuum. This means that gradual changes of compressibility, or of mass density, are present within the tissue volume. These inhomogenities can be characterized by a dimensional parameter: the correlation size, T. Another model, which could be more realistic in the present study, is a discrete scatterer model: the scattering sites are now assumed to be identifyable histologic structures, like blood vessels.

The frequency dependence of the backscattering coefficient for a continuum model with a cylindrical Gaussian correlation function and for a discrete cylinder model is shown in Fig. 2.

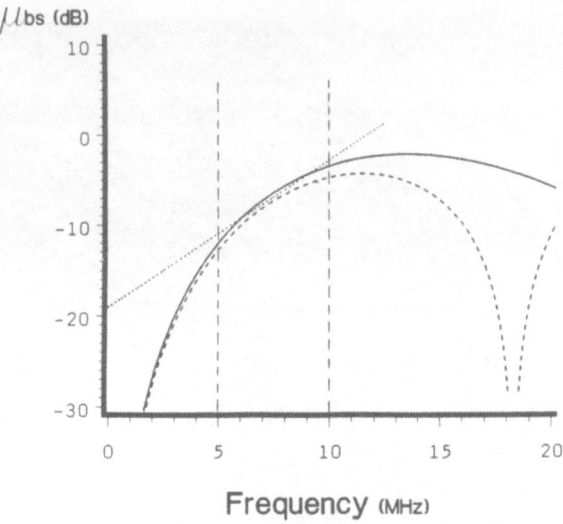

Fig. 2. Backscattering coefficient (in dB) vs. frequency for two scattering models. Solid line: Gaussian-cylindrical Autocorrelation (continuum model), dashed line: discrete cylinder model. Dotted line: linear regression line of Gaussian cylinder model over limited frequency range.

In practice we have selected the Gaussian cylinder model for this study, because of the discontinuities on the curve of the discrete model. The procedure to estimate the scattering dimension T was then: the average backscatter spectrum of the proximal tumour zone was calculated, after segmentation of the RF signals within the ROI. Within the bandwidth of the transducer a linear fit was made by a regression algorithm and the slope and the zero-frequency intercept of this regression line were estimated (c.f. Fig. 2). By this method every scan of a tumour yielded a slope value that was used to estimate the backscatterer size.

Results

The measurement by microscopy of the size of the islets resulted in almost Gaussian histograms with a standard deviation of 30%. The mean values for each tumour were employed in the correlation with the acoustic assessment of mean backscatterer size.

The latter procedure is illustrated by Fig. 3. The backscattered spectra from the tumour were corrected for the beam diffraction and then a straight line was fitted in the plot of the power in dB vs. the frequency. The slope of these regression lines is plotted vs. the zero frequency intercept in Fig. 3. The dots indicate the in vitro measurements and the ones the in vivo

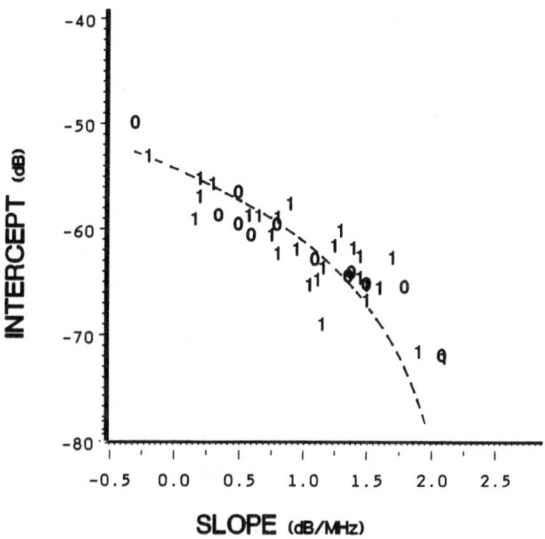

Fig. 3. Dashed line: Zero frequency intercept vs. slope of regression lines as in Fig. 2 for a range of correlation distances (i.e. backscatterer sizes). Data obtained in vivo (1) and in vitro (0) are in close agreement with theoretical curve. Data from 39 scans of 7 eyes.

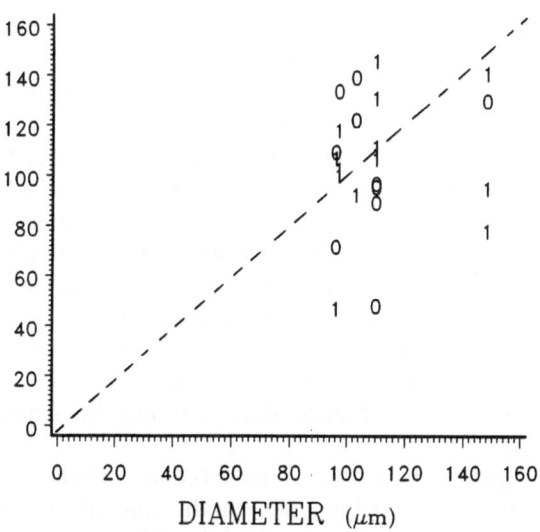

Fig. 4. Scatter diagram of acoustically estimated correlation size against diameter of islets obtained by optical microscopy. Dashed line indicates full correspondence. Data from 22 scans of 5 eyes.

362

obtained results. The dashed line indicates the optimum fit of the Gaussian cylinder model to these data. This fit is rather good, the maximum deviations are of the order of 4 dB and it proves the dominance of the scattering dimension over the backscatter strength in the power spectra.

The data in Fig. 3 was used to determine the backscatter size by employing the slope i.e. estimating the crossing of a vertical line through the data points in Fig. 3 and the theoretical curve. Since each point on this curve corresponds to a certain correlation size (of the Gaussian cylinder) this procedure yields the mean acoustic scatterer dimension T of the RF-B-scan.

The results of this procedure are shown in Fig. 4 where the acoustic size (ordinate) is plotted vs. the histologic diameter of the islets for each of the B-scans performed. As a dimension equivalent to a diameter in microscopy the 3 sd width (-10 dB) of the Gaussian autocorrelation function was taken. It will be evident from Fig. 4 that the mean value of all the acoustic measurements is of the correct order of magnitude as compared to the optical sizes.

The spread in the acoustic measurements is, however, relatively large which has to be attributed to the relatively small tumour volume that could be employed. Nevertheless the main and important conclusion from this study is that the *in vivo* acoustic estimation of the size of histologically distinct microstructures is possible.

Discussion

Although it could be concluded from Fig. 3 that the spectral data constitute the basic idea behind this analysis (c.f. also Lizzi et al., 1987) the large spread in the acoustic dimensions (viz. Fig. 4) needs a further explanation. A reason could be that the observed spread of the optically estimated diameters of the islets within the tumour induces this spread, or a bias in the average correlation size, or both. We undertook a preliminary simulation study (Romijn et al., 1989) in which RF signals were generated from a one-dimensional series of point scatterers with the Gaussian correlation model. The correlation size was randomly chosen from a Gaussian distribution with a 30 μm standard-deviation, and with a mean size of 30 to 100 μm. This variability of sizes produced a bias towards lower correlation size and a decrease in the variability of the estimated mean size values. So the observed spread of the acoustic data can not be explained from this simulation study.

A second explanation could be that the uncertainty of the employed spectral slope value is too high due to the limited acoustic information. When following the strategy described by Lizzi and Laviola (1976) we calculated an uncertainty of 0.2 dB/cm MHz of the slope value per B-scan. This figure yielded a precision of 6 μm of the correlation size which is small when compared to the observed variability of the data in Fig. 4.

In conclusion: this study has shown that *in vivo* estimation of scatterer dimensions is feasible and accurate, but the precision is lower than expected.

Acknowledgements

This work has been supported by a grant from the Netherlands' Cancer Foundation — Koningin Wilhelmina Fonds and was carried out within the framework of the Concerted Action Programme on Ultrasonic Tissue Characterization of the European Community.

References

Cloostermans M J T M, Thijssen J M. 1983. A beam corrected estimation of the frequency dependent attenuation of biological tissues from backscattered ultrasound. Ultrasonic Imag 5: 136–147.

Coleman P J, Lizzi F L, Silverman R H, Helson L, Torpey J H, Rondeau M J. 1985. A model for acoustic characterization of intraocular tumour. Invest Ophthal Vis Sci 26: 545–550.

Feleppa E J, Lizzi F L, Coleman D J, Yaremko M M. 1986. Diagnostic spectrum analysis in ophthalmology: a physical perspective. Ultrasound Med Biol 12: 623–631.

Franken K A P, van Delft J L, Dubbelman T M A R, de Wolff-Rouendaal D, Oosterhuis J A, Star W M, Marynissen H P A. 1985. Hematoporphyrine derivate photoradiation treatment of experimental malignant melanoma in the anterior chamber of the rabbit. Curr Eye Res 4: 641–654.

Lizzi F L, Laviola M A, Coleman D J. 1976. Tissue signature characterization utilizing frequency domain analysis. In: Ultrasonics Symposium Proceedings, J de Klerk, B McAvoy (eds) IEEE Inc., New York, pp. 714–719.

Lizzi F L, Ostromogilsky M, Feleppa E J, Rorke M C, Yaremko M M. 1987. Relationship of ultrasonic spectral parameters to features of tissue microstructure. IEEE Trans UFEC 33: 319–329.

Ossoinig K C. 1974. Quantitative echography—the basis of tissue differentiation. J Clin Ultrasound 2: 33–46.

Poujol J. 1974. Echographic diagnosis of tumours in ophthalmology. In: Ultrasonics in Medicine, M de Vlieger et al. (eds) Excerpta Medica, Amsterdam, pp. 147–165.

Romijn R L, Thijssen J M, Van Beuningen G W J, 1989. Estimation of scatterer size from backscattered ultrasound: a simulation study. IEEE Trans UFFC-36: 593–606.

Romijn R L, 1990. On the quantitative analysis of ultrasound signals and application to intraocular melanomas. Thesis, Nijmegen University.

Silverman R H, Coleman D J, Lizzi F L, Torpey J H, Drillen J, Iwamoto T, Burgess SEP, Rosado A. 1986. Ultrasonic tissue characterizations and histopathology in tumour xenographs following ultrasonically induced hyperthermia. Ultrasound Med Biol 12: 639–645.

Verbeek A M. 1985. Differential diagnosis of intraocular neoplasms with ultrasonography. Ultrasound Med Biol 11: 163–170.

Verhoef W A, Cloostermans M J T M, Thijssen J M. 1985. Diffraction and dispersion effects on the estimation of ultrasound attenuation and velocity in biological tissues. IEEE Trans BME-32: 521–529.

Other ocular pathology

47. A-mode combined with B-mode ultrasonic equipment (Ophthascan S) in ocular and orbital diagnosis

JO FUKIYAMA, SEIJI DEMIZU and ATSUSHI SAWADA

Summary

We have been using Ophthascan S to detect ocular and orbital lesions. We discussed advantages and disadvantages of Ophthascan S showing some illustrative cases we have examined so far. Ophthascan S can be said to be the equipment, in which A-mode and B-mode are most successfully combined without losing the intrinsic advantages of A-mode.

Introduction

In ophthalmic ultrasonic diagnosis A-scan and B-scan are the most important two display modes. Since B-scan provides two dimensional information, it is very easy to clear the shape, the size and the connection to the surrounding tissues.

On the other hand Ossoinig (1979) emphasizes that A-scan provides more useful information than B-scan, because the reflectivity of intraocular and orbital lesions, one of the most significant differential criteria, can be evaluated accurately only with standardized A-scan echography. Therefore both A-scan and B-scan provide different information. So optimal diagnostic results are obtained by combining standardized A-scan and contact B-scan.

Recently modern A- and B-scan equipments have come on the market, Ophthascan series of Biophysic Medical in France is one of these.

Ophthascan S is a remodeled type of Ophthascan B (Fig. 1). It has an extra separate A-probe besides the simultaneous A- and B-mode probe. Using these probes we can perform quantitative echography for optimal tissue diagnosis. The name Ophthascan S is derived from the initial letter of S-curved amplification. The equipment is standardized by Ossoinig in Iowa City. Recently we have had the opportunity to use this equipment. Advantages and disadvantages will be discussed showing several illustrative cases.

Department of Ophthalmology, Miyazaki Medical College Miyazaki, Japan

R. Sampaolesi (ed.), Ultrasonography in Ophthalmology 12, 367–378.
© *1990. Kluwer Academic Publishers, Dordrecht*

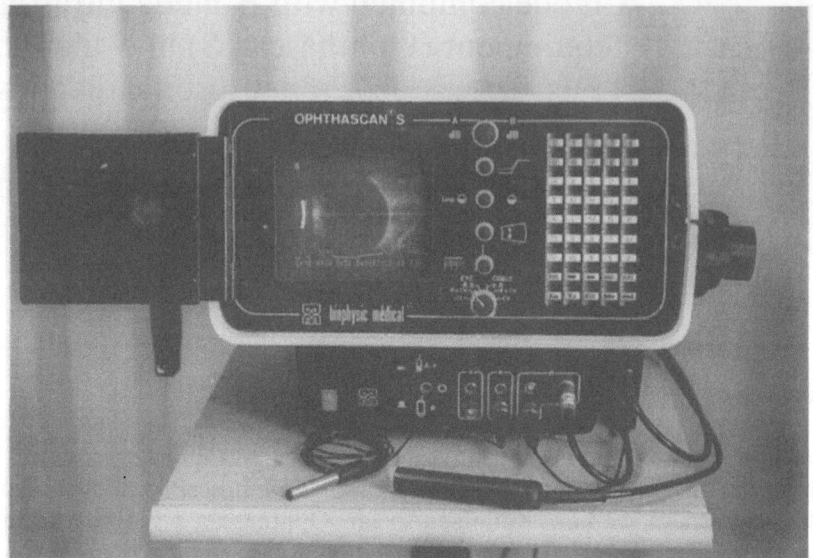

Fig. 1. Outlook of Ophthascan S equipped with A and B probes.

Case presentation

Figure 2 shows echograms of a normal eye with Ophthascan S. The upper is a picture of simultaneous display of B- and cross vector A-mode (abbreviated to B+CV mode) and the lower is cross vector A-mode display, isolated and expanded from B+CV mode (abbreviated to CV mode). In B+CV mode anterior segments such as cornea, iris, anterior and posterior surfaces of the lens are clearly displayed. Optic nerve, and medial and lateral rectus muscles are also distinctly displayed. In CV mode corresponding spikes are shown.

Figure 3 shows a fundus photograph and echograms of Coats' disease. The photograph shows total yellowish coloration of the retina and bullous retinal detachment inferiorly. In B+CV mode bullous retinal detachment and a corresponding high spike are displayed. The lower shows an A-mode echogram of the same direction. The detail is displayed in this echogram.

Figure 4 shows a fundus photograph and echograms of orbital cellulitis. Eye ball is indented in the superotemporal quadrant and choroidal striations are seen beyond the fovea. The upper echogram was taken by a Japanese equipment, Santesomic SSD-121, of which the vector A-scan is fixed in the center of the B-mode image. In the lower echogram with Ophthascan S the cross vector is mobile within the sector angle.

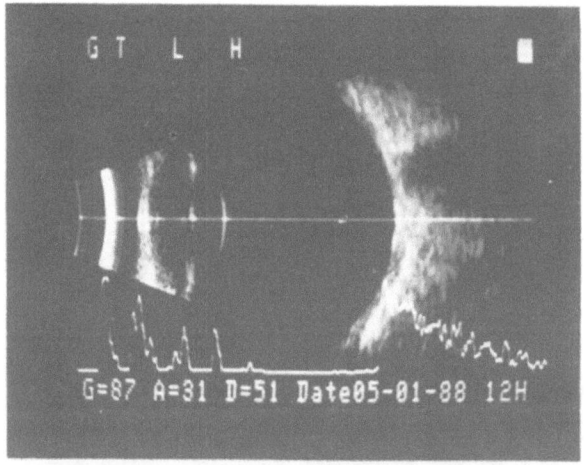

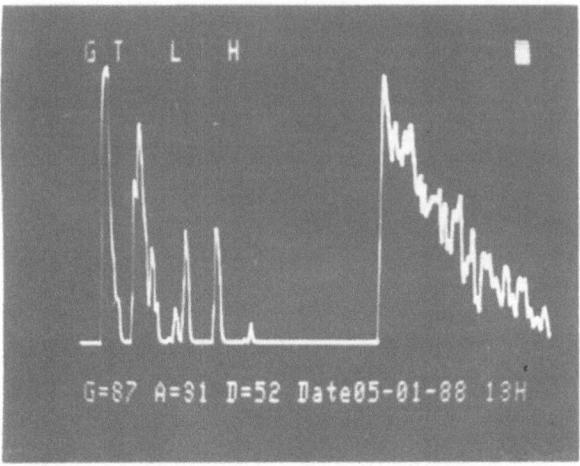

Fig. 2. Echograms of normal eye by Ophthascan S. The upper is a B+CV mode echogram. The lower is a CV mode echogram, isolated and expanded from B+CV mode.

Figure 5 shows a fundus photograph and echograms of preretinal hematoma in a hypertensive patient. In the B-mode echogram, lower left, a hematoma is displayed as a small prominence adjacent to the optic nerve head. Directing of the cross vector A-scan beam to the center of the lesion produces two high reflective spikes in CV mode. The distance between these two spikes is measureable. The upper right echogram shows an expanded CV mode from B+CV mode. In the lower right echogram, using two overlights, one on the spike from the surface of the hematoma and the other on the spike from the retina, the distance can be measured automatically and shown as distance= 0.9 mm.

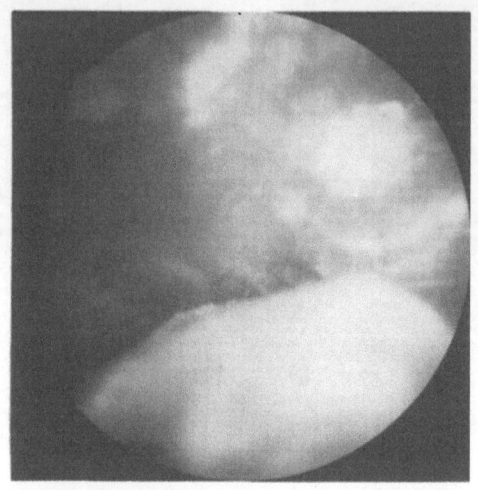

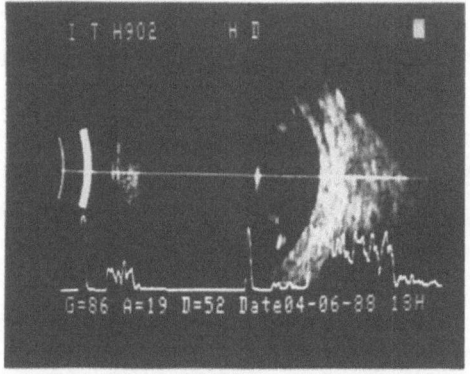

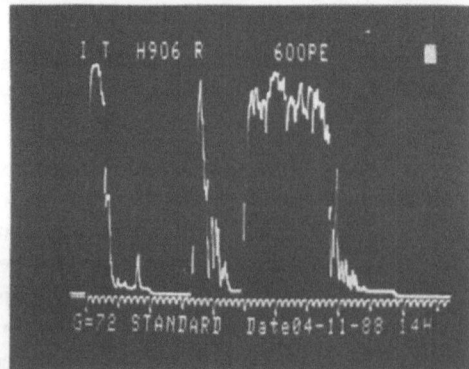

Fig. 3. A fundus photograph and echograms of Coats' disease. The upper B+CV mode echogram is the transverse section of the inferior fundus. The lower A mode echogram was taken by a separate A probe.

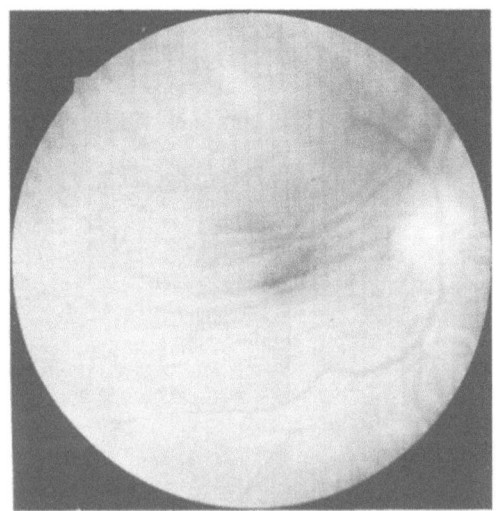

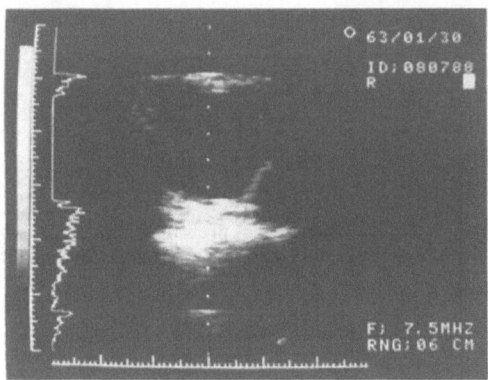

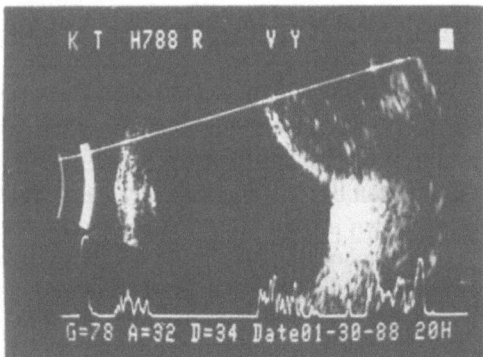

Fig. 4. A fundus photograph and echograms of orbital cellulitis. The eye ball is indented by a huge mass. The upper echogram is taken by Santesonic SSD-121. The alignment of vector A scan is fixed. The lower echogram was taken by Ophthascan S, in which the direction of cross vector A scan is changeable.

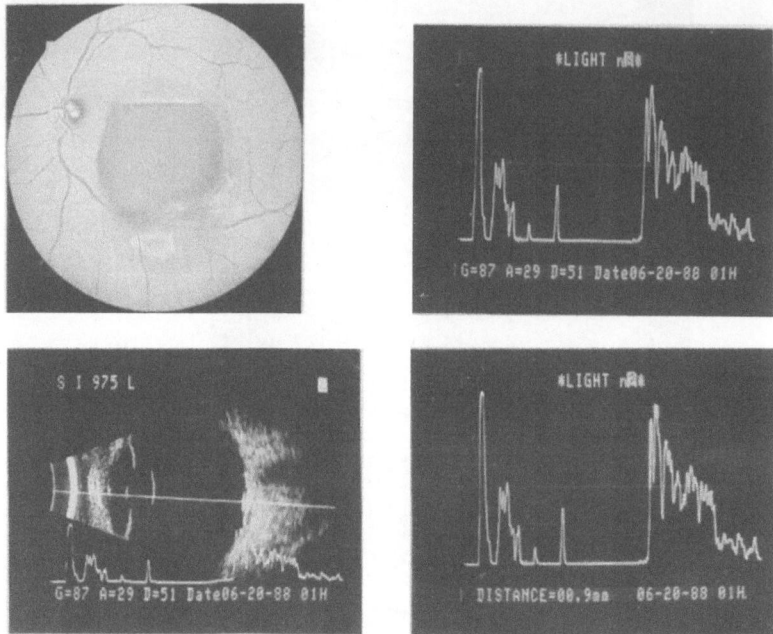

Fig. 5. A fundus photograph and echograms of preretinal hematoma in a hypertensive patient. In fundus photograph preretinal hematoma as well as subretinal hemorrhage and some exudates are seen. The lower left is an echogram of B+CV mode. Two right echograms show how to measure the distance with two overlights. The result is displayed in the lower space.

Figure 6 shows echograms of proliferative vitreoretinopathy. The upper is B+CV mode and the lower CV mode. Using two overlights the reflectivity difference is measured and displayed as difference= 9 dB.

Figure 7 shows echograms of retinal detachment. The upper left is B+CV mode and the lower left is CV mode. Using two overlights the reflectivity difference between the membrane and the sclera can be calculated automatically and the value is shown instantly on the bottom as difference= 3 dB. In the upper right A-scan echogram the maximal echo from the membrane reaches the marker line in the 50% height at the reduced overall gain of 44 dB. When the overall gain is reduced to 30 dB shown as in the lower right, the maximal spike from the sclera reaches the marker line. So the reflectivity difference between the membrane and the sclera is 14 dB, which means the membrane is the detached retina on Ossoinig's criteria in quantitative echography.

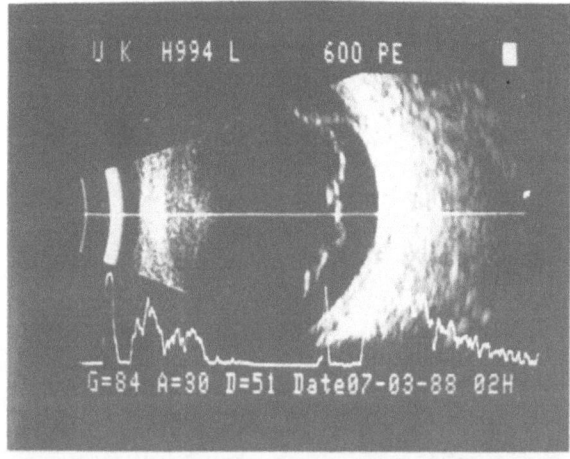

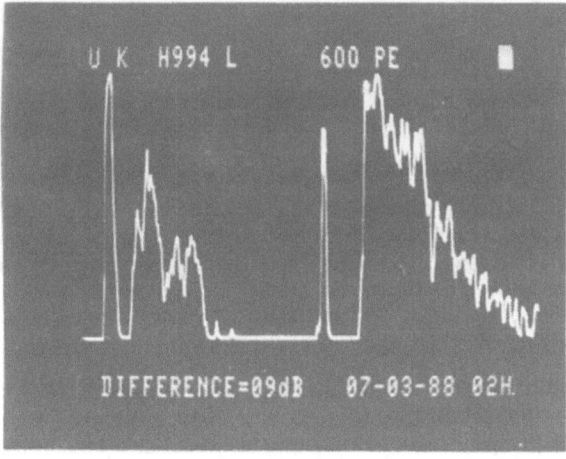

Fig. 6. Echograms of proliferative vitreoretinopathy. The upper is B+CV mode. The lower is CV mode extracted from the upper one. With two overlights, the reflectivity of the membrane to the sclera is measured and displayed in the lower space.

Figure 8 shows echograms of vitreous hemorrhage in a diabetic woman. The upper is a horizontal section and the lower is a transverse section. Several clots and many tiny dots of hemorrhage are dispersed in the vitreous and the thickened posterior hyaloid membrane by hemorrhage is displayed. On performing B-scan spontaneous vitreous movement could be clearly observed. Since the B probe of Ophthascan S is very small, compared with those of other equipments as shown in Fig. 9, we can examine the eye ball and the orbit longitudinally at each meridian.

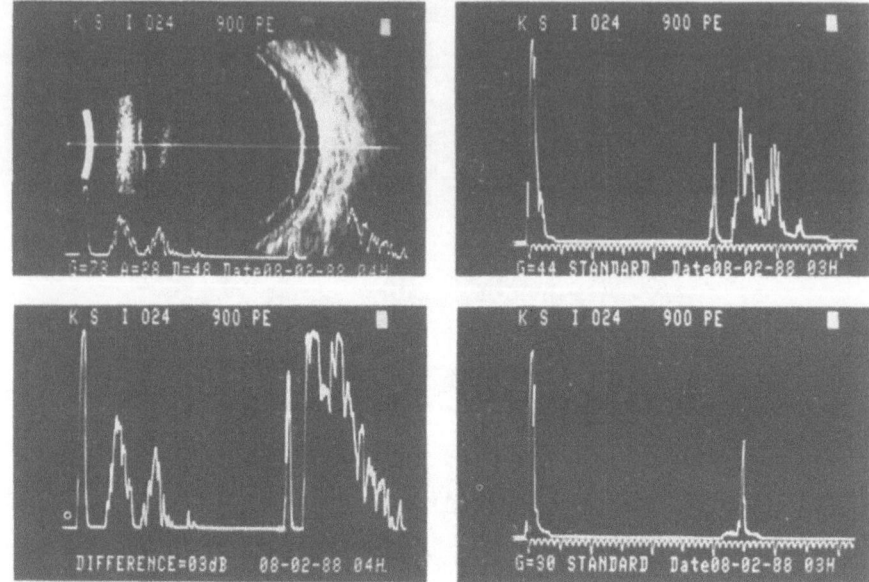

Fig. 7. Echograms of retinal detachment. The upper left echogram is B+CV mode, and the lower left is extracted from the upper left. The reflectivity difference is measured as 3 dB using overlights system. Two right echograms show how to quantify the reflectivity difference between the membrane and the sclera with reduction of the total gain.

Figure 10 shows a fundus photograph and echograms of rhegmatogenous retinal detachment. A fundus photograph of the right eye shows a large tear located in the peripheral superotemporal quadrant. The upper echogram is the longitudinal section of 11 o'clock meridian by Santesonic SSD-121. But the whole image is deviated to the left because the edge of the orbital bone prevents B probe manipulation. In case of Ophthascan S, shown in the lower echogram, the probe is small enough to catch the tear without deviation of the whole image.

Discussion

Most recent ultrasonic equipments have both the functions of A- and B-scan. A-scan is usually equipped with vector A-scan. There are some equipments, in which the distance is measured by two calipers on B-mode image because vector A-scanning does not have the function of measuring the distance. Sometimes we feel difficulty in getting the two calipers set

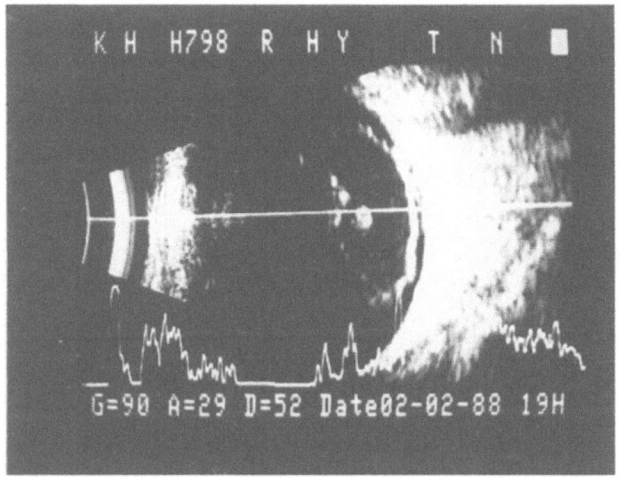

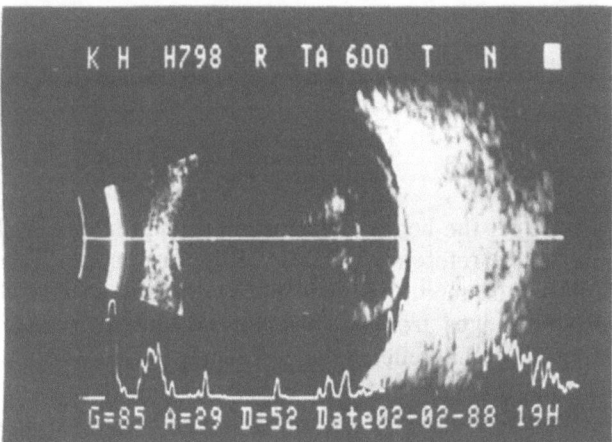

Fig. 8. Echograms of vitreous hemorrhage in a diabetic woman. The upper echogram is taken in the horizontal section and the lower is taken in the anterior transverse section. Many clots and dots of hemorrhage were ascertained to be mobile on kinetic echography.

accurately on the desired points. Therefore it is recommended to use A scan for distance measurement and reflectivity difference. Cross vector A-scan in Ophthascan S, which is visible and mobile on the stored B-mode image, can measure the distance and the reflectivity difference between two or more points along its scanning line, whereas without B-mode display the direction of the sole A-scan beam is often uncertain in detecting lesions.

Cross vector A-scan is very convenient but it does have several problems. The most important one in calculating Δ dB by vector A-scan is that we

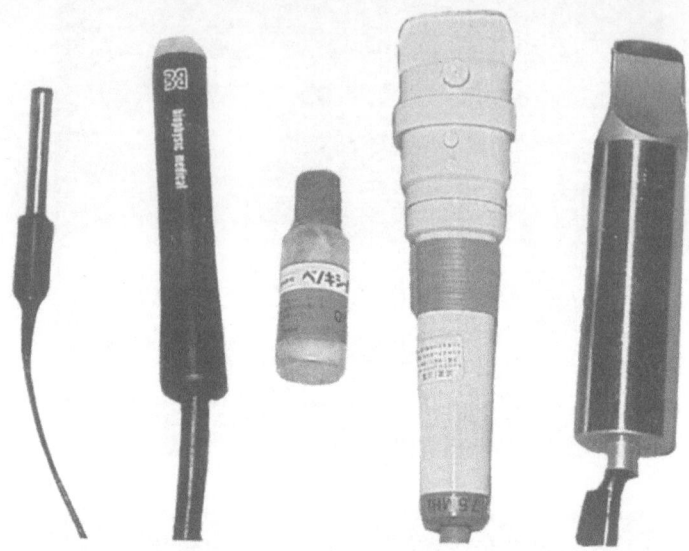

Fig. 9. Several kinds of B probe are compared. The probe of Ophthascan S is the second one from the left end.

sometimes can not get the beam of vector A-scan perpendicular both to the membrane and to the reference tissue (sclera). In quantitative echography perpendicularity to the membrane and the sclera is indispensable and only the maximal echo spikes from the membrane and the sclera should be compared. Therefore the reflectivity difference (Δ dB) of vector A-scan sometimes lacks accuracy.

Recent ultrasonic equipments can display both A- and B-mode simultaneously by B-scan probe alone. Ossoinig emphasizes that advantage of A mode will be lost when A-mode is combined with B-mode, and criticizes the vector A-scan. A-scan beam has non-focused parallel beam, and gooood B-scan probe must producee a focused beam, so the idea of combining both A and B probe itself is mistaken and each probe should have its own design. And it is the best diagnostic method to perform A- and B-mode alternately and to compare image in B-mode (topography) and the reflectivity in A-mode (quantitation). Ophthascan S can display B+CV mode and A-mode alternately, and comparison of both modes is possible. In the sense it has functions of two different kinds of equipment.

As mentioned in the case presentation, quantitative echography can be done by using A probe. After calculating Δ dB by using the cross vector A-scan we can also perform quantitative echography by using A probe alone when perpendicularity to the membrane and the sclera can not be obtained. In Ophthascan series, A-mode has three kinds of amplification; linear,

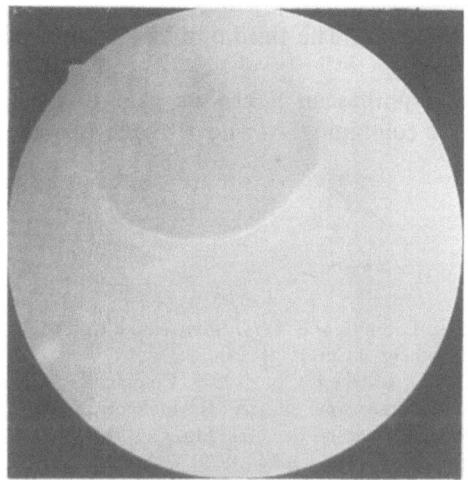

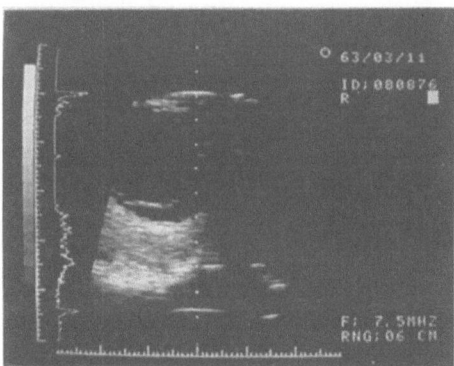

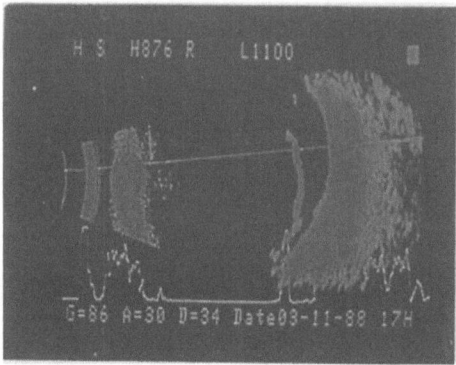

Fig. 10. A fundus photograph and echograms of rhegmatogenous retinal detachment. The upper echogram is taken by Japanese equipment, Santesonic SSD-121, and the lower by Ophthascan S. A large tear can be displayed by either equipment but the image by the former is deviated to the left, due to limited manipulation of the probe.

378

logarithmic and S-curved. The third one affords the wide range of differentiation.

In conclusion, Ophthascan S can be said to be excellent equipment, because even after combining A- and B-mode it possesses their individual advantages fully.

References

Coleman D J, Dallow R L, Smith M E. 1979. Immersion ultrasonography: Simultaneous A-scan and B-scan. Int Ophthalmol Clin 19(4): 67.

Ossoinig K C, Frazier S L, Watzke R C et al. 1977. Combined A-scan and B-scan echography as a diagnostic aid for vitreoretinal surgery. In: McPherson A (ed) New and Controversial Aspects of Vitreoretinal Surgery. St Louis, Mo, C. V. Mosby p. 106.

Ossoinig K C, Standardized Echography. 1979. Basic Principles, Clinical Applications and Results. In: Dallow R L (ed) Ophthalmic Ultrasonography: Comparative Techniques Int. Ophthal. Clin., 19/4 Little, Brown & Co., Boston.

48. Echo-ophthalmography in children

ANNA BERTÉNYI

There are some differences between the echo-ophthalmography of children and of adults. The methods of ultrasonography are similar, however, the diagnoses and diseases are not the same.

Methods and material

A-mode equipment Kretztechnik 7000 and 7100 MA were used with transducers of 6, 8 and 10 MHz frequencies and of 5 mm diameter.

The age of our patients was between 1 month and 14 years. Local anesthesia was used but small children were usually examined through the eyelids. We performed general anesthesia only in exceptional cases, when it was necessary for an other examination or operation.

The axial length of the globe was measured in every case, sometimes repeatedly.

Most of the children referred to echo-ophthalmography had a *leukokoria* (a white pupillary reflex) caused by different congenital or acquired diseases such as retinopathia prematurorum (ROP) and retrolental fibroplasia (RLF), uveitis, cataract, retinitis exudativa externa (Coats' disease), pseudoglioma, persistent hyperplastic primary vitreous (PHPV), retinitis proliferans or — the most dangerous of all — retinoblastoma.

Intraocular echography

Our foremost task is to rule out or demonstrate the presence of retinoblastoma. Differential diagnosis is based upon the following echographical characteristics:

Budapest, Hungary

R. Sampaolesi (ed.), Ultrasonography in Ophthalmology 12, 379–385.
© *1990. Kluwer Academic Publishers, Dordrecht*

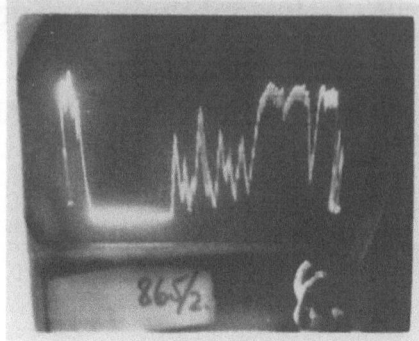

Fig. 1. Echogram of retinoblastoma. Prominency 12 Dioptr. Low system sensitivity.

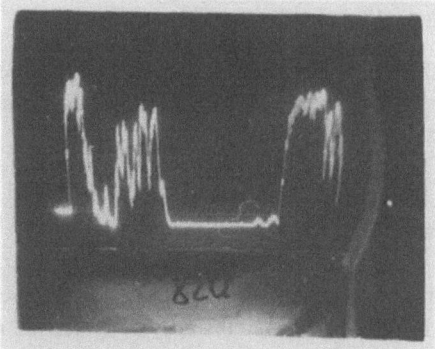

Fig. 2. Echogram of PHPV.

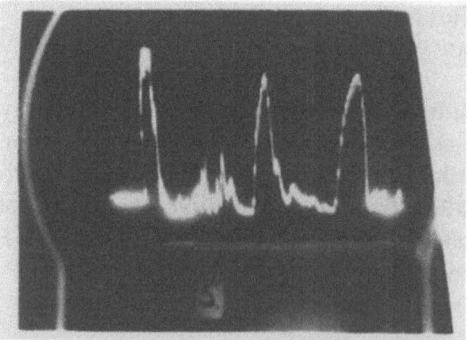

Fig. 3. Echogram of persistent hyaloid artery.

This malignant tumor is detected usually in the eyes of children younger than three. The echogram shows multiple echoes of high amplitudes connected with the sclera (Fig. 1). Its attenuation is significant (Poujol, 1973). Microphthalmos is found very rarely in eyes with retinoblastoma (Till and Ossoinig, 1975).

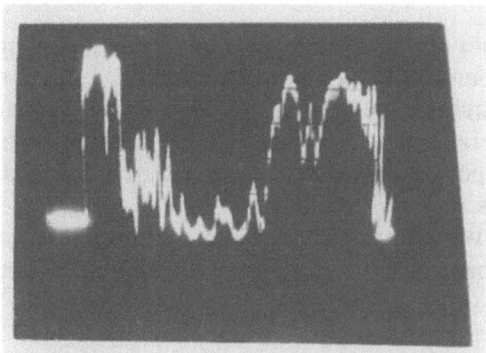

Fig. 4. Echogram of Coats' disease.

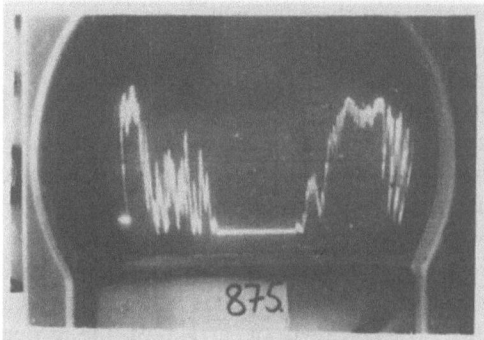

Fig. 5. Echogram of uveitis. Maximal system sensitivity.

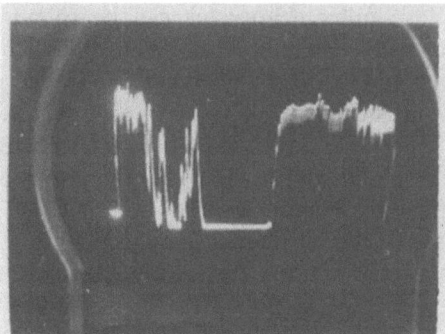

Fig. 6. Echogram of RLF.

In cases of congenital or traumatic cataracta the echograms are normal if no other disease is present.

Persistent hyperplastic primary vitreous (PHPV) is a monocular congenital disorder. Pathological multiple echoes can be seen just behind the lens, in the anterior part of the vitreous (Fig. 2).

Persistent hyaloid artery in itself does not cause leukokoria but is sometimes incidently found in leukokoric eyes as well. The characteristic echogram shows a sagittal fascicle of high reflectivity in the vitreal space (Fig. 3).

Retinitis proliferans may cause pathological echoes of medium or high amplitudes in the posterior part of the vitreous. Differential diagnosis from a retinoblastoma is sometimes difficult.

Retinitis exudativa externa (Coats' disease). Multiple echoes are reflected from the vitreal space and if reflectivity is high enough, it can be misinterpreted as a tumor (Fig. 4).

In cases of uveitis pathological echoes may arise from any part of the vitreal space, however, their amplitudes never reach those of a tumor (Fig. 5).

Pseudoglioma is a collective term for white masses in the vitreal space, which are of different — mostly unknown — etiology. Localization and amplitude of the echoes may greatly vary, but sound attenuation never reaches that of a retinoblastoma.

Retinopathia prematurorum (ROP) and its advanced form retrolental fibroplasia (RLF): 10–15 years ago the incidence of ROP and RLF were 33% of all the leukokoric eyes among our patients (Bertényi and Fodor, 1981). Recently this proportion has been decreasing significantly.

The eyes of premature babies with an advanced RLF are microphthalmic in 36% (Bertényi et al., 1980). By means of repeated measurements we proved that the increase of the visual axis was prognostically a favourable sign. However, the slowing-down or arrest of the growth of the globe indicates the severity of RLF. The characteristic echogram (Fig. 6) shows many echo-peaks with high amplitudes behind the lens, while the posterior part of the vitreal space is acoustically clear except there is a retinal detachment (Fig. 7). Similar echograms can be found in Coats' disease, PHPV or uveitis but never in retinoblastoma.

The frequency of injuries in children makes them important for the echo-ophthalmologist. Contusions as well as perforations of the globe may cause a hemophthalmos which makes ophthalmoscopy impossible. In these cases retinal detachment often has to be ruled out or demonstrated by ultrasound.

Sometimes we have to localize the lens whether it is normally located, subluxated or luxated in the vitreous.

For a short time after the injury the lens is moving in the vitreous, so we can detect it by the following method: We are examining the patient both in a lying and then in a sitting position. As long as the lens is not fixed in the vitreous we can registrate its movement even by A-mode echography (Fig. 8).

Echographic localization of foreign bodies is similar in children and in grown-ups. An X-ray photo should be taken prior to the echo-ophthalmography, but we can renounce it in very small children or in cases of suspected X-ray negative foreign bodies. A maximal acoustical impedance is characteristic of all foreign bodies (Figs. 9, 10, 11).

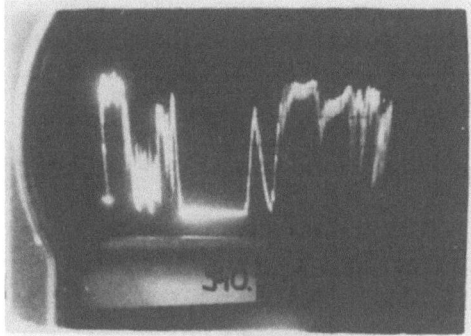

Fig. 7. Echogram of RLF with retinal detachment.

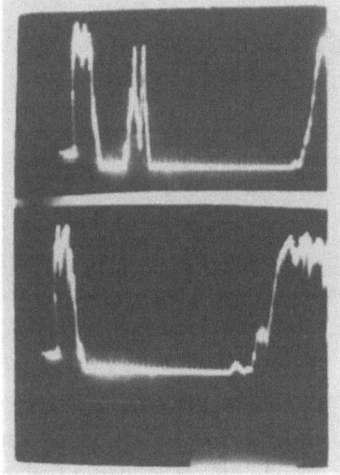

Fig. 8. Echograms of a lens luxated in the vitreous. Above: lying position. Below: sitting position.

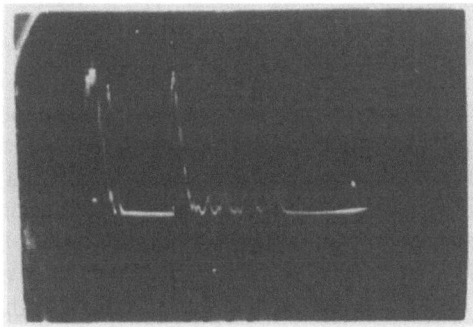

Fig. 9. Echogram of an intraocular foreign body. Minimal system sensitivity.

384

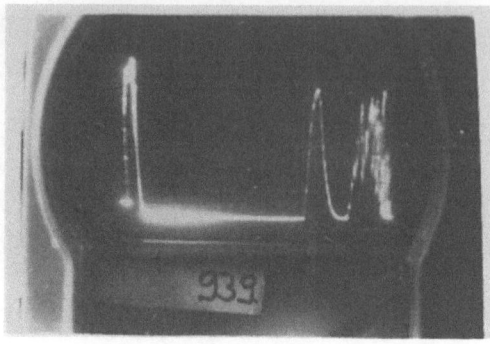

Fig. 10. Echogram of an orbital foreign body. Minimal system sensitivity.

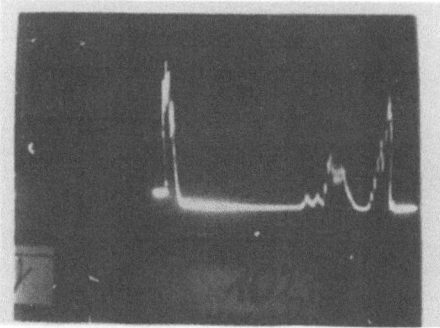

Fig. 11. Echogram of an intrascleral foreign body. Minimal system sensitivity.

Late consequences of injuries make echo-ophthalmography necessary because of blurred media. In the background of an uveitis in adults echography often reveals a juvenile injury or an undetected foreign body.

Orbital echography

Unilateral exophthalmos and injuries are the most frequent indications of orbital echography. An orbital foreign body may suggest a double perforation if there is a penetration in the anterior segment of the globe too. Retrobulbar hematomas are mostly caused by contusions. Hemangioma is found rarely in the orbit and it is very seldom intraocular in children (Fig. 12). However, its characteristic echogram helps the differential diagnosis. The high-reflectivity echopeaks are extremely kinetic on the A-scan.

Most of the congenital lesions and tumors of the orbit can be demonstrated by echography except for those which are far behind the globe, because of limits of ultrasound penetration.

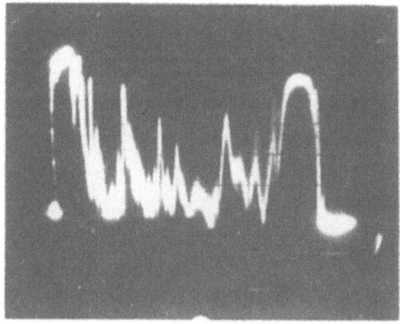

Fig. 12. Echogram of hemangioma chorioideae. Low system sensitivity.

Echo-biometry

The advantages of echographic measurements are as follows:
- it is an exact, quick and painless method without any danger
- opacity of refractive media does not cause any difficulties
- parts of the sagittal axis can be measured separately
- not only the sagittal, but some other axes are measurable too.
  The most frequent clinical applications of echo-biometry in children:
- Congenital and juvenile glaucoma (control of therapy).
- ROP and RLF (microphthalmos, prognostical value of growth).
- Ametropia (progression of myopia, control of antimyopic surgery: Kolozsvári et al., 1988).
- Lens thickness (Marfan's syndrome).
- Phthisis bulbi (all axes shortened).
- Tumors, cysts.
- Foreign bodies (localization).
- Exophthalmos.
- Intraocular lens implantation.

References

Bertényi A, Fodor M. 1981. Docum. Ophthal. Proc. Series, Dr. W. Junk Publishers, The Hague 29: 97–102.
Bertényi A, Véli M, and Fodor M. 1980. Ultrasound in Med. & Biol., 6: 19–24.
Kolozsvári L, Nagy Z, Alberth B. 1988. Szemészet 125: 59–62.
Ossoinig K C. 1965. Wiss. Z. Humboldt Univ. Berlin, Math. Naturwiss. 14: 185–191.
Poujol J. 1973. Bull. Soc. d'Ophthal. France, Rapp. annuel, No. spec. pp. 85–113.
Till P, Ossoinig K C. 1975. In: Ultrasonography in Ophthalmology. Karger, Basel, pp. 49–62.

49. Radio frequency echographical study of pseudophakodonesis

P. E. GALLENGA*, G. CENNAMO**, G. LIGUORI**,
B. PIGNALOSA** and P. DAPONTE***

Summary

A study of pseudophakodonesis of the IOL in anterior and posterior chamber was performed using the Radio frequency (RF) echographic signals. The results were similar but more accurate than those previously obtained using M mode echography: iridodonesis and firm IOL in the case of AC IOL implantation; no inertial movements of the iris and the IOL in the case of PC IOL implantation.

The authors outline the advantages presented by the echographic techniques in comparison with the optic and cinematographic methods, i.e.: less complex and more reproducible technical apparatus, easier practical execution and in particular the possibility of studying the inertial movements in IOL implantation in PC. Other advantages offered by the RF signals analysis are outlined.

The importance of the preparative evaluation of phakodenesis, by RF signals analysis in the choice of the type of implantation to be performed is stressed. IOL mobility has long been considered the main cause of long term ocular complications.

The rotation of an eye with an IOL induces a series of aftermovements of aqueous, iris and vitreous, which may be intensified or diminished by the implant itself; thus, the degree of severity of the endophthalmodonesis will be proportionally related to that of the pseudophakodonesis. Jacobi and Jagger used a film framing rate of 64 frame/sec to analyse IOL oscillations in patients who had undergone extracapsular or intracapsular IOL extraction with IOL in AC or fixed iris.

The study was performed by observing the light reflex from the front surface of the lens to track its tilt. As with any reflection from a smooth surface, the angular swing of the reflected beam is effectively doubled relative to the tilt of the lens [1].

* Department of Ophthalmology, University of Chieti, I.66700 Chieti, Italy
** Department of Ophthalmology, II School of Medicine, University of Naples, Italy
*** Department of Elettrotecnica, University of Calabria, Italy

R. Sampaolesi (ed.), Ultrasonography in Ophthalmology 12, 387–392.
© 1990. Kluwer Academic Publishers, Dordrecht

This study confirmed that iris supported intraocular lenses in eyes that had undergone an intracapsular cataract extraction exhibited much greater tilting for longer duration immediately after each saccadic globe rotation than eyes that had undergone an extracapsular cataract extraction.

Miller and Doane (1984) studied implant nature and extent and iris movements after intracapsular cataract extraction by using a high speed camera capable of picture rates up to 500 frame/sec. However 200 frame/sec, prove adequate in most cases [2].

Several types of anterior chamber and iris supported lenses were examined. None of the anterior chamber lenses examined showed any significant motion during ocular movement. However all eyes containing such lenses showed an iridonesis characteristic of an intracapsular cataract extraction. Whereas the lens remained still the iris moved and probably striked the stationary implant, under appropriate conditions. The iris supported IOLs showed an extensive, violent movement that can stretch and compress the iris extensively.

In 1983–84 we performed an ultrasonographic study of IOL induced aftermovements (pseudophakodonesis) by using M mode ultrasonic systems (Ophthalmoscan 200 by Sonometrics) [3, 4]. M mode systems have been

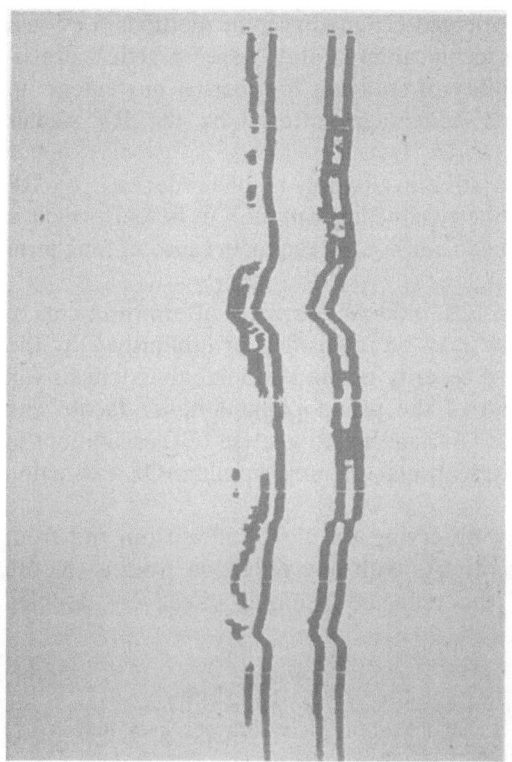

Fig. 1. Intraocular lens in posterior chamber examined with M mode. No significant after-movements of the IOL was observed, where at the same time significant endoophthalmodonesis was present. A: anterior and posterior surfaces of the cornea B: anterior surface of the IOL. C: anterior surface of the vitreous.

developed to examine temporal variation in tissue dimensions. In M mode operation a transducer is aligned along a selected axis within the eye. Then a transducer remains fixed while processed echo voltages intensity modulate an oscilloscope screen. If all tissue structures remain stationary, a series of parallel lines is displayed. If tissue position fluctuates with time, corresponding variations occur in the distances between these [5] lines so that a complete time history of tissue position is portrayed.

The IOL aftermovements study was obtained by having the patient move his eye to a given position and then immediately returning to the starting position while maintaining the probe in the same direction.

Thus it was possible to pinpoint inertial motions within the global structures after each ocular movement [3, 4]. In the group with iris supported IOLs, significant aftermovements of the IOL were observed. In this group we also observed significant iridodonesis. In the group with PC IOL in the sulcus no significant aftermovements of the IOL and iris were observed (Fig. 1).

Over the last years we have studied phakodonesis and pseudophakodonesis by means of radiofrequency (RF) echographic signals. In order to obtain, process and store the R. F. echographic signals we set up a measurement system composed of Sonometrics Ophthalmoscan 200, a 15 MHz focused probe, a Data 6000 Universal Waveform Analyzer with MHz 8 Bit sampling plug in PC-AT IBM personal Computer. The multiple acquisitions were of 7 frame/sec (7 μsec/frame) [6].

Signals from the anterior and posterior surface of the cornea and from the anterior surface of the lens or of the IOL after each saccadic globe rotation were examined.

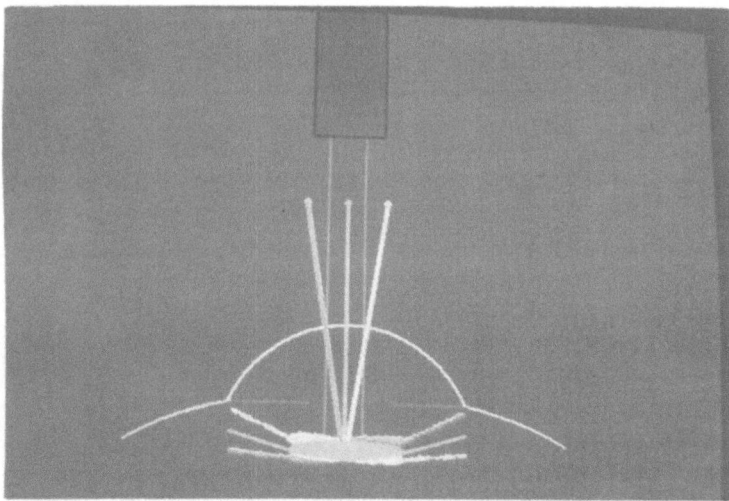

Fig. 2. Smallest variations in the incidence of the ultrasound beam give rise to modifications in the reflectivity of the peaks from the IOL.

The variations in reflectivity of the peaks from the single surfaces were evaluated. Even smallest variations in the incidence of the ultrasound beam, give rise to modifications of the reflectivity of the single peak from the interfacies under examination (Fig. 2).

Anterior and posterior surfaces of the cornea were taken as the steady parameter for eventual inertial movements of the structures under examination (Fig. 3). The RF signals and the results obtained using M mode echography confirm those obtained with the optic and cinematographic methods, regarding the inertial movements in IOL implantation in AC, after intra and extracapsular extraction. RF echographic signals and M mode examination showed the same results with respect to IOL implantation in A.C. and in P.C. in the sulcus (Figs. 4, 5).

The possibility of examination of PC IOL inertial movement is undoubtably the major advantage presented by echographic technique in comparison with the optic and cinematographic methods. This examination is impossible with the latter methods if a good mydriasis is not achieved which however changes the physiological conditions.

Considering that the great majority of IOL implantation is actually performed in PC then this advantage is fundamental. Other advantages are:
– a less complex and therefore more reproducible technical apparatus.
– an easier practical execution.

We wish to outline here, some features of the RF signal examination which, in our opinion, render this technique elective in phako- and pseudophakodonesis study.

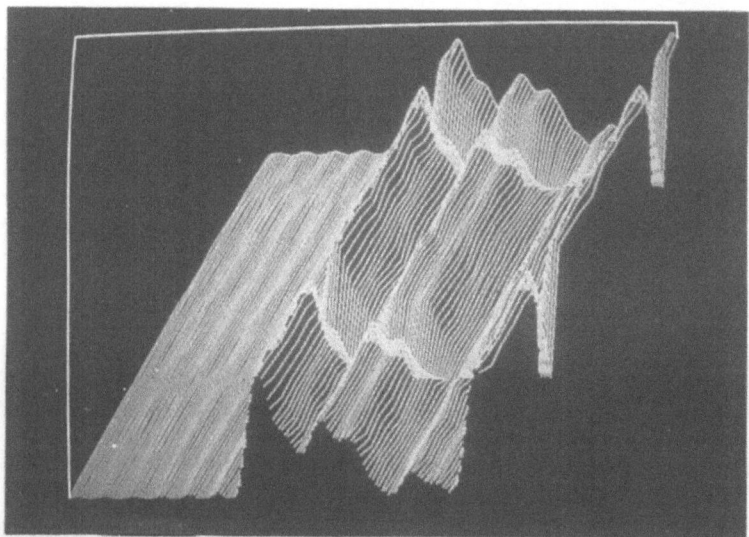

Fig. 3. Multiple acquisitions from the anterior and posterior surfaces of the cornea are taken as the steady parameter for eventual inertial movements of the IOL.

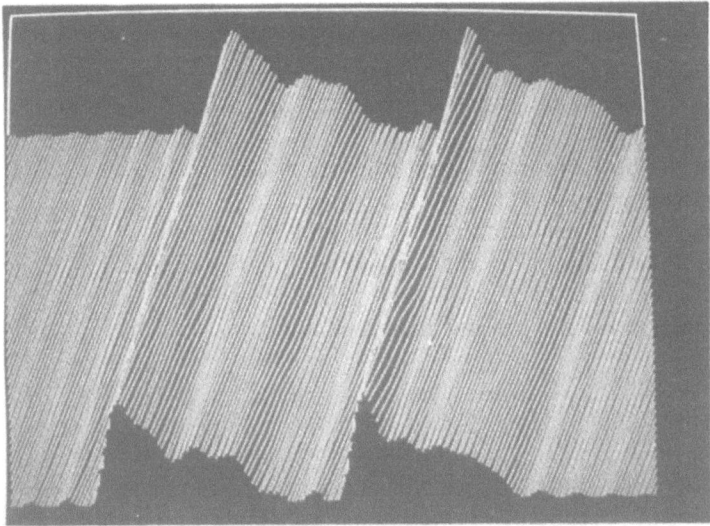

Fig. 4. Multiple acquisitions from the anterior and posterior surfaces of the PC lens placed in the sulcus; no modification in the reflectivity of the peaks indicate absence of pseudophakodonesis.

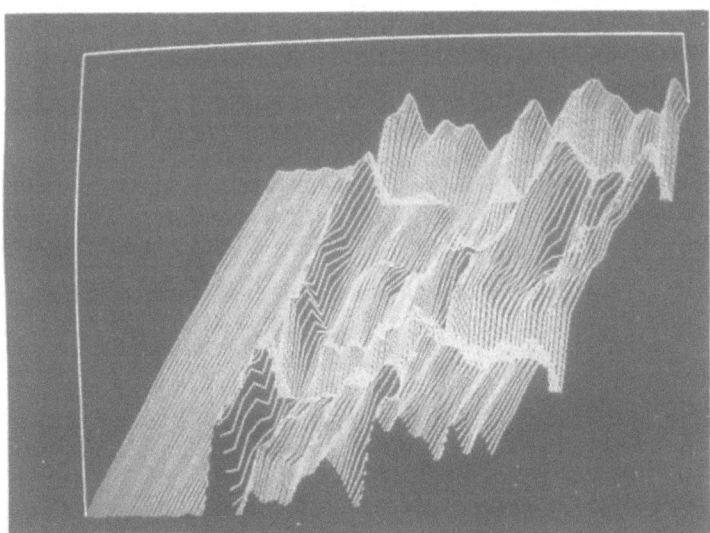

Fig. 5. Multiple acquisitions from the anterior and posterior surfaces of the PC lens; the modifications in the reflectivity of the peaks from the IOL indicate the presence of a pseudophakodonesis.

RF signals analysis:
- discloses even the slightest degree of lens tilt (5–10°)
- permits the direction of the ultrasound beam to every point of the surface in object; M mode examination requires that the beam shuns the center of rotation of the IOL
- permits the contemporaneous study of the inertial movements of the iris, IOL and, in particular, the vitreous.

The efficacy of the technique is not diminished by the low number of frame/sec used. The optic and cinematographic studies demonstrate, that the mean timelength of an oscillation is about 160 msec, while the minimal maximizable with RF signals is about 140 msec.

Conclusion

Undoubtedly the study of pseudophakodonesis is important for its clinical implications but preoperative evaluation of phakodonesis with the RF signals analysis assumes the same importance in the choice of the type of implantation to be performed which will be effected in AC, in the sulcus or in the capsular bag according to the degree of phakodonesis.

References

[1] Jacobi K W, Jagger W S. 1981. Physical forces involved in pseudophakodonesis and irridodonesis. Albrecht von Graefes Arch Klin Exp Ophthalmol 216 I: 49–53.
[2] Miller D, Doane Marshall G. 1984. High-speed photographic evaluation of intraocular lens movements. Am J Ophthalmol 97: 752–759.
[3] Bonavolontá A, Cennamo G, D'Avanzo M. 1983. Endoftalmodonesi e cristallino artificiale: studio ecografico. Atti LXIII Congresso Societa' Italiana di oftalmologia.
[4] Gallenga P E, Cennamo G. 1984. Pseudophakodonesis as a major cause of late corneal and retinal complications in IOL surgery . Tenth Biennal Congress of the International Society for Ophthalmic Ultrasound, SIDUO X, St Petersburg, Florida.
[5] Coleman D J, Lizzi F L, Jack R L. 1977. Ultrasonography of the eye and orbit. Lea and Febiger Philadelphia. pp. 79–81.
[6] Cennamo F, Cennamo G, Daponte P et al. Ocular Tissue Characterization *in vivo* by Radio Frequency Signal Analysis.
XXV International Congress of Ophthalmology Kugler Publications e Ghedini Editore Roma.

50. Uveal effusion and nanophthalmos

HUGO QUIROZ and EDUARDO MORAGREGA

Uveal effusion and nanohthalmos

Uveal effusion, which is a fluid leakage from the choriocapillaris into the choroid, is classified by Brockhurst in idiopathic, inflamatory, and hydrostatic (Table 1) [3].

Nanophthalmic eyes, are small eyes, with an extremely thick sclera, which may decrease venous drainage of the vortex veins [3, 9]. This anatomic variation could produce a different spectrum in ultrasound examination [9]. Choroidal thickening and detachment, even when in an incipient form, are best evaluated with ultrasound. We report herein the most important ultrasonographic features of three patients with nanophthalmos.

Case reports

Case 1

A 36 year old man, with a one year history of decreased vision in his right eye, was referred for treatment of an exudative choroiditis. The patient had undergone subretinal fluid drainage in 1985, after a four months regimen of systemic steroids. In January 1986, when he was first seen, his visual acuity was: RE: HM, with a + 13.00 diopters correction, and LE: 20/60, with a +13.50 diopters correction. Corneal diameter was 10×10 mm, both horizontally and vertically. Gonioscopy revealed a open angle, grade 3–4, bilaterally. Anterior chamber depth was slightly decreased, mainly in his left eye. The fundi in his right eye showed a total retinal detachment with smooth convex ballooning elevations of the retina, without breaks. Areas of choroidal detachment were also identified. The fundi in the left eye dis-

Retina Service, Hospital Asociación Para Evitar la Ceguera en México. Vicente García Torres # 46, Coyoacán México D. F., C. P. 04030. Mexico

R. Sampaolesi (ed.), Ultrasonography in Ophthalmology 12, 393–400.

Table 1. Classification of uveal effusion.

1. Idiopathic.
2. Inflammatory
    Trauma, intraocular surgery.
    Autoimmune uveitis.
    Scleritis, infected scleral buckle.
    After panretinal photocoagulation.
3. Hydrostatic.
    Dural arteriovenous fistula.
    Hypotony.
    Nanophthalmos.

closed some retinal folds on the macular area, and the disc appeared small. Echographic examination of the RE showed diffuse thickening and detachment of the choroid, as well as retinal detachment in a small eye. (Figs. 1 and 2) The ultrasound of the LE disclosed choroidal thickening in a small eye (Fig. 3). The patient refused vortex vein decompression surgery. In December 1986, the retina reattached spontaneously, and visual acuity improved to 20/100. The pigment epithelium showed a leopard spot mottling (Fig. 4). The patient has had no further changes after 16 months follow up (Fig. 5).

Case 2

A 5 year old girl was examined because of decreased vision. In both eyes her visual acuity was 20/20 with +5 diopters correction. Corneas were 10 mm in diameter, both horizontally and vertically. Gonioscopy and anter-

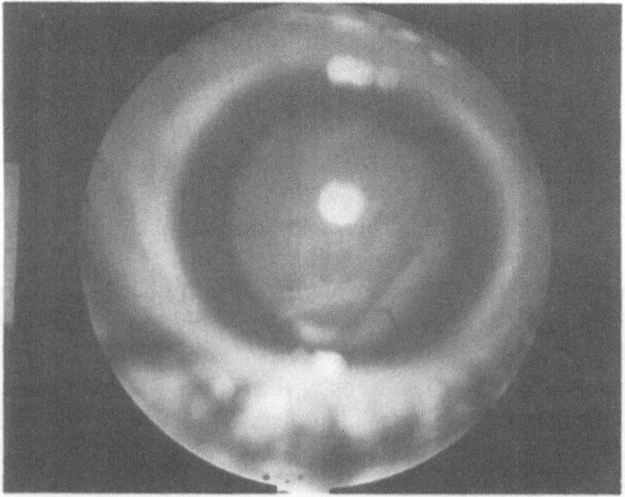

Fig. 1. Case 1. Complete retinal detachment in right eye.

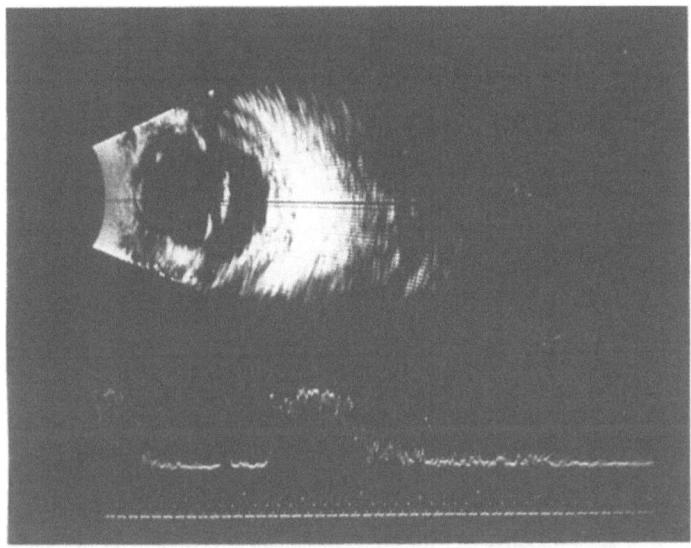

Fig. 2. Case 1. A- and B-scan echography representing choroidal and retinal detachment in right eye.

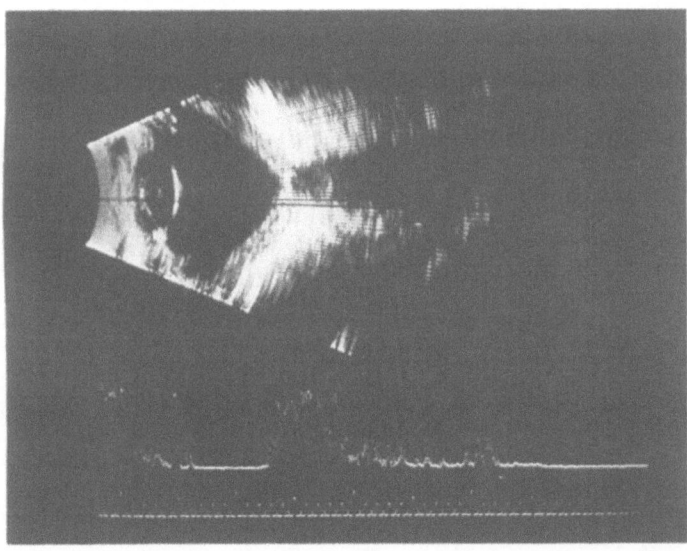

Fig. 3. Case 2. A- and B-scan ultrasonography showing diffuse thickening of the choroid in left eye.

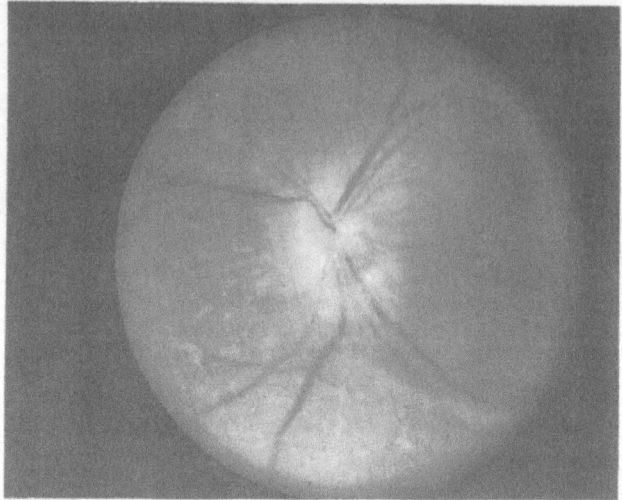

Fig. 4. Case 1. Spontaneous retinal reattachment after 10 months in right eye.

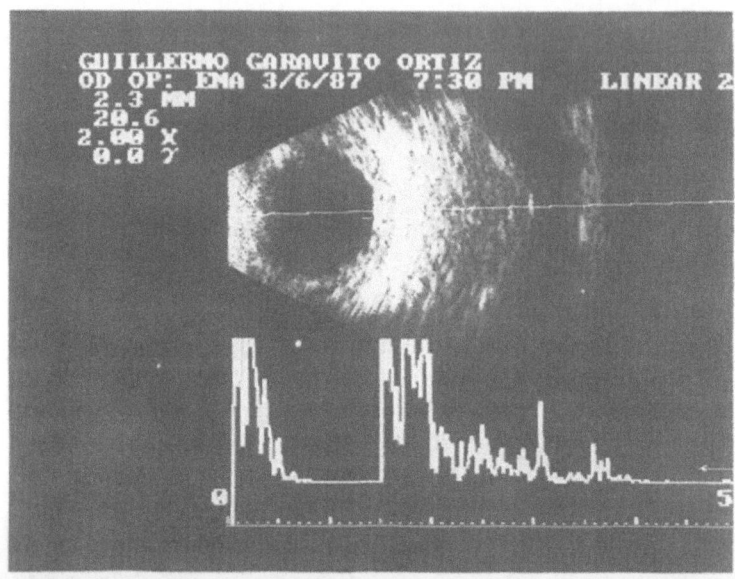

Fig. 5. Case 1. A- and B-scan echography of the right eye after spontaneous retinal reattachment. Choroidal thickening is evident.

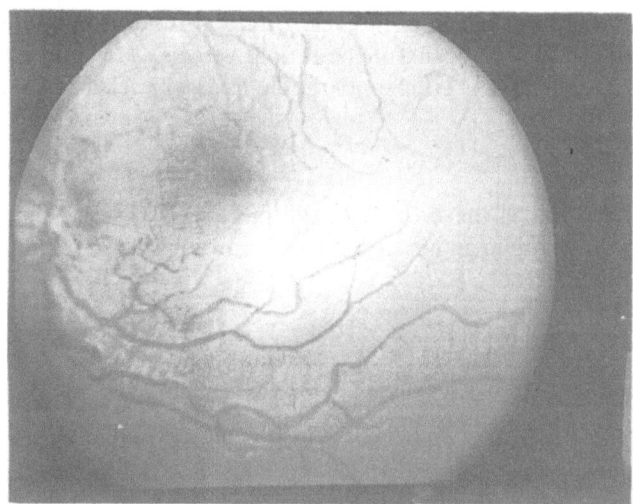

Fig. 6. Case 2. Macular striae and venous tortuosity.

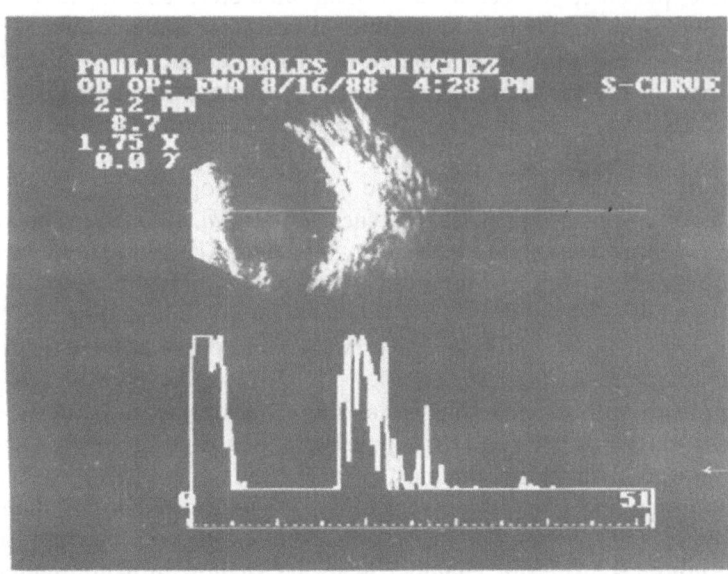

Fig. 7. Case 2. A- and B-scan echography showing A-P axis of 15.6 mm and choroidal width of 2.2 mm.

ior chamber were normal in both eyes. Bilateral fundi examination showed hyperopic disc, mild tortuosity of the retinal vessels, and some retinal striae on macular area (Fig. 6). Ultrasonographic findings are shown on Fig. 7.

Case 3

This 3 year old boy is the brother of the patient on case 2. The fundi were identical to those found in his sister. His ultrasound was also similar in both eyes (Fig. 8).

Discussion

Nanophthalmos is a rare entity in which the eye is pathologically small but otherwise morphologically relatively normal. Uveal effusion accompanies many diseases, when it is not secondary to trauma or surgery, it is often related either to the idiopathic, or to the autoimmune form, like patient in case 1.

Nanophthalmos has some characteristic features that include the following: a very small eye, high hyperopia with thick aphakic-style glasses in phakic patients; a decreased corneal diameter, and a shallow anterior chamber. One of the less common forms of presentation in uveal effusion is that associated with nanophthalmos. This entity should be suspected when the patient has the characteristic features of nanophthalmos [5].

Ecography is a highly sensitive and specific test for detecting the choroidal abnormalities that are seen in nanophthalmos [8]. This entity may result in blindness if it is not recognized and treated appropriately. Decompression of the vortex veins has proven to be successful [6, 3]. Remissions and exacerbations without treatment, have been reported, [7] like patient in case one, who refused surgery and remitted spontaneously. Treatment for glaucoma in nanophthalmic eyes is actually standarized, [9] but timing for vortex decompression in nanohthalmic eyes with uveal effusion has not been established.

Patients with longstanding uveal effusion sydrome, might have decreased antero-posterior axis, and hyperopic correction (Fig. 9), but corneal features are different. In nanophthalmos, corneal diameter is often reduced, whereas in longstanding idiopathic uveal effusion syndrome, corneal diameters are normal, and Descement striae are commonly seen because of chronic hypotony [3]. Anterior chamber is always shallow in nanohthalmos, meanwhile in idiopathic uveal effusion it is always deep [1, 2].

The echographic features in cases 1, 2 and 3 are characteristic of nanohthalmos, these patients should be followed for life to prevent complications, and given adequate treatment if they appear.

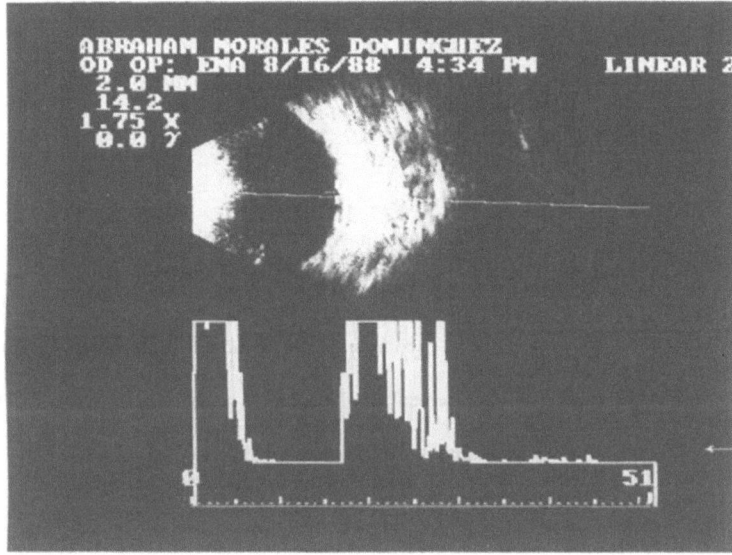

Fig. 8. Case 3. A- and B-scan ultrasonography showing A-P axis of 17.1 mm and choroidal width of 2.0 mm.

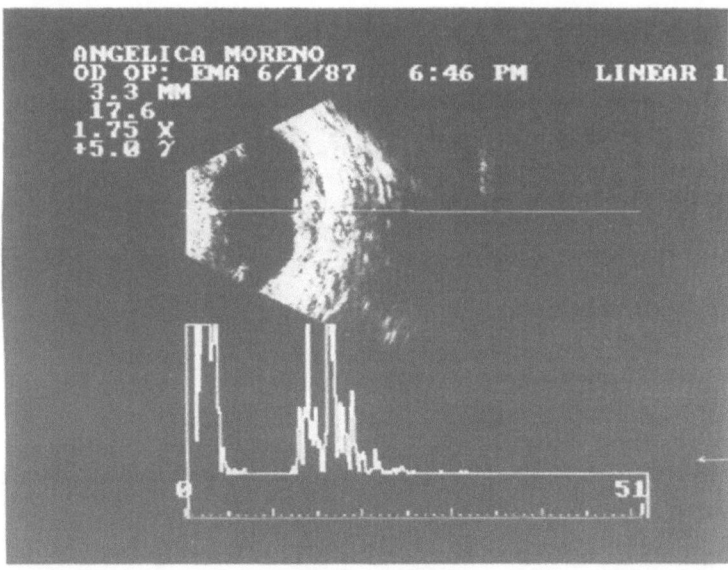

Fig. 9. Patient with idiopathic uveal effusion disclosing choroidal thickening (3.3 mm) and decreased A-P axis (17.6 mm).

Nanophthalmos may occur in an sporadic form as in patient from case 1, who had no positive family history, or as in case 2 and 3, where a recessive autosomic inheritance is the most likely explanation reported [8, 5].

References

[1] Bellows A R, Chylack L T Jr, Hutchinson B T. (1981). Choroidal detachment: clinical manifestations, therapy and mechanisms of formation. Ophthalmology 88: 1107.
[2] Brockhurst R J. 1975. Nanophthalmos with uveal effusion: a new clinical entity. Arch Ophthalmol 93: 1289.
[3] Brockhurst R J. 1980. Vortex vein decompression of nonophthalmic uveal effusion. Arch Ophthalmol 98: 1987.
[4] Calhoun F P, Jr. 1975. The management of glaucoma in nanophthalmos. Am Ophthalmol Soc 73: 97.
[5] Cross H E, Yoder F. 1976. Familial nanophthalmos. AM J Ophthalmol 81: 300.
[6] Gass J M D 1983. Uveal effusion syndrome: a new hypotesis concerning pathogenesis and technique of surgical treatment. Trans Am Ophthalmol Soc. 81: 246.
[7] Gass J M D. 1987. Stereoscopic atlas of macular diseases. The C. V. Mosby Co., St. Louis, Mo. ed. 5, p. 166.
[8] Ryan E A, Swaan J, Chylack L T, Jr. 1982. Nanophthalmos with uveal effusion: clinical and embryologic considerations. Ophthalmology 89: 1013.
[9] Singh O S, Simmons R J, Brockhurst R J, Trempe C L. 1982. Nanophthalmos: a perspective on identification and therapy. Ophthalmology 89: 1006.

51. 'Monstrous' deformations (myopic staphyloma) detected by ultrasound

LEONARDO FALCO*, CINZIA MAZZINI**, STEFANO ESENTE*,
NICOLA PASSARELLI*, and PAOLA SANTORO***

Summary

Some 'monstrous' images of the eye (myopic staphyloma), examined by
ultrasound, are presented. Different grades of staphyloma are presented and
discussed. Some clinical considerations are made.

Introduction

When pathological lesions or congenital abnormalities reduce scleral resistance, intraocular pressure can lead to a weakening (ectasia) of the ocular
bulb. Ectasia, accompanied by uveal adhesion and resulting pigmentation is
known as staphyloma (Toselli and Miglio, 1979).

Curtin (1985) ophthalmoscopically described five varietes (Types 1 to 5)
of primary posterior staphyloma and five compound varietes (Types 6 to 10)
of posterior staphyloma that are essential variations of primary Type 1
combined with Types 2 and 5. Each, he says, affects a different area of the
fundus, and while one or two are oddities, all are important... Curtin
(1985) further reports that observation of myopic staphyloma is directly
proportional to the axial length of the myopic eye. This statement contradicts
Tsuboi's studies which do not correlate staphyloma to the axial length of the
myopic eye (Tsuboi et al., 1981).

Echographic descriptions of myopic staphyloma have been presented by
Coleman, 1977; Hassani, 1978; Poujol, 1981; Mazzeo, 1987; Stefani, 1987.
An interesting ultrasound study was done by Inoue et al. (1982) who made
objective measurements of the shape of the posterior staphyloma in high
myopia. They reported that depth rather than axial length should be
considered when comparing functional disturbances and morphologic variations of staphyloma.

* Centro Oculistico. Via Pietro Dazzi N.g, 50141, Firenze, Italy
** II Clinica Oculistica, Università di Firenze Firenze, Italy
*** I clinica Oculistica, Università di Firenze, Firenze, Italy

R. Sampaolesi (ed.), Ultrasonography in Ophthalmology 12, 401–403.
© 1990. Kluwer Academic Publishers, Dordrecht

402

In this paper, we present different types of ultrasonograms in myopic staphyloma and our survey's results concerning the incidence of staphylomatose ectasia in relation to the axial length of the myopic eye.

Materials and methods

139 patients who came under our observation at two different clinics underwent ultrasound tests. These patients were referred primarily for echobiometric testing and IOL calculation.

Two different ultrasonograps were used: a Sonometrics 400 (Sonometrics System) and a Sonomed B 3000 (Sonomed Technology, Inc.).

Patients who presented an antero-posterior axis greater than 27 mm were considered. Five ultrasonographic projections of each myopic eye were done: one antero-posterior, one superior, one lateral, one inferior and one medial.

The patients were divided into two groups:
Group 1: patients who did not present any ultrasonographically evident ectasic modifications of the ocular wall;
Group 2: patients who did present ultrasonographically evident modifications of the ocular wall.

Patients were evaluated as belonging to the first or second group by two examiners on two separate occasions.

Results

Results are shown in Fig. 1:
The data obtained show a relationship, though not directly proportional, between the axial length of the myopic eye and the existence of staphyloma.

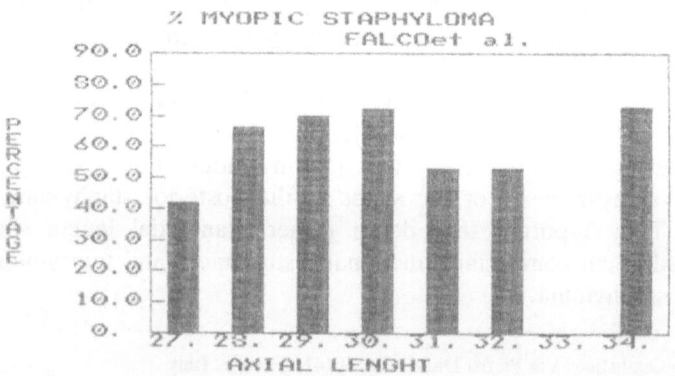

Fig. 1. Percentage of staphiloma found in eyes of length in the range from 27 to 34 mm.

Objective, ophthalmoscopic findings of myopic staphylomatose ectasia, were 26% of the total number of eyes examined.

Discussion

The findings presented in this study, are not the result of ophthalmoscopic tests, but rather ultrasonographic objectivity, and differ percentage-wise from the data reported in the literature. This is particularly evident in the 'shorter' myopic eyes. The percentage incidence of staphyloma in the 'longer' myopic eyes is consistent with the values reported in the literature.

This percentage deviation can be attributed to the fact that the ultrasound images can reveal a slight weakening of the eye more readily than an ophthalmoscopic examination. We believe that the B-scan ultrasound image can reveal ectasis nearly as well as an anatomic section.

Initially, our data were a source of perplexity, however, Curtin's reports did lend them credence: '... It is our current impression at the Myopic Clinic of the Manhattan Eye, Ear and Throat Hospital that probably all cases of pathologic myopia have a posterior staphyloma of some type at some stage of development. It is the quintessential lesion of pathologic myopia.' We believe that Curtin's statements can in some way substantiate the findings of this survey.

References

Coleman D J, Lizzi F L, Jack R L. 1977. Ultrasonography of the eye and orbit. Lea & Febiger, Philadelphia. pp. 301.

Curtin B J. 1985. The myopias. Basic science and clinical management. Harper & Row, publishers. Philadelphia. pp. 301–308.

Hassani S N. 1978. Real time ophthalmic ultrasonography. Springer–Verlag, New York. pp. 126–127.

Inoue H, Tokoro T, Muramatsu T. 1983. The objective measurement of the shape of the posterior staphyloma in high miopia. Acta: XXIV International Congress of Ophthalmology. J B. Lippincott Company, Philadelphia. pp. 1183–1185.

Mazzeo v. 1987. Ecografia dell' apparato oculare. Fogliazza ed., Milano. pp. 224–226.

Poujol J. 1981. Echographie en ophtalmologie. Mosson, Paris. pp. 20, 47.

Stefani F H, Hasenfratz G. 1987. Macroscopic ocular pathology. Springer–Verlag, New York. pp. 23, 60.

Toselli C, Miglio M. 1979. Oftalmologia clinica. Monduzzi (ed) Bologna. pp. 280.

Tsuboi S, Nuhata T, Tanaka Y, Manabe R. 1981. Posterior staphyloma and fundus changes in high myopia. Folia Ophthalmol Jpn 32: 1771–1778.

52. Echographic findings in malignant glaucoma

DANIELE DORO, ENRICO MANTOVANI, MICHELE SALA
and FERRUCCIO MORO

Summary

A case is presented of bilateral non-simultaneous malignant glaucoma in a 57 year old woman. Contact B-scan and standardized A-scan echography respectively evidenced low reflective dots with apparently continous curved veils and single echo spikes consistent with interfaces between aqueous and anterior vitreous of the left eye one week after trabeculectomy. Only low reflective dispersed opacities fading with time could be evidenced after successful medical therapy. Contact B-scan echographic finding was similar in the right blind eye with long-standing malignant glaucoma. A slow mixture of aqueous and vitreous might explain our echographic results. According to our experience aqueous-vitreous interfaces can be echographically detected in the early malignant glaucoma only. The abnormally thick lens found in both eyes of our patient can be a key factor of ciliary block.

Echography can provide useful information in diagnosing malignant glaucoma.

Introduction

Shallow or flat anterior chamber and elevated intraocular pressure after filtering glaucoma surgery are the well-known hallmarks of malignant glaucoma. Cilio-lens or cilio-vitreal block in phakic and aphakic eyes respectively is thought [8] to cause misdirection of the aqueous flow into the vitreous.

A-scan evidence of an echo-free space between two low reflective vitreous echoes was interpreted by Buschmann [1] as aqueous pockets in the vitreous of eyes with malignant glaucoma. A single low to medium reflective vitreous echo indicating a vitreous-aqueous interface was found by means of standardized A-scan echography in four phakic eyes with malignant glaucoma [7]. According to these Authors the finding of a single vitreous echo

University Eye Clinic of Padua, Padua, Italy

R. Sampaolesi (ed.), Ultrasonography in Ophthalmology 12, 405–409.

indicated that the pockets of aqueous touched the retina; on A-scan examination it was difficult or impossible to distinguish a posterior vitreous detachment from an aqueous-vitreous interface. Actually, Frezzotti et al. [3] reported an echographic A-scan diagnosis of vitreous detachment in an eye with absent anterior chamber and high intraocular pressure after filtering procedure.

To our knowledge, both A- and B-scan examination of eyes with malignant glaucoma have never been reported.

Case report

A 57 year old woman had a history of acute angle closure glaucoma in the right eye. Surgical iridectomy had been performed elsewhere, but postoperatively intraocular pressure remained elevated.

When we saw the patient about one year after surgery the right eye was

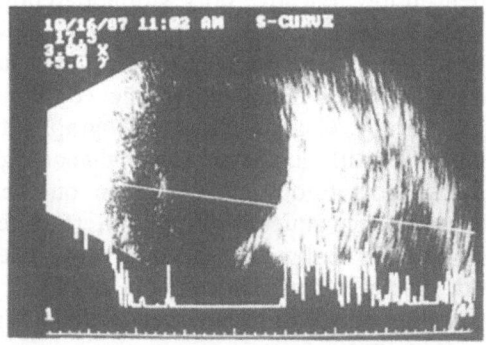

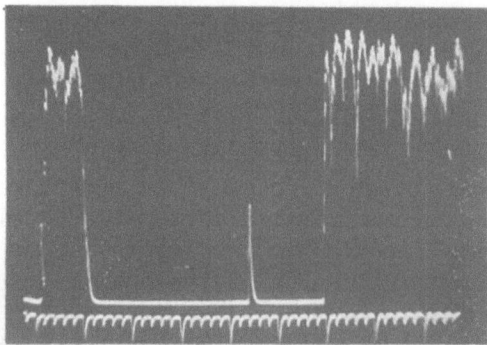

Fig. 1. Echography of the left eye with malignant glaucoma a week after trabeculectomy. A) Contact A-/B-scan: low reflective dots and an apparently continous curve-shaped veil in the nasal anterior vitreous. B) Standardized A-scan echography: low reflective unstable echo spike in the nasal anterior vitreous. The findings are consistent with aqueous-vitreous interface.

blind, painless, with flat anterior chamber and high (40 mmHg) intraocular pressure. A dust-like image was evident in the anterior vitreous on contact B-scan examination (Ultrascan Digital IV B — Coopervision; 10 MHz probe); on standardized A-scan (Kretztechnik 7200 MA) no vitreous echoes were displayed at T + 6 dB setting sensitivity. Contact automatic ultrasound biometry showed an increased (4.7 mm) thickness of the lens and short (21.32 mm) axial length.

Ultrasound biometry of the left eye curiously gave the same measurement of lens thickness and similar (21.03 mm) axial length. This eye had a full visual acuity and was affected with chronic narrow (grade I) angle glaucoma; applanation intraoculàr pressure with beta-blocking therapy ranged between 24 and 29 mmHg. The eye underwent trabeculectomy according to Cairns' technique modified by Moro [6]. Postoperatively the anterior chamber failed to reform and intraocular pressure was around 30 mmHg with steroid and mydriatic-cycloplegic drops and systemic acetazolamide. Low reflective dots and apparently continous curve-shaped veils (contact B-scan) (Fig. 1A) and single low reflective unstable echo spikes (standardized A-scan at T + 6 dB setting) (Fig. 1B) were found in the 360 degree anterior vitreous chamber a week after trabeculectomy. No aftermovements of the lesions in the anterior vitreous could be evidenced on B-scan examination. These findings were consistent with interfaces between anterior vitreous and aqueous; interfaces were more evident nasally. Medical treatment was successful in restoring a deeper anterior chamber and normal intraocular pressure without hypotensive agents in two weeks.

In the following months a clear separation between aqueous and vitreous faded but diffuse low reflective dispersed opacities in the anterior vitreous persisted on contact B-scan examination (Fig. 2); no vitreous echoes could be displayed on the screen of the Kretz unit at T + 6 dB sensitivity.

1% atropine drops were administered in the left eye once a day. However, a sudden flattening of the anterior chamber with mild corneal de-

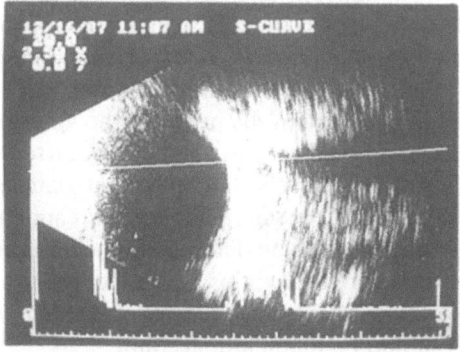

Fig. 2. Contact A-/B-scan echography of the left eye two months after trabeculectomy: diffuse low reflective dispersed opacities in the anterior vitreous with no clear evidence of aqueous-vitreous interface.

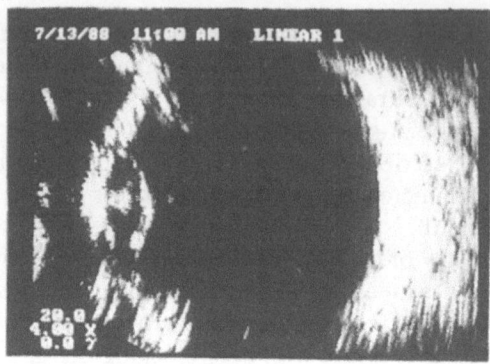

Fig. 3. Immersion B-scan echography of the right eye with longstanding malignant glaucoma: flat anterior chamber and no noteworthy vitreous abnormalities.

compensation, cortico-nuclear cataract and intraocular pressure between 16 and 22 mmHg was observed seven months after trabeculectomy. No clear evidence of aqueous pockets was detectable by standardized echography in the anterior vitreous. The patient underwent uneventful intracapsular cataract extraction in the left eye. Postoperatively, the anterior chamber remained moderately shallow, intraocular pressure was normal without medication and corrected visual acuity was 20/30; only rare dust-like opacities of the anterior vitreous could be displayed at high system sensitivity setting of the B-scan unit both in the left and the right eye. Mini-bath immersion B-scan of the right eye showed no noteworthy vitreous abnormalities (Fig.3).

Conclusions

The reported case enables us to draw some remarks.
1) Interfaces between aqueous and vitreous can be evidenced with both standardized A-scan and contact B-scan echography only shortly after the onset of malignant glaucoma. Interfaces are better displayed when the B-scan probe is aimed at the anterior nasal vitreous; obviously the nose makes it difficult to aim the probe at the anterior temporal vitreous.
2) Both after successful medical treatment, as occurred in the left eye of our patient, and in advanced untreated malignant glaucoma, as in the right eye of our patient, no clear interfaces between aqueous and vitreous but only dust-like opacities can be detected in the anterior vitreous by means of contact B-scan echography; this finding indicates a possible slow mixture of aqueous and vitreous. However, artifacts due to the contact B-scan probe should be taken into account.
3) A single echo spike originating from vitreous detachment or interface between aqueous and vitreous, which show a similar reflectivity on

standardized A-scan, may be differentiated by means of topographic and kinetic criteria of the two conditions on contact B-scan examination.

4) The eyes of our patient with malignant glaucoma had abnormally thickened lenses, which can favour ciliary-lens block. We cannot confirm the data of normal or reduced ultrasonically measured thickness of the lens in eyes with malignant glaucoma as found by Leroux-Lesjardins et al. [4], but we agree with the same Authors about the short axial length of eyes with malignant glaucoma.

5) Only rarely, due to hazy media, can aqueous pockets be seen in the anterior vitreous by contact goniolens examination [9]; standardized echography provides a nice evidence of aqueous vitreous interfaces shortly after the onset of malignant glaucoma so that affected eyes can be treated with adequate medical or surgical therapy [2, 5].

References

[1] Buschmann W. 1978. Special techniques. In: Handbook of Clinical Ultrasound. M De Vlieger et al. (eds) John Wiley & Sons, New York, 842.

[2] Chandler P A, Simmons R J, Grant W M. 1968. Malignant glaucoma: medical and surgical treatment. Am J Ophthalmol 66: 495–502.

[3] Frezzotti R, Bardelli A M, Nuti A, Casini P. 1981. Follow-up a distanza della nostra casistica di glaucoma atalamico. Boll Oculist 60: 829–840.

[4] Leroux-Lesjardins S, Massin M, Poujol J. 1977. Etude biométrique du glaucome malin. Arch Ophthalmol 37 (8 – 9): 523–530.

[5] Luntz M H, Rosenblatt M. 1987. Malignant glaucoma. Surv Ophthalmol 32: 73–93.

[6] Moro F, Borellini S, Cavallaro N. 1978. Antiglaukomatose Trabeculektomie. Klin Mbl Augenheilk 172: 670–676.

[7] Perrone S, Steindler P, D'Ermo F, Doro D. 1983. Preoperative echographic localization of aqueous humor deposits in malignant glaucoma: experimental and clinical study. In: Acta XXIV International Congress of Ophthalmology (San Francisco, 1982), P Henkind (ed) J. P. Lippincott & Co., Philadelphia. pp. 119–121.

[8] Shaffer R N, Hoskins H D Jr. 1978. Ciliary block (malignant) glaucoma. Ophthalmology 85: 215–221.

[9] Simmons R J. 1979. Current problems in malignant glaucoma. Docum. Ophthalmol. Proc. Series 22: 195–199.

53. Ultrasound findings in brawny scleritis

VINCENZINA MAZZEO, PAOLO PERRI and PAOLA MONARI

Introduction

Brawny or nodular scleritis is a relatively rare disease which is not always easy to diagnose clinically. Up to the present only seven cases of this disease have been described in the echographic literature (Chang et al., 1980; Ossoinig and Harrie, 1983; Green, 1987).

This report deals with two cases we have examined during the last five years. The echographic findings are quite unusual and are extensively described in order to explain the interpretation of the images which allow an accurate diagnosis.

Case reports

Case 1

DPG a 45-year-old Caucasian man was referred to the University Eye Clinic of Ferrara to undergo an echographic examination with the clinical suspicion of a choroidal melanoma in his RE. His clinical history dated back to 1967 when he was operated on for a small subconjunctival nodule in the inferior part of his RE. At that time hystological diagnosis of 'Micronodular lympho-hyperplastic scleritis' was made. A year later another scleral biopsy was performed and a diagnosis of 'Sclerosing chronic phlogosis' was reported.

From 1968 to 1983 he did well except for some recurrent redness of the eye. In 1983 a new nodule was discovered in the external third of the inferior conjunctival sac. He immediately visited an ophthalmologist, who discovered a liquid retinal detachment in the inferior temporal quadrant. In the inferior nasal quadrant a solid subretinal mass was present, which reached the equator. At the periphery of the mass a pigmentary dispersion

University Eye Clinic, Ophthalmic Department U.S.L. Ferrara, Italy

411

R. Sampaolesi (ed.), Ultrasonography in Ophthalmology 12, 411–417.
© *1990. Kluwer Academic Publishers, Dordrecht*

was found. In october 1983 he underwent his first echographic examination which was consistent with a nodular scleritis.

A month later he was hospitalized and a new biopsy was performed. The hystological diagnosis was 'Lymphoid pseudotumour'. He was then treated with general and local steroids. In the meantime the serous retinal detachment had disappeared spontaneously. Since then he has had several echographic examinations. No change has occurred in the echographic and ocular findings.

Case 2

BW Caucasian woman 83 years old. Personal history was positive for mastectomy when she was 73. Instable hypertension had LED to a temporary left side paresis. When she was 70 years old she had undergone successful retinal surgery for a retinal detachment in her LE. The patient did not remember the type of surgery. For many months she complained of blurred vision in both eyes. A private practitioner diagnosed a complete retinal detachment in her right eye and an almost complete cataract in the left one. When she was admitted to the hospital, in her own city, ocular findings were as follows.

Visual acuity was finger counting in both eyes with no improvement with lenses. Anterior segments of both eyes were normal except for a slight reduction of the direct pupillary reaction to light on the right side. The lens of the RE showed subcapsular peripheric opacities and sclerosis of the nucleus while the lens of the LE was almost completely opaque. IOP was: shiøtz RE 9.5/5.5 grs, LE 7/5.5 gr. Ophthalmoscopic examination of the RE revealed an almost complete retinal detachment. The retina was more elevated in the inferior quadrants with a few areas of periretinal proliferation. Under the retina, just below the disc, a large area of choroidal degeneration was present. It had a mottled appearance with pigment clustered in small dots and it appeared to be slightly elevated. Because of her previous personal history she was sent for an ultrasound examination in both eyes.

Ecographic findings

A-scan (Kretztechnik, 7200 MA, 8 MHz). While perfoming topographic echography a solid zone was found. The anterior surface of the mass gave origin to a steeply rising echo of high reflectivity, even if the retina was detached. It had a wide base and two spikes and was followed by a series of low to medium echoes. The pathological area finished with a high echo (Figs. 1 and 2). An analysis of the significance of the different echoes is carried out in the discussion.

B-scan (Contact and immersion. Ophthalmoscan 200, Sonometrics

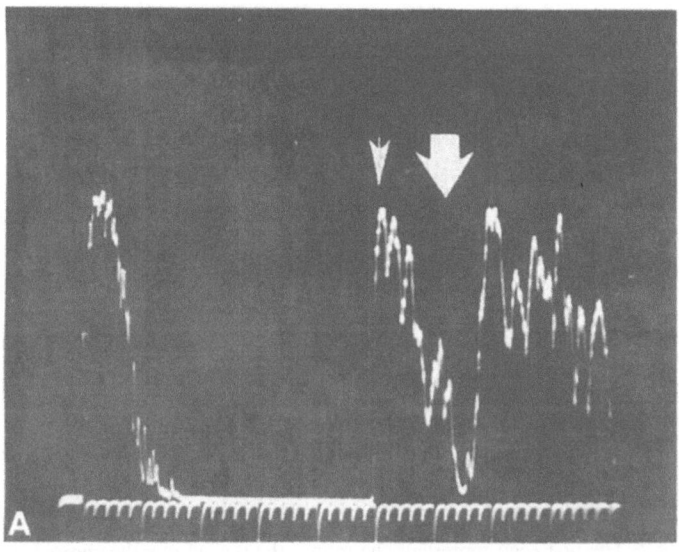

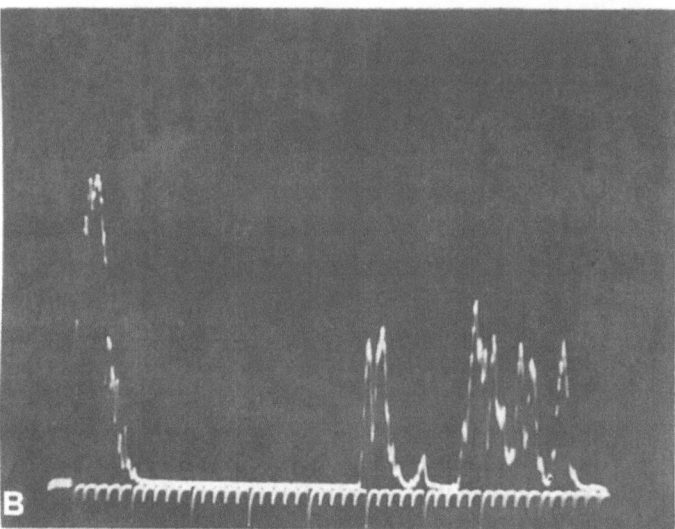

Fig. 1. Case 1. A: A-scan trace at Tissue Sensitivity; B: same trace at TS −24 dB. Thin arrow: vitreo-retinal interface, thick arrow: sclera.

Systems, 7.5 and 10 or 15 MHz). The echographic findings on the B-scan vary according to the characteristic of the equipment. With a B-stable technique a solid area with a hollow space inside was found. It strongly attenuated the sound, thus simulating choroidal excavation (Fig. 3A). With the grey-scale the empty space was no longer empty and a certain deform-

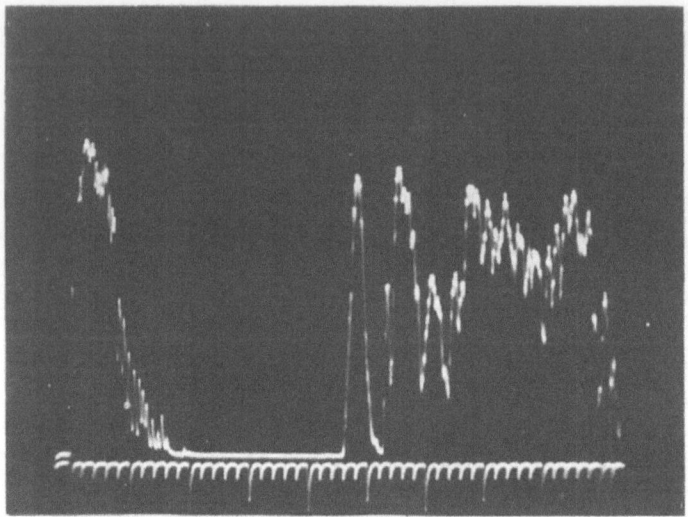

Fig. 2. Case 2. The first echo represents the retina, the second one the choroid, the medium spikes the sclera. Sound attenuation is also present.

ation of the ocular wall was noticed (Figs. 3B, 4A and B) by lowering the system's sensitivity (Fig. 4C) or increasing the probe frequency, the thickness of the anterior surface of the mass became evident (Fig. 3C).

Discussion

The diagnostic key-criteria on the A-scan mainly depends on topographic echography. Particular attention must be paid to the distances of the different echoes which are to be related to the different ocular coats. A measure of the ocular diameters is to be performed in every case but in general the average transverse diameter of an emmetropic eye is around 29–30 μsec. If we consider the A-scan images, especially in Fig. 2, where the retina is detached, the second echo is the anterior surface of the mass.

Therefore the third one should be the sclera, but this possibility is unlikely because if this were the case the sclera would be in a anomalous position as occurs in posterior staphilomas.

In nodular scleritis the anterior echo originates from the retina and choroid together as in choroidal detachment, while the sclera is swollen and gives origin to the series of low spikes. The last echo of the pathological zone represent the interface between the sclera and the Tenon's fascia.

The appearance on the B-scan is that of a 'choroidal mass' but if we compare the acoustic interface of a real choroidal tumour with that of the

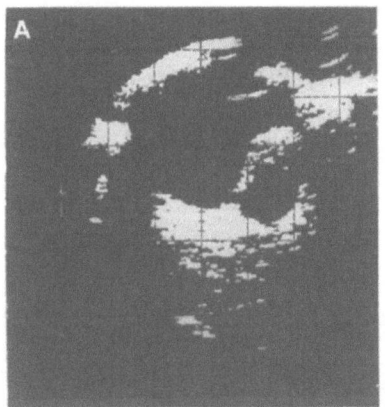

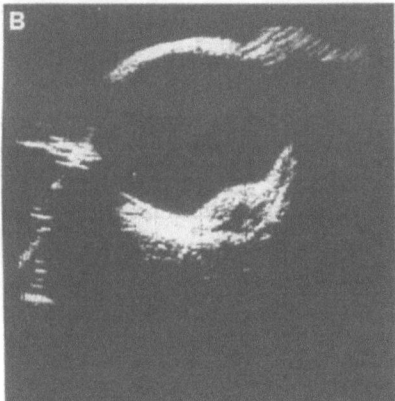

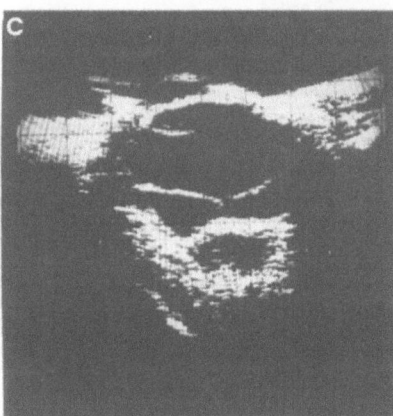

Fig. 3. A: case 1 (B-stable). The sclera is represented by the empty space that simulates a very deep choroidal excavation. B: same case (manufacturer grey-scale at 15 MHz). The mass is not scanned in its thickest aspect. C: case 2 (manufacturer grey-scale at 10 MHz) the choroid is elevated under the total retinal detachment.

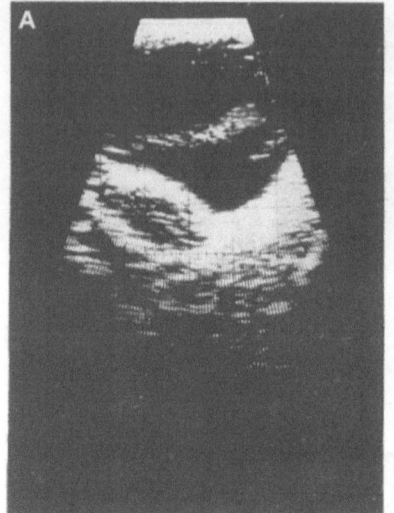

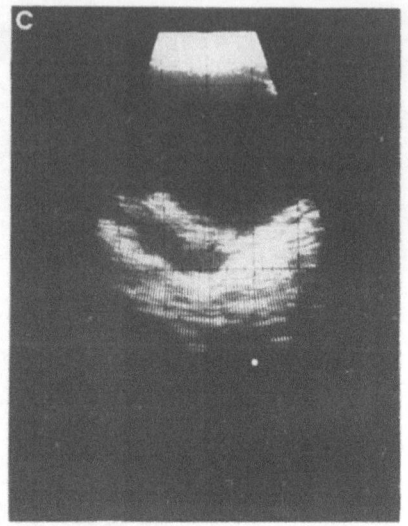

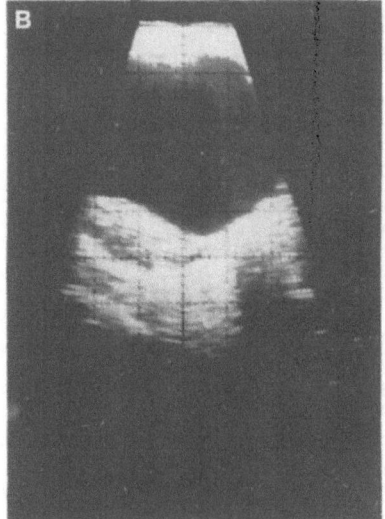

Fig. 4. A: case 2, the ocular wall curvature is altered in the site of
the lesion. B and C: case 1
(Home made grey-scale). On
the left side the image is taken
with the maximum amplification,
on the right at W10 dB.

mass we clearly see that the first echo of the lesion is too thick to be an
interface only (Ossoinig, 1982; Coleman et al., 1977).

In fact it is a normal or thickened choroid. Under this layer the ocular
wall is seen to be deformed by the fusiform enlargement of the sclera. No
other pathology can be echographically confused with brawny scleritis other
than malignant melanoma. Both pathologies have some common pattern
such as the sound attenuation and the 'false' and 'true' choroidal excavation
respectively.

References

Coleman D J, Lizzi F L, Jack R L. 1977. Ultrasonography of the eye and orbit. Lea and Febiger. Philadelphia.

Chang S, Coleman D J, Dallow R. 1980. Trends in ophthalmic ultrasonography. In Kuryak A. Progress in Medical Ultrasound. Excerpta Medica. Amsterdam. p. 279.

Green R L. 1987. Ecographic diagnosis of posterior scleritis. Docum Ophthal. Proc Series 48: 515–519.

Ossoinig K C, Harrie R P. 1983. Diagnosis of intraocular tumors with standardized ecography. In: Lommatzsch P K, Blodi F C (eds.) Intraocular Tumors. Springerverlag, Berlin. p. 154.

Ossoinig K C. 1982. Advances in diagnostic Ultrasound. Proceedings of the 20th International Congress of Ophthalmology. Lippicot Co., Philadelphia, p. 89.

54. Echographic findings in lymphoid hyperplasia of the choroid

VINCENZINA MAZZEO, LUCA RAVALLI and PAOLO PERRI

Introduction

In 1977 Coleman et al. (1977) wrote 'Lymphoid hyperplasia of the choroid may be ultrasonically indistinguishable from an "en planque" melanoma but may be suspected due to greater sound absorption by inflammatory tissue'.

Through a comparison of reports already published in the literature we have tried to discuss the significance of the echographic finding of a case of Benign Reactive Lymphoid Hyperplasia (BRLH) which we have been following.

BRLH is a very rare disease and on our knowledge only two cases have been published (Desroches et al., 1983; Escoffery et al., 1985) since the very extensive paper by Ryan et al. (1972) and Shields' book on tumours (1983).

Because of the rarity of the disease the history and the clinical findings will be widely reported.

Case report

A 55-year-old white woman was referred in August 1987 to undergo an echographic examination. Five months previously she had complained of a painless reduction in visual acuity, a diminished palpebral fissura and redness of her right eye.

In a previous consultation an increased intraocular pressure (IOP) had been found and she was given timolol 0.50% twice a day.

Another ophthalmologist later found a retinal cyst at the pars plana at 1 o.c. in the same eye.

When seen for the first time visual acuity was 6/10 with correction in her right eye and 10/10 in her left one.

IOP was 19 mmHg in the right eye. No proptosis was present.

The palpebral fissura in the right side was reduced.

University Eye Clinic, University of Ferrara, Ferrara, Italy

R. Sampaolesi (ed.), Ultrasonography in Ophthalmology 12, 419–425.

420

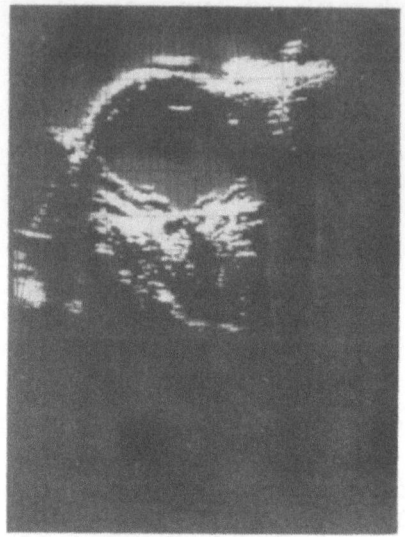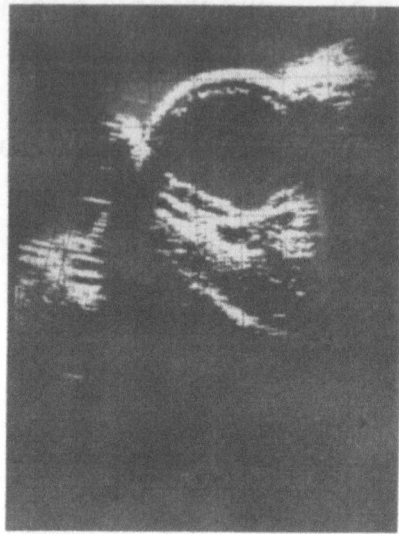

Fig. 1. BRLH. Immersion B-scan technique (Ophthalmoscan 200, 10 MHz). On the left: shallow anterior chamber. Anteriorly thick choroid resembles a shallow choroidal detachment. Posteriorly the choroid is irregularly thickened. On the right side: in this section the extrascleral areas are clearly depicted.

The episcleral veins were dilated and two subconjunctival nodules were present on the upper half of the globe. They were of a salmon colour.

The anterior chamber was shallow. No other pathologic change was present in the anterior segment.

Fundoscopic examination showed a slight nasalization of the retinal vessels at the disc.

There was a diffuse yellowish thickening of the choroid. Some point pigmented line followed the papillo macular bundle. At the periphery some patches of choroidal pigment were present. At the biomicroscopic examination of the fundes the ora serrata could clearly be seen and the choroid was also thickened. At 1 o.c. a cyst of the pars plana was present.

The left eye was normal.

Fluorescein angiography showed a choroideal hyperfluorescence due to alteration of the pigment epithelium temporal to the disc and in the superior temporal quadrant. In late phases fluorescence from deep layers was present along with multiple radiating lines of blocked fluorescence. The echographic examination is widely described in the text. CT scanning showed a thickening of the ocular walls especially in the temporal side and around the optic nerve that was normal. No contrast enhancement existed.

The clinical findings led us to suspect the diagnosis of BRLH. Systemic evaluation revealed only an increase in T lymphocytes in the circulating blood; a lowering of the ratio T4/T8 due to an increase of the T8 component and a mild lymphoid infiltration of the bone marrow. A biopsy of the subconjunctival nodules revealed well differentiated mature lymphocytes.

She was then prescribed oral Dexametazone to be tapered rapidly. At the end of the therapy only minor changes were noticed both on echography and fluorescein angiography. After that two follow-ups were made at a distance of 2 and 3 months respectively. After the second one it was decided to try local steroids. Two doses of 80 and 60 mgr of retrobulbar Dexametazone retard were given with an interval of 15 days. Again only a slight amelioration was noticed. In February 88 a worsening of the clinical signs and of the echographic findings was noticed. The situation remained unchanged for 4 months then the patient underwent radiation therapy. Only after 1000 rads did the situation improve in a very satisfactory way.

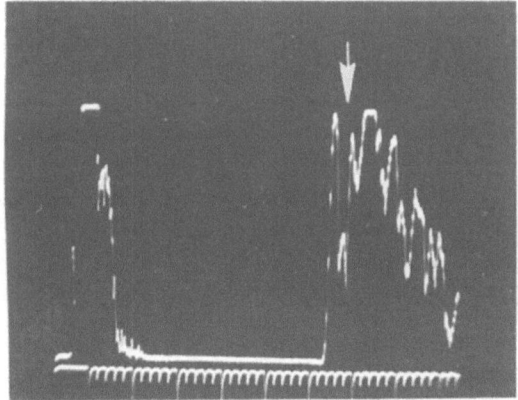

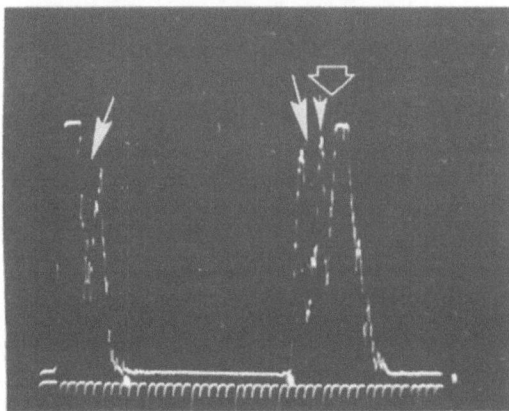

Fig. 2. BRLH. A-scan (Kretztechnik 7200 MA, 8 MHz). On the top: the thickened choroid shows medium reflectivity (thick arrow). At the bottom: the choroidal thickening is shown by the thick arrows, the sclera and the extrascleral extensions by the thin and the empty arrows respectively.

Echographic findings

In our opinion B-scan images were more useful for diagnostic purposes in our case. In fact with the immersion technique (Ophthalmoscan 200. Former Sonometrics SSI NY) it was possible to visualize immediately the thickening of the whole choroid from the ciliary body to the disc (Fig. 1 left). The thickening was slightly irregular. In fact the choroid was thicker near the disc where a 'pseudo cupping' of the disc occurred (Mazzeo, 1987). Two extrascleral zones were seen around the optic nerve and one was present on the temporal side (Fig. 1 right).

On the A-scan (Kretztechnik 7200 MA. Former Kretztechnik Austria). The choroidal thickening was also visible (Fig. 2—(top) and (bottom)). Only a slight amelioration was visible after general and local steroids so, when an increase of the extrabulbar involvement was seen, (Figs. 3 and 4) radiation therapy was started. After only 1000 rads a reduction in the choroidal thickening and the extrabulbar involvement was found (Fig. 5).

Discussion

Ocular involvement in BRLH changes from case to case as Ryan et al. (1972) amply demostrated on their 19 cases (22 eyes).

The lymphoid tissue invades in a different way one or more sites of the uvea and/or the orbit immediately outside the eyewall.

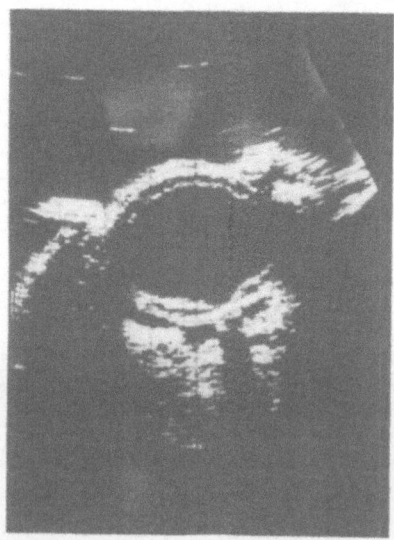

Fig. 3. BRLH. Examination dated February 1988. In comparison with the image of Fig. 1 an enlargement of the extrascleral extensions is noticed.

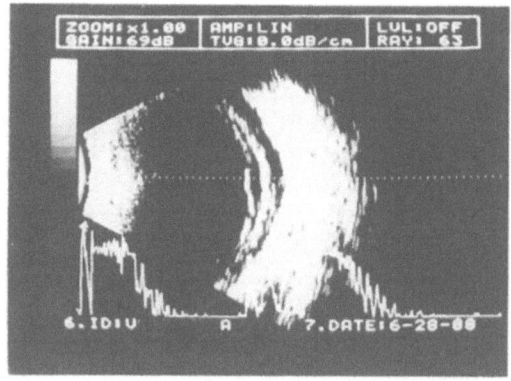

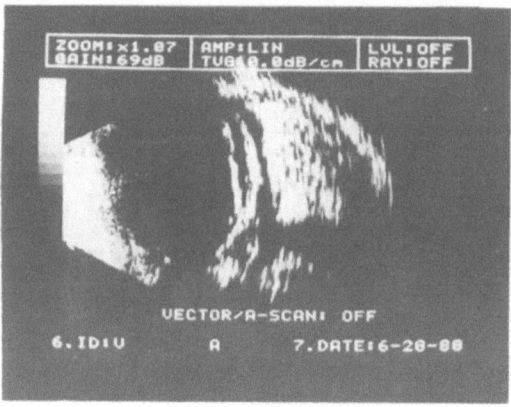

Fig. 4. BRLH. Examination dated February 1988. (Sonomed Mod. B 3000 Sector scan, 10 MHz).

The more cited differential diagnosis of BRLH is that of diffuse melanoma of the choroid, more or less amelanotic and/or a ring melanoma.

In fact Ryan et al. (1972) based their paper on the pathologic specimens of eyes enucleated because they were suspected of harbouring a choroidal melanoma.

Many other differential diagnosis are cited in the literature, especially those with the malignant forms of lymphomatous tumors, but the latter is only made on the bases of biopsies and clinical course.

From a strictly echographic point of view it seems the we cannot confirm the already cited description by Coleman et al. (1977).

In the only other case described by Desroches et al. (1983) it seems that ultrasound while useful cannot completely rule out a malignant melanoma (mm) in the sense that on both echographic techniques some patterns characteristic of mm were present whereas others were not. On A-scan a

424

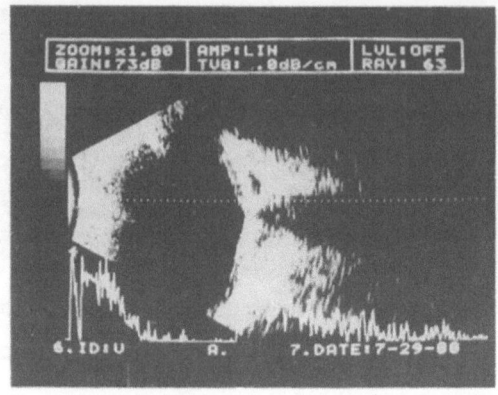

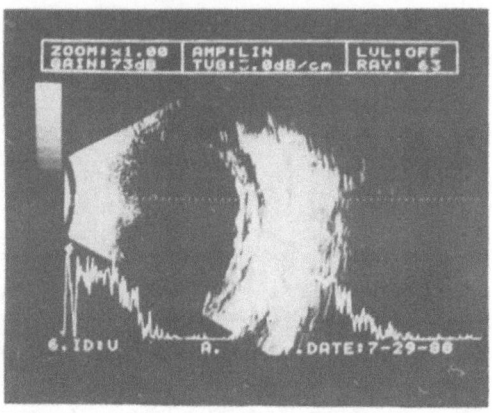

Fig. 5. BRLH after radiation therapy. Same sections of Fig. 4. A noticeable reduction of the choroidal thickening and the extrabulbar tissue is present.

low and regular internal reflectivity was present in both internal and extra-bulbar areas, on B-scan the areas were empty when examined with the Bronson Equipment and low reflective when examined with the Ocuscan. No spontaneous vascular activity was seen and the sclera seemed intact on both A- and B-scans.

In our case, instead, only one A-scan echogram was thick enough to evaluate the internal reflectivity of the lesion that appeared to be medium. On B-scan the images of the total ocular involvement and of the extrascleral areas were so well depicted that we believe these images to be of diagnostic significance if the ocular involvement occurring in BRLH is taken into consideration.

References

Coleman D J, Lizzi F L, Jack R L. 1977. Ultrasonography of the eye and orbit. Lea and Febiger. Philadelphia.

Desroches G, Abrams G W, Gass J D. 1983. Reactive lymphoid hyperplasia of the uvea. Arch Ophthalmol 101: 725–728.

Escoffery R F, Bobrow J C, Smith M E. 1985. Exudative retinal detachment secondary to orbital and intraocular benign lymphoid hyperplasia. Retina 5: 91–93.

Mazzeo V. 1987. Ecografia dell'apparato oculare — Testo Atlante. Fogliazza Editore, Milano.

Ryan S J, Zimmerman L E, King F M. 1978. Reactive lymphoid hyperplasia. Tr Am Acad Ophth & Otol 76: 652–671.

Sheilds J A. 1983. Intraocular Tumors. Mosby St. Louis.

55. Diffuse lymphoid infiltration of the uvea and periocular tissues

A. LOMBARDI*, J. O. CROXATTO*, and A. ZAMBRANO

Introduction

In 1967, Gass [7], described the clinical presentation and histopathology of an apparently non-neoplastic inflammatory pseudotumor of the uveal tract whose main characteristic was its diffuse thickening due to a lymphoplasmacytic infiltration which extended to the retrobulbar tissue and the optic nerve.

Later, in 1971, Ryan et al. [11], made a retrospective study of 21 eyes in 19 patients from the files of the Registry of Ophthalmic Pathology of the AFIP and set down the more common clinical signs, the histopathologic characteristics and the most frequent misdiagnoses of an entity they called reactive lymphoid hyperplasia.

In 1982 Desroches et al. [5], presented the clinical findings resulting from ultrasonographic and computed tomographic studies of a patient who presented that disease and whose correct diagnosis avoided enucleation.

In more recent studies, this entity, which had previously been considered inflammatory in nature, has been considered of neoplastic nature [8–9]. Consequently, Jakobiec proposes calling it lymphoid infiltration or lymphoid tumor of the uvea.

We wish to present here the clinical and echographic findings of two patients who presented this disease, both of whom were diagnosed by histopathologic means — in the first case, through the study of an enucleated eyeball with a supposed diagnosis of diffuse malignant melanoma of the choroid; in the second, through a study of the material of an iridocyclectomy performed because a ciliary body melanoma was suspected.

Case 1

A 65 year-old man consulted his ophthalmologist in March 1974 complaining of a decrease in vision in his right eye. His visual acuity was 20/40 in the

* Centro Oftalmológico Malbran and Fundación Oftalmólogica, Argentina Jorge Malbran. Parera 162, Buenos Aires, Argentina.

R. Sampaolesi (ed.), Ultrasonography in Ophthalmology 12, 427–437.
© 1990. Kluwer Academic Publishers, Dordrecht

right eye and 20/20 in the left. The right eye had a posterior subcapsular cataract while the anterior chamber, fundus and intraocular pressure reported normal. The left eye was normal. In April 1975 the patient returned for a check-up. His visual acuity had decreased in the right eye to light perception. The cataract was now total, the anterior chamber narrower, and the intraocular pressure by applanation tonometry was 26 mm Hg in the right eye and 16 mm Hg in the left. The left eye remained normal. The intraocular pressure improved with medication and the patient underwent an uneventful intracapsular cataract extraction in June 1975. During the immediate post operative period, a partial exudative non-rhegmatogenous retinal detachment was observed and the pars plana could be seen without scleral depression. Intraocular pressure without medication was 20 mm Hg in the right eye and 14 mm Hg in the left, 8 mg of dexamethasone acetate and 3 mg of dexamethasone phosphate were administered during three weeks, producing a partial improvement of the retinal detachment. The ophthalmoscopy showed a yellow-white diffuse choroidal infiltration which was more elevated at the posterior pole leaving the optic disk of normal appearance, recessed. Scattered at the posterior pole, there were pigmentary clumps with clear edges and a retinal detachment in the lower quadrants. Fluorescein angiography disclosed patches of early hyperfluorescence mixed with small spots of hypofluorescence corresponding to the pigmentary clumps, and leakage into the vitreous cavity in the venous phase of angiogram (Fig. 1).

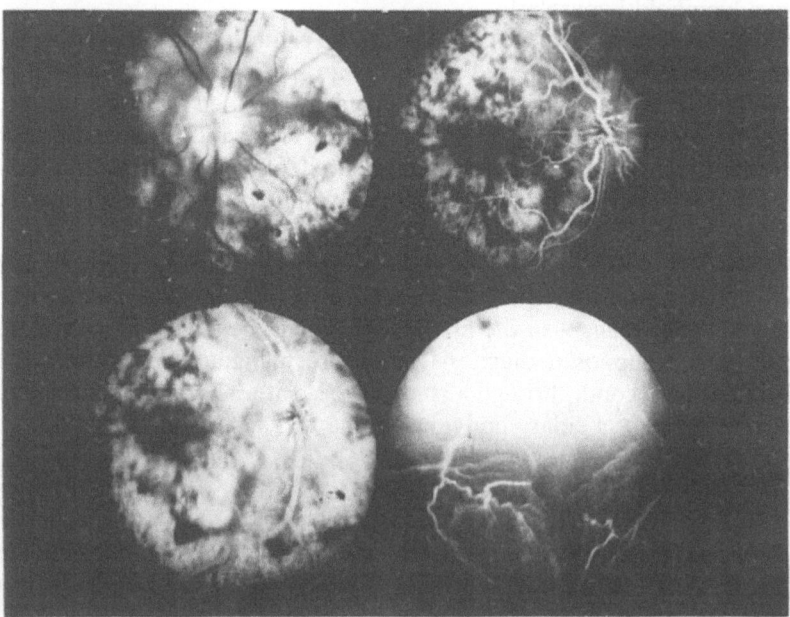

Fig. 1. Fluorescein angiography discloses patchy early hyperfluorescence mixed with small spots of hypofluorescence, retinal detachment, and leakage into the vitreous cavity.

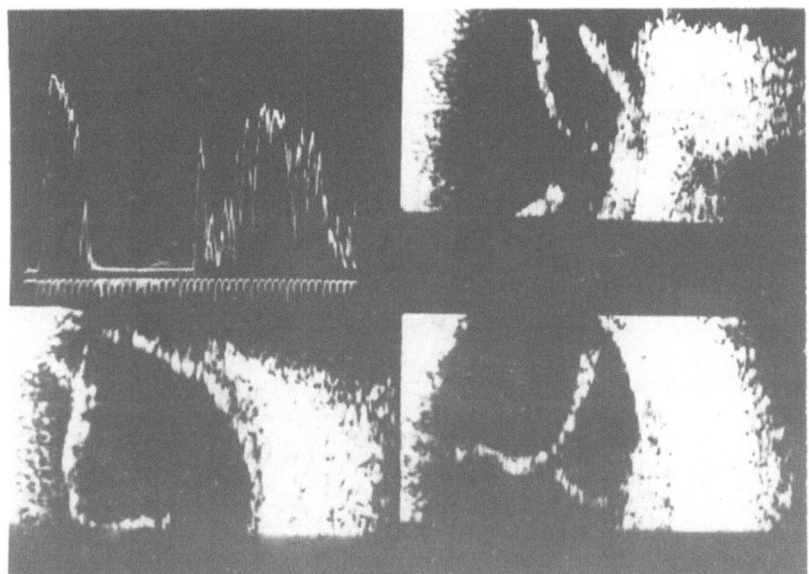

Fig. 2. B scan shows solid choroidal thickening and bullous retinal detachment. Standardized A mode reveales regular, low reflectivity echoes without spontaneous vascular movements.

In August 1977, the retinal detachment was total, the anterior chamber had become narrow and the intraocular pressure had risen to 24 mm Hg in the right eye. At this time an ultrasonography was requested. The B-scan examination with the Bronson Turner unit showed a solid diffuse choroidal thickening which was more pronounced at the posterior pole and gradually got thinner as it reached the periphery while in front of it there was a mobile, bullous retinal detachment. Standardized A-scan examination with the Kretztechnick 7200 MA confirmed the solid nature of the lesion which had low reflectivity and regular echoes with no spontaneous vascular activity (Fig. 2). Faced with the belief that it was a diffuse choroidal melanoma, the eye was enucleated by the referring ophthalmologist, who, during surgery, found a jelly-like tissue adhering to some parts of the episclera. Gross examination of the eye showed an aphakic right eye with a bullous retinal detachment and a diffuse thickening of the choroid which was greater at the posterior pole (Fig. 3).

Light microscopy examination revealed that the lesion was made up of a diffuse proliferation of lymphocytes, plasma cells, plasmacytoid lymphocytes, Russel and Dutcher bodies. The extrascleral extension had occurred in two different ways: one, by means of emissaries; the other, through a direct invasion of the sclera which had become disrupted by the lymphocytic infiltrate (Fig. 4). The patient has been followed to date with periodical examinations, with no systemic disease ever having been found.

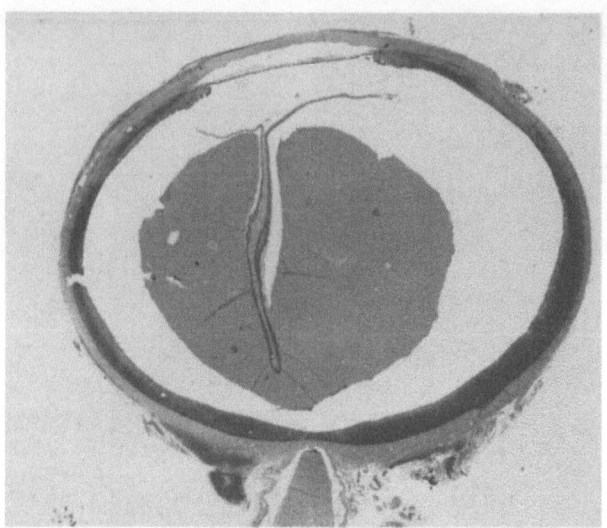

Fig. 3. Low power view of the enucleated eye disclosing diffuse choroidal infiltration and retrobulbar extension. The retina is totally detached.

Case 2

A 30 year-old woman consulted her ophthalmologist in March 1983 complaining of redness of her right eye. Examination revealed a thickening and congestion of the anterior episcleral tissue which extended from the lower sclerocorneal limbus to the fornix. It was painless to the touch and the conjunctiva slid over it freely. Her visual acuity in both eyes was 20/20 and the rest of the exam proved normal. She was prescribed topical Dexamethasone but when no improvement was seen, a biopsy was performed revealing a lymphoid infiltrate of unknown nature. Since the patient lived 1600 km away from the place of treatment, she could only make sporadic return visits.

In March 1984 she returned after noticing some blurring in the vision of her right eye. During biomicroscopy, a ciliary body tumor was detected at 6 o'clock which narrowed the anterior chamber angle and displaced the lens upward and forward. Her visual acuity was 20/25 and 20/20 in the right and left eyes respectively and the fundus was normal.

Two months later an iridocyclectomy was performed in order to extirpate the tumor, and the histophathologic study disclosed reactive lymphoid hyperplasia. The medical workup, blood chemistry and bone marrow biopsy were all normal.

In December 1984, she noticed a decrease in the visual acuity of her right eye, now only 20/70, and the fundus examination disclosed a dark yellowish choroidal thickening encircled by the temporal vascular arcades. Fluorescein

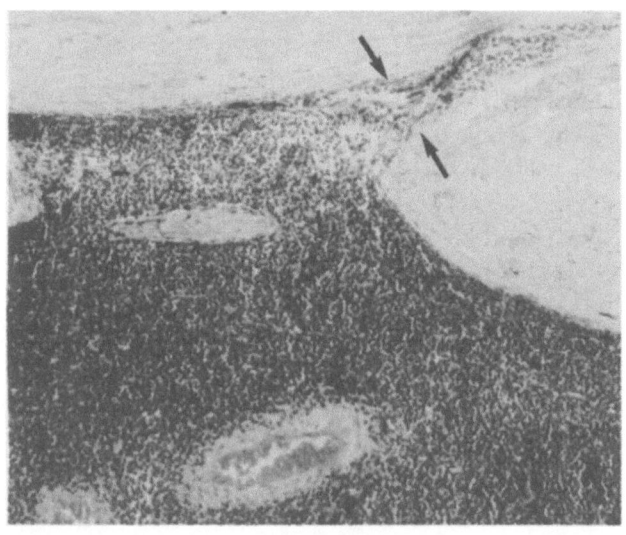

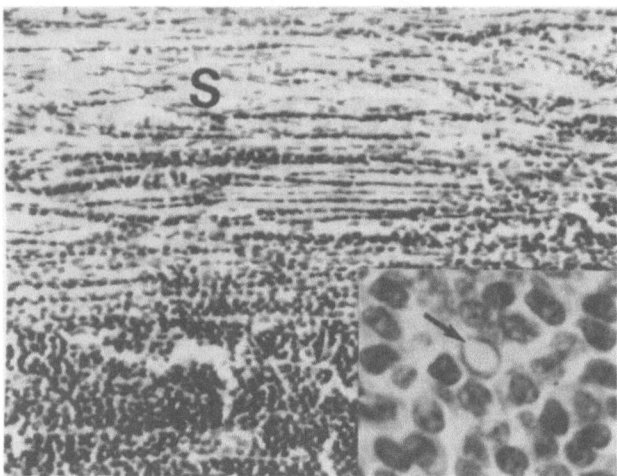

Fig. 4. (Top) lymphocytic infiltrate extending to the orbit through scleral emissaries (between arrows).
Bottom: lymphocytes infiltrating the sclera (S) at the ecuator. Inset, the infiltrate is composed by lymphocytes and plasma cells disclosing Dutcher bodies (arrow).

angiography revealed, in the early stages, an irregular filling of the choroid in the affected area, which was encircled by fine choroidal folds, a mottled hypofluorescence in the papillomacular bundle which extended under the lower temporal arcade, and a retinochoroidal anastomosis of a branch of the lower temporal artery. In the late phases there was neither leakage nor dye retention (Fig. 5). The patient was medicated with 24 mg of methylpredni-

432

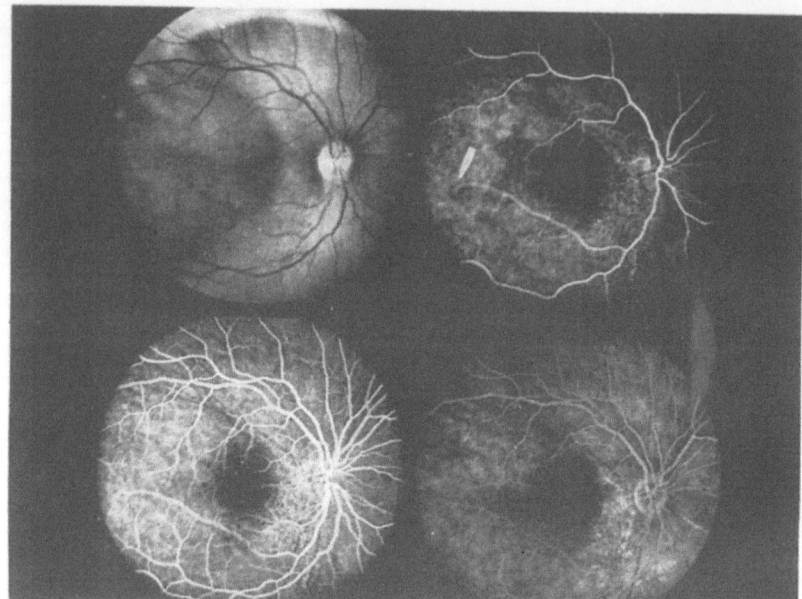

Fig. 5. (Top left) Red free photograph highlights the lesion. (Top right) Fluorescein angiography shows an irregular filling of the choroid in the affected area, which is encircled by fine choroidal folds, and a retinochoroidal anastomosis (arrow). (Bottom right) Nor dye retention or leakage is seen.

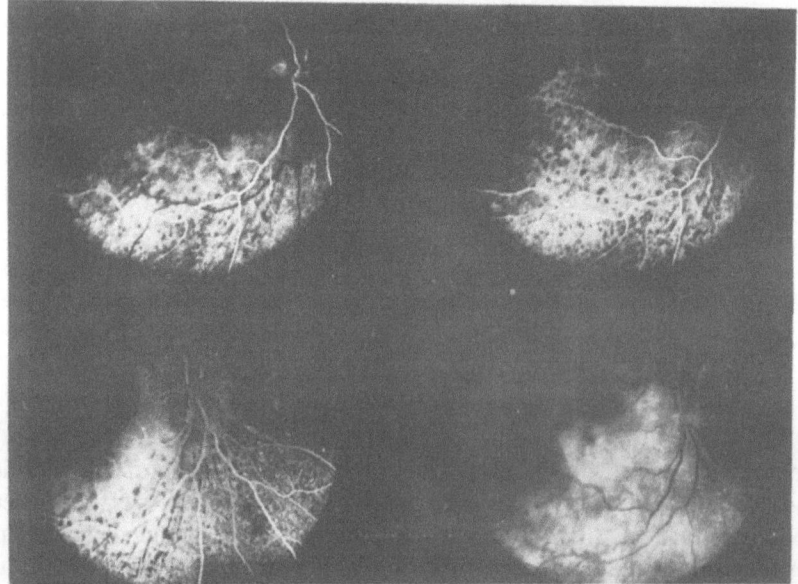

Fig. 6. Fluorescein angiography shows pigmentary disturbances throughout the posterior pole and late dye retention with leakage in the macular area.

solone daily but she quit taking it after a month due to gastritis with no improvement in her condition.

Her condition slowly deteriorated until her visual acuity was 20/400 in the right eye and 20/20 in the left by July 1986. Fluorescein angiography showed a manifest worsening: the pigmentary disturbances extended throughout the posterior pole and in the macular area, late dye retention with leakage was observed (Fig. 6). Three months later a computed tomography was performed, with and without contrast enhancement, revealing a diffuse thickening of the posterior scleral-uveal rim. In July 1987, fluorescein angiography registered little change and macular cistoid degeneration was found. Ultrasonography was performed with an Ophthascan S. The B-mode revealed a diffuse solid choroidal thickening which was more pronounced at the posterior pole, with an area of retrobulbar sonolucency surrounding the optic nerve, while at the equator a line of sonolucency occupying Tenon's space was also found. Standardized A-mode confirmed the solid nature of the choroidal thickening, of low to medium reflectivity, with regular echoes and no spontaneous vascular movements, as well as the retrobulbar infiltration (Fig. 7). The choroidal thickening measured 3.5 mm at the posterior pole and 2.7 at the equator.

The CT scan remained unchanged while in a new clinical workup cervical adenopathy was discovered. Histopathologic examination of the biopsy

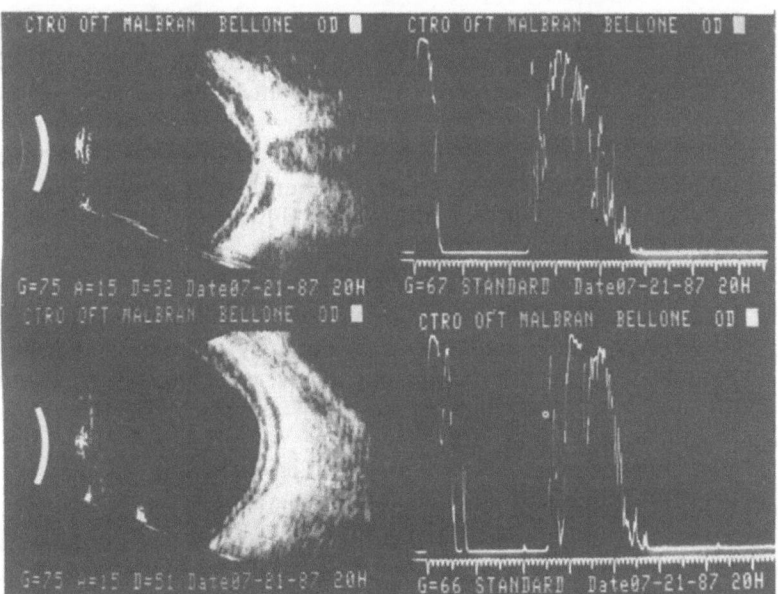

Fig. 7. (Top left) B scan revealed a diffuse solid choroidal thickening with an area of retrobulbar sonolucency surrounding the optic nerve. (Bottom left) a line of sonolucency occupies the Tenon's space at the equator. (Top and Bottom right) Standardized A mode shows the lesion with low to medium reflectivity.

434

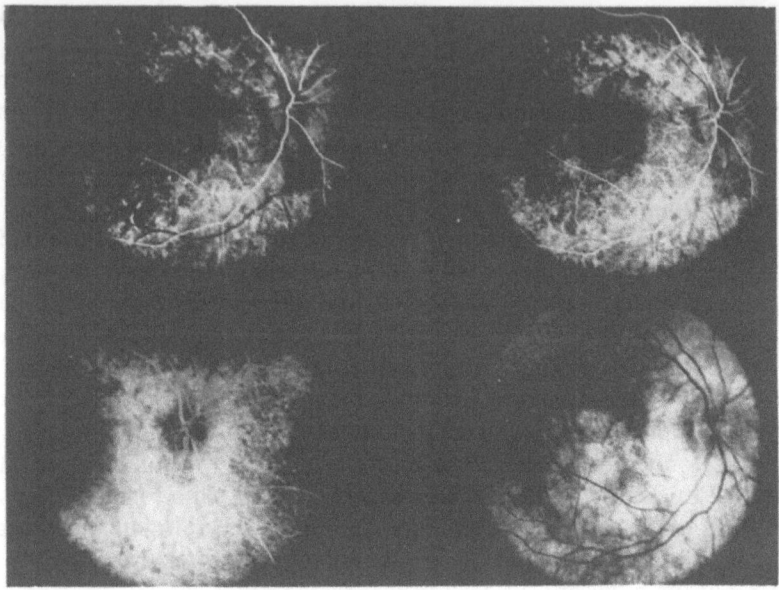

Fig. 8. Fluorescein angiography reveales resolution of late dye retention and leakage.

specimen revealed a lymphoid hyperplasia. Six months later, the patient returned evidencing a spontaneous improvement in the anterior epibulbar component while fluorescein angiography also registered an improvement since the late dye retention and the leakage had diminished even though the diffuse alteration of the pigment epithelium persisted (Fig. 8).

Her visual acuity remained at 20/200, probably due to the cistoid macular edema.

Her last check-up was July 19, 1988, at which time further improvement in the fundus was seen although some yellowish infiltrates persisted in the macular and inframacular areas. Ultrasonography revealed a reduction in the choroidal thickening to 1.5 mm, the almost complete disappearance of the retrobulbar infiltration, and an increase in choroidal reflectivity over the previous echographic findings (Fig. 9).

Discussion

Lymphoid infiltration of the uvea and periocular tissues is a highly infrequent entity considered inflammatory in nature prior to studies by Mauriello et al. and Jakobiec et al. in which it was described as neoplastic in nature since, in the cases studied, the uveal infiltrates presented morphological and immunohistological characteristics of well differentiated lymphoplasmacytic malignant lymphomas [9] or low grade tumors [8]. There are, however,

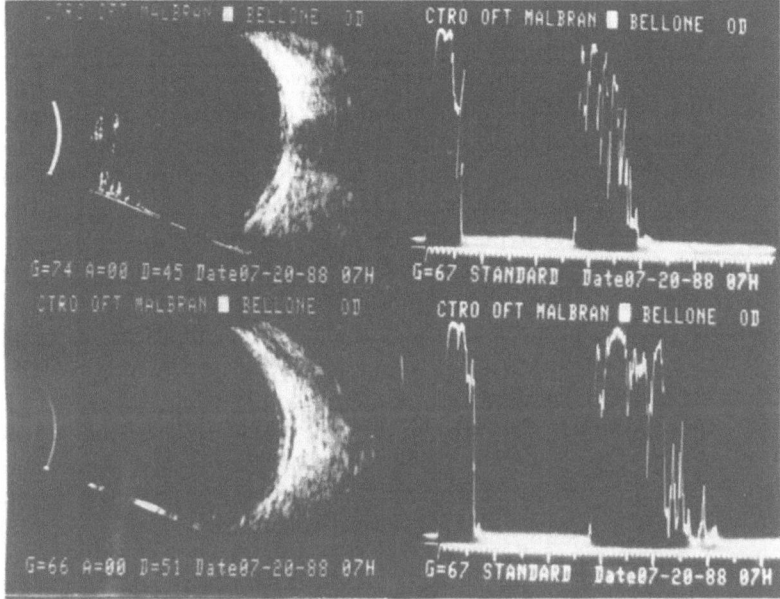

Fig. 9. B mode shows reduction of the choroidal thickening and almost complete disappearance of retrobulbar infiltration. Standardized A-mode shows that the choroid is thinner and more reflective.

certain doubts about its nature due to the fact that it is rarely associated with any systemic disease, and the prognosis is good.

This entity is usually unilateral with the first symptoms appearing in middle age; the youngest case reported is that of a 30 year-old woman [11], an age which coincides with the second case we have reported.

The most common initial symptom is reduced visual acuity, which could be due to the choroidal infiltration itself, to the secondary retinal detachment or, as Gass suggests [7], to the cellular infiltration of the optic nerve. The choroidal infiltration generally becomes manifest in the form of multiple yellowish patches with indistinct edges at the posterior pole, and which may be confluent, adopting the appearance of a creamy diffuse choroidal thickening. While the presence of these infiltrates is one of the outstanding characteristics of this entity, in some cases we feel that the earliest sign may be the anterior epibulbar infiltration witnessed in 2 of the 3 cases presented by Jakobiec and in the second case we have presented.

When the lymphoid infiltration invades the anterior choroid, the pars plana can be seen without scleral depression; likewise, when this infiltration invades the ciliary body, can be mistaken for a ciliary body melanoma. Exudative retinal detachment is present in a high percentage of the cases [6] and, in more than half of them, is associated with glaucoma. Some patients can present proptosis due to the retrobulbar infiltration but its absence does not leave out this possibility as has been demonstrated in the cases we have presented as well as those presented by Ryan, Jakobiec, Desroches, etc.

The most common ancillary tests employed are the computed tomography, the fluorescein angiography and the ultrasonography. In the computed tomography with injection of contrast material, a thickening of the scleral-uveal rim, a reduction in the size of the vitreous cavity due to the infiltrate and the presence of extraocular foci can be seen. The fluorescein angiography shows early hyperfluorescence, pigmentary mobility, dye retention in the lesions and, occcassionally, leakage causing cistoid macular edema. In the second case we have presented, chorioretinal anastomosis was also found.

Without a doubt, the most useful ancillary test for a correct diagnosis is the ultrasonography. The findings are as follows: 1) solid choroidal thickening of low reflectivity with regular echoes which indicate homogeneous infiltration. There are no spontaneous vascular movements. Jakobiec et al. using immersion technique, showed a thickening of the ciliary body and of the anterior ocular tunics. 2) Extrascleral foci were seen like retroscleral sonolucent spaces generally located in the vecinity of the optic nerve and presenting the same reflectivity as the choroidal infiltrate. In the equatorial region, they adopt a linear shape and occupy Tenon's space. 3) Normal sclera: Although this finding has been commonly reported as a characteristic of this entity histopathologically we could observe in case 1 that, at the equatorial level, the sclera was disrupted by the lymphocytic infiltrate. Therefore, from now on, a more careful search should be made to determine if such a scleral invasion is present.

Two types of treatment have been used: local and systemic therapy with corticosteroids [5–8], and low doses of ocular radiotherapy [6–8]; both with good results. In the second case we have presented, the patient suspended the corticotherapy, with a progressive worsening of her condition during a year and a half. After another year and a half, there was spontaneous improvement without any type of treatment.

Differential diagnosis

Diffuse malignant melanoma

Angiographically it is possible to see intratumoral vascularization and echographically, spontaneous vascular movements. The state of the sclera is not a distinctive sign since intrascleral and transcleral invasion may be seen in both diseases.

Scleritis

The anterior epibulbar extension may be mistaken for anterior scleritis but the absence of pain is distinctive. When posterior scleritis adopts the shape of a localized mass, it is the same color as the neighbouring tissue and has a normal choroidal vascular pattern. Ultrasonography with the B-mode shows flattening of the normal posterior concavity of the eyeball, thickening of the posterior layers of the eye and edema of Tenon's space. A mode ultrasonography shows scleral thickening with high amplitude internal spikes and retrobulbar edema [2, 3, 4, 10].

Acute multifocal placoid pigment epiteliopathy

In the posterior pole, yellowish white multifocal placoid lesions are also seen but this disease is bilateral, generally affects young people, evolves in a few weeks and does not contain choroidal thickening or extraocular extension.

References

[1] Beasley H. 1961. Lymphosarcoma of the choroid. Am J Ophthalmol 51: 1294–1296.
[2] Benson W E, Shields J A, Tasman W et al. 1979. Posterior scleritis. A cause of diagnostic confusion. Arch Ophthalmol 97: 1482–1486.
[3] Benson W E. 1988. Posterior scleritis. Surv Ophthalmol 32: 297–316.
[4] Cappaert W E, Purnell E W, Frank K E. 1977. Use of B sector scan ultrasound in the diagnosis of benign choroidal folds. Am J Ophthal. 84: 375–379.
[5] Desroches G, Abrams G W, Gass J D M. 1983. Reactive lymphoid Hyperplasia of the uvea a case with ultrasonographic and computed tomographic studies. Arch Ophthalmol 101: 725–728.
[6] Escoffery R F, Bobrow J C, Smith M E. 1985. Exudative retinal detachment secondary to orbital and intraocular benign lymphoid hyperplasia. Retina 5: 91–93.
[7] Gass J D M. 1967. Retinal detachment and narrow angle-glaucoma secondary to inflammatory pseudotumor of the uveal tract. Am J Ophthalmol 64: 612–621.
[8] Jakobiec F A, Sacks E, Kronish J W, Weiss T, Smith M. 1987. Multifocal static creamy choroidal infiltrates. Opthalmology 94: 397–406.
[9] Mauriello J A Jr, Langloss J, Weiner J, Zimmerman L. 1982. A clinico-pathologic and immunohistologic study of lymphoproliferative lesions of the uveal tract. ARVO Abstracts. Invest Ophthalmol Vis Sci 22 (Suppl): 171.
[10] Rochels R, Reis G. 1980. Echography in posterior scleritis. Klin Monatsbl Augenheilkd 177: 611–613.
[11] Ryan J R, Zimmerman L E, King F M. 1972. Reactive Lymphoid Hyperplasia. Trans Am Acad Ophthalmol Otolaryngol 76: 652–671.

Physics and techniques

56. In vivo determination of sound velocity in eye media

G. L. VAN DER HEIJDE, J. WEBER and G. TIESINGA

Introduction

Echography is an important technique to characterize tissue in the eye. Acoustic parameters provide information about the attenuation of the ultrasound and reflectivity of bounderies between tissue of different acoustic impedance. The velocity of sound in the lens is of special interest and may be used for calculation of axial length needed for preoperative determination of intraocular lens power. Several authors found that the velocity of ultrasound in the lens was not a fixed value, as in the anterior chamber or vitreous (1532 m/sec, Jansson and Kock, 1962), but varied depending on its opacity. Coleman et al. (1975) presented a study on 50 cataractous human lenses, in which the velocity of sound was found to be 1629 m/sec on the average, 11 m/sec slower than that of normal adult lenses. They also postulated a trend of decreasing sound velocity in the lens with increasing age. Pallikaris and Gruber (1981) measured the velocity of ultrasound in 37 human lenses shortly after intracapsular lens extraction and related pre-operatively made slit lamp photographs of the cataract to the velocity of ultrasound in the excised lenses. Their results show a velocity of 1641.35 m/sec on the average, a decrease of sound velocity in lenses with nuclear sclerosis and an increase in lenses with opacity of the posterior capsule. In contrast with these findings, Loffredo et al. (1983) observed, in an analogous experimental set-up, an increase of the ultrasound velocity in cataracts with nuclear sclerosis. Measurements of the forementioned authors were performed in vitro: the time for sound to travel through the excised lens supported in saline bath was compared with the time for sound to travel through an equivalent thickness of saline alone. Furthermore, it has been shown by Willard (1947) that ultrasound velocity is extremely sensitive to temperature changes. Therefore, special care must be taken to keep the excised lens in condition and to control temperature and other physical

Department for Medical Physics, Free University, Van der Boechorststraat 7, 1081 BT Amsterdam, The Netherlands

R. Sampaolesi (ed.), Ultrasonography in Ophthalmology 12, 441–447.

parameters which might influence the measurement. Measurements of ultrasound velocity in the intact eye are difficult to perform and are, up to now, not described in the literature. In this paper we present a method to determine the velocity of ultrasound in the living eye. A necessary condition is that the subject has at least a minimum of accommodation left.

Methods

Our method is based on comparing the time needed for sound to travel through the eye in the accommodating and non accommodating eye.

During accommodation the thickness of the lens increases maximally about 0.5 mm. This process is accomplished by rearranging elastic fibers within in the lens (Koretz and Handelman, 1982). One may suppose therefore that sound velocity in the lens does not change during accommodation.

The increase in lens thickness (Δd), can be expressed as the product of the sound velocity in the lens (v_2) multiplied by the incremental time to travel through the lens (Δt_2) and equals the decrease of the length of the occupied aqueous humour (sound velocity v_1). Or, remembering that tissue thickness should be multiplied by two to obtain transit time:

$$v_2 \cdot \Delta t_2 = v_1 \cdot \Delta t = 2 \cdot \Delta d. \qquad (1)$$

The transit time Δt in aqueous cannot be measured directly but can be obtained by a roundabout way. During accommodation also other intraocular distances will change: the anterior chamber depth (AC) and to a less extent the length of the vitreous decrease. For a complete mathematical description also alterations of the axial length during accommodation are taken into account. Comparing two accommodation settings, differences in transit time in AC (Δt_1), lens (Δt_2), vitreous (Δt_3) and axial length (ΔL) should fulfil the following equation:

$$v_1 \cdot \Delta t_1 + v_2 \cdot \Delta t_2 + v_3 \cdot \Delta t_3 = 2 \cdot \Delta L. \qquad (2)$$

Sound velocity in vitreous (v_3) is equal to that in aqueous (v_1) (Jansson and Kock, 1962). Rearranging Equation (2), one obtains:

$$(\Delta t_1 + \Delta t_3) = -\frac{v_2}{v_1} \Delta t_2 + \frac{2 \cdot \Delta L}{v_1}. \qquad (3)$$

Substitution of the last part of Equation (1) results in:

$$(\Delta t_1 + \Delta t_3) = -\frac{v_2}{v_1} \cdot (1 - \frac{\Delta L}{\Delta d}) \Delta t_2 \qquad (4)$$

When axial length does not change during accommodation, so $\Delta L = 0$, Equation (4) will reduce to (1). In that case the slope of the regression line of the transit time of (AC + vitreous) versus transit time through the lens will give v_2/v_1. Sound velocity in aqueous of 1532 m/sec is generally accepted as a standard by most investigators, so regression analysis with help of Equation (4) will give the sound velocity in the lens.

In the discussion the implications for $\triangle L \neq 0$ will be given.

Changes of intraocular transit times during accommodation were measured using high resolution A-scan echography. Figure 1 shows the principle of our technique. After an adjustable time delay following the moment an echo of interest exceeded a trigger level, elapsed time was linearly transformed into a voltage until the next echo. In such a way small changes corresponding to about 2 μm tissue thickness may be registered. Technical details of this method are described elsewhere (De Vries et al., 1987).

A mini ultrasound transducer with a frequency of 10 MHz was built in an eye cup that could be sucked to the sclera.

The subject voluntary changed the fixation of his contralateral eye. Because accommodation of both eyes is coupled, thickness of the lens in the

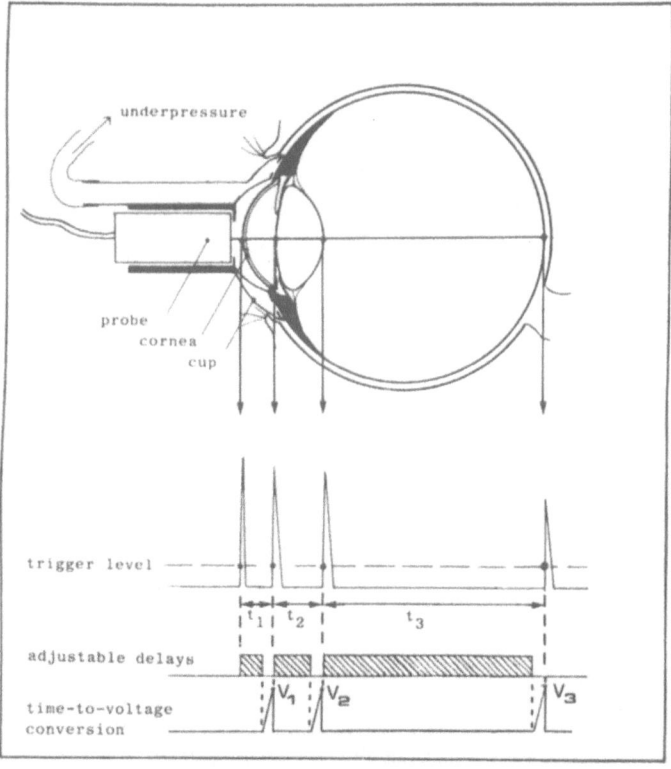

Fig. 1. Principle of applied echographic technique. The upper panel shows the eye with ultrasound probe mounted in contact glass. In the lower panel signal detection and further processing is shown. The voltages V1, V2 and V3 are proportional to transit time variations of intraocular media.

eye with cup will also change. The exact amount of accommodation does not matter; the only condition to use our method is that the lens in the measured eye is able to alter its thickness. Nevertheless, to improve signal-to-noise ratio, it is recommended to take advantage of the entire accommodation range of the subject.

In our set-up the subject made maximal accommodation excursions during 30 sec. Transit times of AC, lens and vitreous were simultaneously sampled with a frequency of 250 Mz using a personal computer with 12 bit A/D conversion.

Results

Figure 2 shows an example of simultaneous recordings on the same scale of transit time variations of AC, lens and vitreous. The subject, aged 26 and having an accommodation range of 8 D, made voluntary accommodation

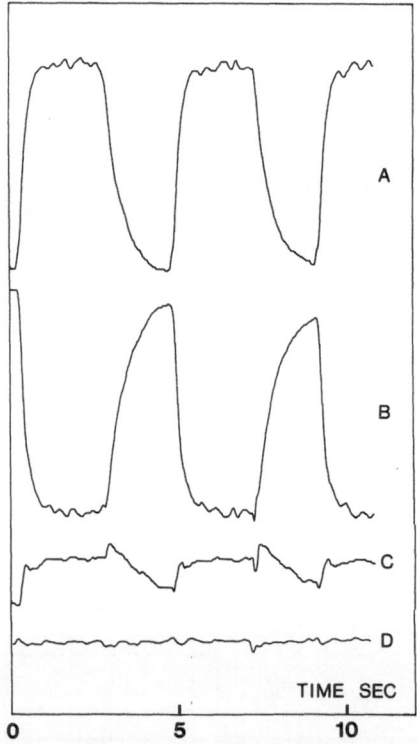

Fig. 2. Simultaneous recordings during accommodation step stimuli of 8 D. Trace A, B and C correspond with the transit time in the anterior chamber, lens and vitreous respectively (same scale). Trace (D) shows the axial length of the eye obtained by multiplying transit times with the appropriate velocities of sound.

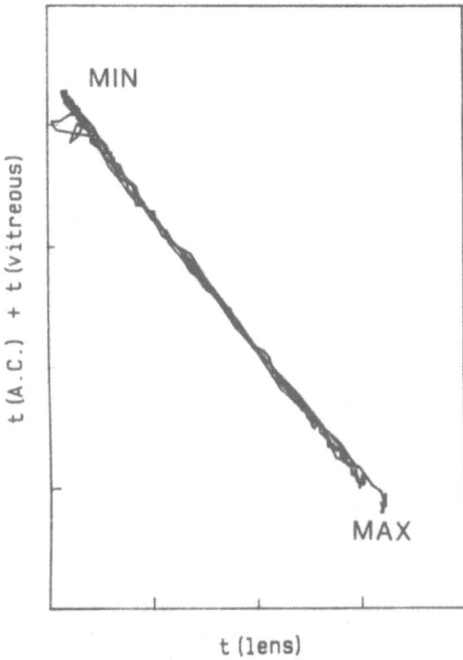

Fig. 3. Scatter diagram of transit time in AC + vitreous (ordinate) and lens (abscissa) at the same scale. MIN and MAX denote respectively minimal and maximal accommodation.

steps of maximal amplitude. As described, transit times were plotted in a scatter diagram (Fig. 3). Horizontally the time t (lens) is plotted and vertically t (AC) + t (vitreous). The top left corner corresponds to the situation where the eye does not accommodate. For increasing accommodation datapoints 'move' in a more or less linear way to the bottom right corner. Results show in all cases a linear relationship over the entire range of accommodation.

The high correlation between the transit times, viz. 0.995 or more, implies an accurate determination of sound velocity. The mean standard deviation of the velocity determined in this way turned out as 8 m/sec that is 0.5% of the value in water. No systematic investigations are performed yet.

Discussion

Our method to determine the velocity of sound in the lens can be applied when a few conditions are fulfilled. The most important factor is that at least some thickness variation can be achieved in the eye to be measured. Accuracy of our measurements show that changes in accommodation larger than about 0.01 D can be registrated. Experimentally, a necessary condition is that fixation of the ultrasound probe with respect to the optical axis is maintained. We have checked this by instructing the subject to make horizontal eye movements at a fixed distance. No effect could be found of eye movement or pupillary contraction on the results of our measurements.

Changes in the eye occurring during accommodation, for instance the transit time in the lens, may influence the amplitude of the echoes. Because our method makes use of amplitude detection this would implicate that lens thickness variations influence the signal amplitude and consequently also the moment of detection of the echo. Results of experiments using a reflector mounted on a micrometer in a waterbath, showed that the effect of absorption on the moment of detection can be ignored. At first sight, axial length variations during accommodation cannot be ruled out. Equation (4) shows that a linear relation between transit times is also obtained when axial length changes in proportion with the thickness of the lens. Our preliminary results indeed show this linear behaviour, but on physiological grounds it cannot easily be understood that axial length is exactly proportional to the increase in lens thickness over the entire accommodation range.

In literature axial length changes during accommodation are not clearly demonstrated. The classical experiment of Young (1801) subjectively showed that axial length does not play a part. Coleman et al. (1969) found an equally distributed enlargement and reduction of the axial length, possibly by limiting the range of accepted axial length variations. Resolution of digital counting systems as used by them and other investigators (Lepper and Trier, 1987) is insufficient to detect these small variations. In addition, because the ciliary muscle pulls the ora serrata anteriorly during accommodation (Moses, 1970), a possible change will be manifested in only one direction. Evidence whether axial length changes during accommodation can be obtained by doing experiments on subjects with no crystalline lens. Such experiments on young unilateral aphakes and pseudophakes and currently being performed in our laboratory.

References

Coleman D J, Wuchinich D, Carlin B. 1969. Accommodative changes in the axial dimension of the human eye. In: Gitter (ed) Opthalmic ultrasound. Mosby St Louis, pp. 134–141.

Coleman D J, Lizzi F L, Franzen L A, Abramson D H. 1975. A determination of the velocity of ultrasound in cataractous lenses. Bibl Ophthal 83: 246–251.

De Vries F R, Van der Heijde G L, Goovaerts H G. 1987. System for continuous high-resolution measurement in the eye. J Biomed Eng 9, 32–37.

Jansson F, Kock E. 1962. Determination of the velocity of ultrasound in the human lens and vitreous. Acta Ophthalmol Kbh 40, 420.

Koretz J F, Handelman G H. 1982. Model of the accommodative mechanism in the human eye. Vision Res 22, 917–927.

Lepper R D, Trier H G. 1987. Measurement of accommodative changes in human eyes by means of a high-resolution ultrasonic system. In: Ossoinig (Ed) Ophthalmic echography, pp. 157–162.

Loffredo A, De Lellis A, Cennamo G. 1983. Ultrasound velocity in different types of lens opacities. Ophthalmic Ultrasonography, Dr W. Junk Publishers, The Hague, pp. 257–260.

Moses R A. 1981. Accommodation. In: Moses (ed) Physiology of the eye, The C. V. Mosby Company, St Louis.

Pallikaris I, Gruber H. 1981. Determination of sound velocity in different forms of cataract. Docum Ophthal Proc Series 29: 165–169.

Young T. 1801. On the mechanism of the eye. Phil Trans B, pp. 23–88, cited in Davson H. (1962). The eye, vol 3, Academic Press, New York.

57. Two and three dimensional image processings applied to ophthalmic region

M. ITO*, T. SHIINA*, Y. SUGATA** and Y. YAMAMOTO**

Summary

For qualitative and quantitative diagnosis, related information should be extracted and displayed in two and three dimensions as much as possible. In this report much effort is devoted to useful ultrasound image processings such as detection of weak echoes, reconstruction of sectional images with interpolation, C-mode imaging, and three dimensional (3D) display. Furthermore, two three dimensional scans are introduced for comparison; single transducer and an array transducer.

Introduction

For two and three dimensional displays, image processings are indispensable. In ultrasound imaging such processes as near and far gain controls including time gain compensation, fast time constant, and others have already been established.

When reflected echoes are weak, simple amplification is not enough because of noises and saturated amplitudes of other echoes. We introduced here the moving average technique to the weak echoes from lesions in the vitreous body and fairy good results are obtained.

There are some cases where tissue information can be obtainable from a reconstructed image of non-scanned plane or surface better than a cross-sectional B-mode image. Here we try to construct images of eyeground using a large number of successive echo signals, which are similar to the conventional C-mode image technique.

Finally some progresses of 3D display will be discussed from the view point of image processings.

* Tokyo University of Agriculture and Technology, Department of Electronic Engineering, Koganei-shi, Tokyo 184, Japan
** Tokyo Metropolitan Komagome Hospital, Department of Ophthalmology, Bunkyo-ku, Tokyo 113, Japan

R. Sampaolesi (ed.), Ultrasonography in Ophthalmology 12, 449–453.

Principles

Extraction of weak echoes

When a lesion of small reflections exist, it is hard to detect and display it with a normal B-mode scan, because the echo level is small and it often moves owing to experation and other causes. In this experiment $n(\leq 128)$ B-mode images are taken within ten seconds with the array transducer set at the same position by immersion method. Now let the collected B-mode images be $B(i)$ $(i = 1,2,...n)$ and the digitized original echo level of a point (x, y) in $B(i)$ be $b(x, y)$ (i).
Then the moving average of the point (x, y) is

$$MA(x, y)\,(p) = \frac{1}{2N + 1} \sum_{i = p - N}^{i = p + N} b(x, y)\,(i)$$

where N is the number of neighbour sampling points with respect to the center point p. Next we calculate the average value (Av) of echo levels in the vitreous body of a selected B-mode image, say m th image $(1 \leq m \leq n)$. Final image (B) is composed of pixels, each of which is a maximum value, say bx, y(km), among pixels satisfying the condition that $MA(x, y)\,(p) \geq$ c.Av, i.e.,

$$bx, y = \begin{cases} \text{max among bx, y(p)'s for all p such that } MA(x, y)\,(p) \geq \\ \qquad c.Av\ (1 \leq p \leq n) \\ \\ 0, \text{ otherwise.} \end{cases}$$

This process is carried out for all coordinates (x, y) in the vitreous body. Main parameters are thus the values of c, N, and n.

Construction of surface image of the eyeground

Echo signals reflected at the surface of the eyeground constitute the image of the eyeground. Since it is difficult to identify the echo signals from the surface, if the tissue in the vitreous body is not uniform. Here we treat a case only where no reflected echoes can be observed from the vitreous region. Echoes from the surface are collected by the spiral scan of single transducer and by the linear scan of an array transducer.

Reconstruction of ultrasonograms

Spirally driven single transducer draws loci such as circular, square, and octagonal, and others. The direction of each ultrasound line is set by the corresponding two step angles. The minimum angle is 7.5°/80 per one step.

In any above methods, the total number of sampled ultrasound lines along the scanning locus is about 7,500 points. The total amount of digitized raw echo data is accessed in 23 sec in this system.

Ultraonogram of any cross section can be constructed as follows.
1. All the echo data corresponding to the specified plane are ontained from the intersections of ultrasound lines and the plane.
2. Interpolate the data free points of the image of step 2.
3. Smooth the interpolated image after step 3, if necessary.
4. Display it as a quasi-colored image of 256 × 256 × 8 bits.

Experimental results

For the extraction of weak echoes from the vitreous region, three parameters n, N, and c are evaluated. Opitimum values under the experiment are each found to be $n = 100 \sim 128$, $N = 10$, $c \approx 2$. $c = 1$ results in noises in the image and $c = 3$ excludes some echoes. Smaller values of N give noises and fairly large values, say $N = 15 \sim 20$ result in smaller display of a tissue than expected. For comparison, we constructed two images by other methods; one in which each pixel is the largest value among the n pixels of the same coordinate (x, y) and are above a threshold level c.Av, the other one in which each pixel is the average value of the n pixels of the same coordinates.

A proliferative diabetic retinopathy with recurrent vitreous hemorrhages is shown on the photograph (Fig. 1). The conventional B-mode image by an array transducer with maximum gain hardly discloses a weak echo of vitreous membrane. By the moving average method weak echoes from the vitreous

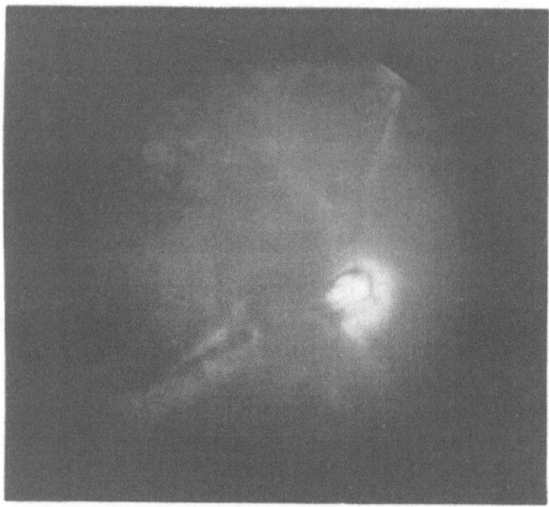

Fig. 1. A diabetic retinopathy with recurrent vitreous hemorrhages.

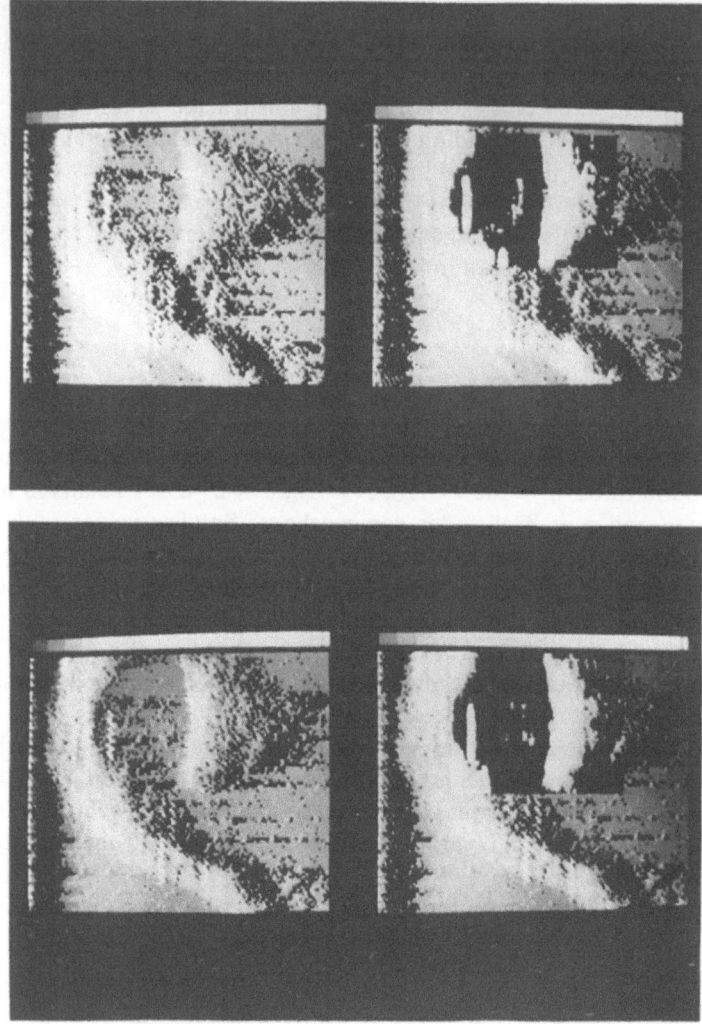

Fig. 2. Detected weak echoes from the vitreous body (n = 128, N = 10, c = 2.0).

membrane or hemorrhage can be detected as shown in Fig. 2(a, b). The plane image of fundus of surface is reconstructed from the stored echoes. Optic disc seems to be detected on the plane as a small area with slightly high echo levels.

Conclusion

We described a method to detect a weak echo using the so called moving average technique, in which a lesion is applied in the vitreous body. We also

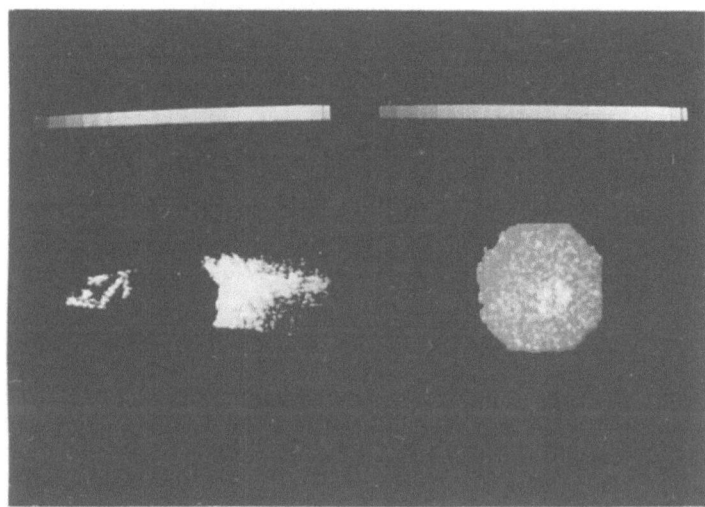

Fig. 3. Reconstructed image of fundus surface.

showed that a reconstructed ultrasonogram, which is different plane from the scanned crosssection, say, the echogram of the surface of an eyeground, is useful for diagnosis. In addition two and three dimensional display methods are discussed and a progress report is presented.

References

Ito M, Yamamoto Y, Sugata Y. 1985. Proc. WFUMB, 555.

Ito M, Yamamoto Y. 1986. Jap. J. ME & BE 24, 7, 43.

Ito M, Aizu J, Shuu K, Yamamoto Y, Sugata Y. 1987. Reconstruction of ultrasonogram and three dimensional image of a tissue, Proc. China-Japan Joint Conf. on Ultrasonics, May, Nanjing.

58. Three dimensional scan using a single transducer and image construction

YUKIO YAMAMOTO*, YASUO SUGATA*, MICHIKO TOMITA*, and MASAYASU ITO**

Summary

This paper describes data accessing methods for obtaining ultrasonogram of any specified section and displaying the contour of a tissue in ocular region. Three 3D scanning methods, which are suitable for a large quantity of echo signals, are proposed to extract qualitative information on any cross section from the stored data. A single probe is used here just because it has better resolution than an array transducer and versatile scan.

Introduction

A series of successive B-mode images yield total information of a tissue of interest. Thus any scanning method will serve as long as echo signals are collected uniformly even from a tissue of small volume. This paper discusses some data accessing methods, using a single transducer, to obtain ultrasonograms of any specified section and extention to a three dimensional display of a tissue in ocular region. For this purpose three scanning methods, which are suitable for a large quantity of echo signals, are proposed. A single probe or transducer is used here because of better resolution than an array type. Flexible scan makes the space density of echo data fairy uniform.

A series of echo signals accessed by a selected scan are stored successively in the buffer memory for further processings such as reconstruction of ultrasonograms of any crosssection and echo enhancement display of vitreous body, and others. Several image processings together with experimental results are discussed.

* Department of Ophthalmology, Tokyo Metropolitan Komagome Hospital, Japan
** Department of Electronic Engineering, Tokyo University of Agriculture and Technology, Japan

R. Sampaolesi (ed.), Ultrasonography in Ophthalmology 12, 455–460.

456

Scanning methods

This system consists of ultrasound diagnostic equipment, and the subsystem including the scanner, image processing and display unit as shown in Fig. 1. Two stepping motors are jointly controlled so that the ultrasound beam be directed toward the eye to be scanned in several fashions. By the control unit (or 3D scanner), we can make scans such as spiral scans, single sector scan, sector-sector scan, and manual scan. Clinical data are obtained by the immersion method supine.

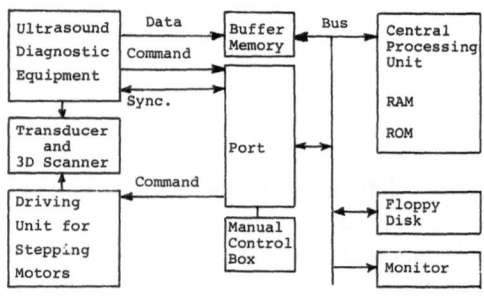

Block diagram of the system

Fig. 1. Block diagram of the system.

A series of echo signals are sampled, synchoronized with both beam movement and sampling time for echo signals. Echoes are digitized in 8 bits, of which upper 4 bits are displayed.

The ultrasound lines draw the circular, square, and octagonal loci. The direction of each ultrasound line is set by the corresponding two step angles. The minimum angle is 7.5°/80 per one step. Note here that ultrasound lines are almost perpendicular to the paper. The adjacent lines in the square and octagonal scannings never cross each other, but they intersect at some points in the sprial scanning, yielding the same sampling points. This is due to the digital control of motors in generating a spiral line. But this gives rise to a feature in which data free points tend to be interpolated easily by the irregular sample points. The simple square scan gives farely uniform and dense data. Some part of the plane parallel to the line becomes difficult to be interpolated, however. Octagonal scan produces effects half way between the spiral scan and the square one.

Reconstruction of ultrasonograms

The total number of sampled ultrasound lines along the spiral line is about 7500 points. Maximum scanning angle is about 8 to 45 deg depending on the present number of steps of two motors.

For a depth of 5 cm, 66.7 μ s of echoes are stored, giving 256 samples per ultrasound line for detected signals. This device uses 8 bits for video output and 4 bits for display. The total amount of raw data, about 1 M bytes is obtained in 23 sec. Ultrasonogram of any cross section can be constructed as follows.

1. Give a plane on the monitor, observing a reference ultrasonogram say, initially constructed horizontal or vertical image as shown in Fig. 3.
2. All the echo data corresponding to the specified plane are obtained from the intersections of ultrasound lines and the plane.
3. Interpolate the data free points of the image of step 2.
4. Smooth the interpolated image after step 3, if necessary.
5. Display it as a quasi-colored image of 256 × 256 × 8 bits.

Three dimensional (3D) image

Abnormal tissues in the vitreous body and the posterior region can be identified on an ultrasonogram even if one can not identify it by observing through the lens of an eye.

The contour of the cross section of interest can be extracted by binarizing the corresponding digital image of ocular region. The total shape is displayed as a three dimensional image, which is the overlay of the contours of sliced sections. Colored ultrasonogram of any section can be overlayed on the B/W 3D image to examine pathological relations between the section and the shape.

The effect of different viewing directions is observed by generating a 3D image, which can be seen in three dimensional rotation transformation.

Experimental results

The residual retinal detachment after closed vitrectomy to a proliferative diabetic retinopathy is shown in a fundus photograph (Fig. 2). The U-shaped retinal detachment outside of the vascular archade extending to the equator is well represented in a reconstructed image on CRT (Fig. 4(c)). Rotated images are shown in a series of photographs (Fig. 4(a), (b)).

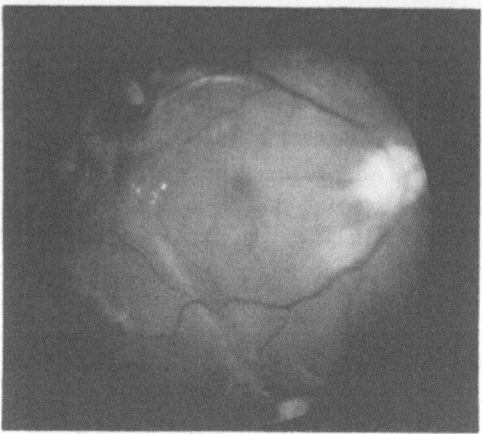

Fig. 2. Fundus photograph of residual retinal detachment.

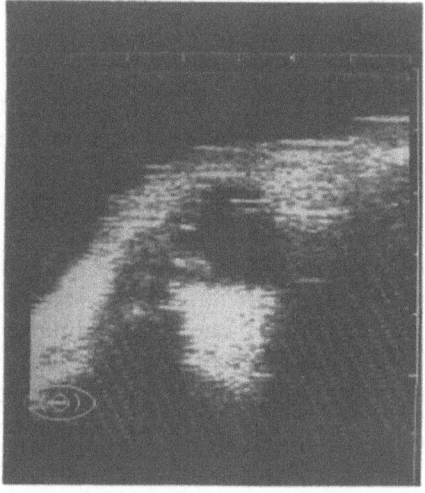

Fig. 3. B-mode image of the retinal detachment.

Concluding remarks

Useful scanning methods are introduced to store a large capacity of tissue information, from which the tissue is diagnosed in a 3D way. It takes about two minutes to construct an ultrasonogram, but this time can be shortened by specially-designed hardware.

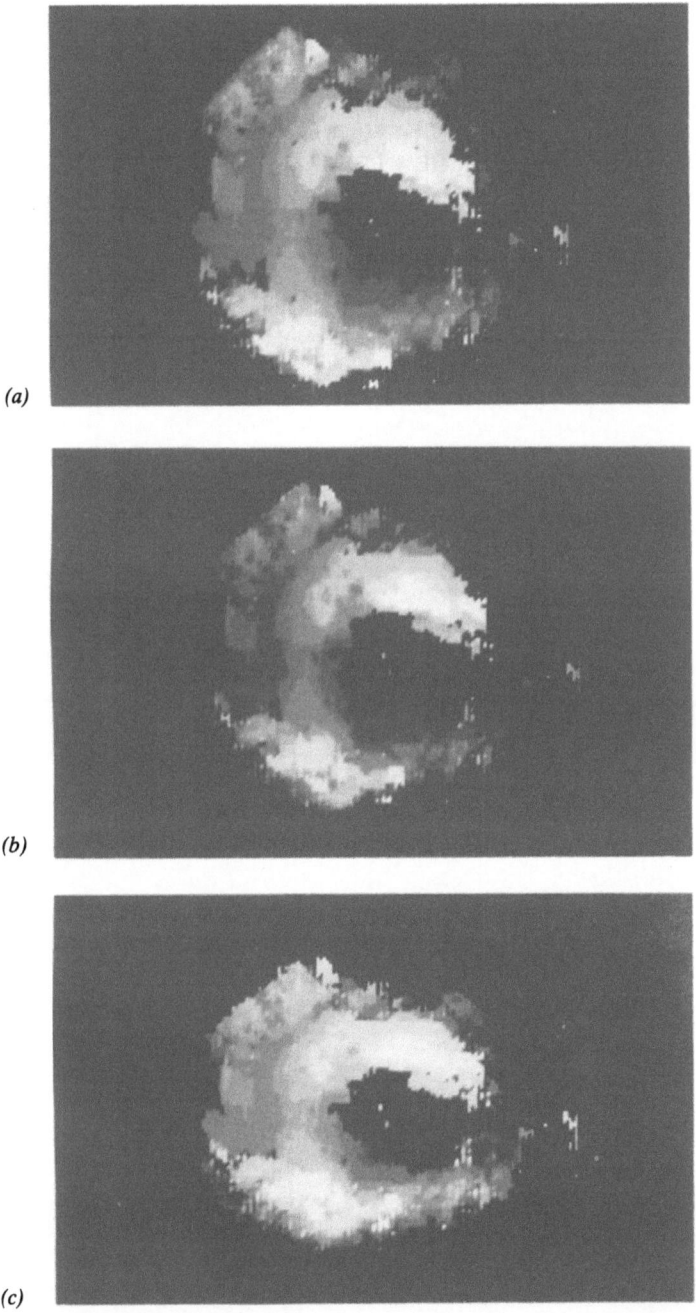

(a)

(b)

(c)

Fig. 4. 3D images of retinal detachment, with different viewing directions.

460

References

Hill CR, Carpenter DA. 1976. Ultrasonic echo imaging of tissues: instrumentation, British Journal of Radiology 49: 238–243.

Ito M, Yamamoto Y, Sugata Y. 1985. Proc. WFUMB, 555.

Ito M, Yamamoto Y. 1986. Jap. J. ME & BE,24,7,43.

Yamamoto Y, Sugata Y, Tomita M, Ito M. 1987. Three-dimensional display of the ocular region. Improvement of scanning method. In: K C Ossoinig (ed) Ophthalmic Echography pp. 207–214.

59. Three dimensional display of ocular region using an array transducer

YASUO SUGATA*, YUKIO YAMAMOTO* and MASAYASU ITO**

Summary

We report here a three dimensional (3D) display system for the ocular region, using an array transducer. The prototype system consists of real time diagnostic equipment, real time rotation process unit, and other units such as mechanical probe-scanner and joystic. Personal computer is interfaced to the system for further complex processes and experiments.

The 10 MHz linear array transducer is moved linearly by the scanner and the successive echo data are stored in the memory, and the extracted contour data are then transfered to the rotation process unit to display the total shape in a three dimensional fashion.

Introduction

Ultrasound diagnostic equipments, in which two dimensional images or ultrasonograms are mainly used for diagnosis are prevalent nowadays. In order to obtain as much information as possible about a tissue one requires not only cross-sectional images but also three dimensional information such as the shape and the relative location of the cross-section to the tissue itself.

In this paper we wish to present a real time 3D display hardware system using an array transducer together with some pertaining problems and techniques such as high-speed operations to display the shape, viewing angles, and image construction methods. Experimental but useful results in ophthalmic lesions are also demonstrated.

* Department of Ophthalmology, Tokyo Metropolitan Komagome Hospital, Japan
** Department of Electronic Engineering, Tokyo University of Agriculture and Technology, Japan

R. Sampaolesi (ed.), Ultrasonography in Ophthalmology 12, 461–466.

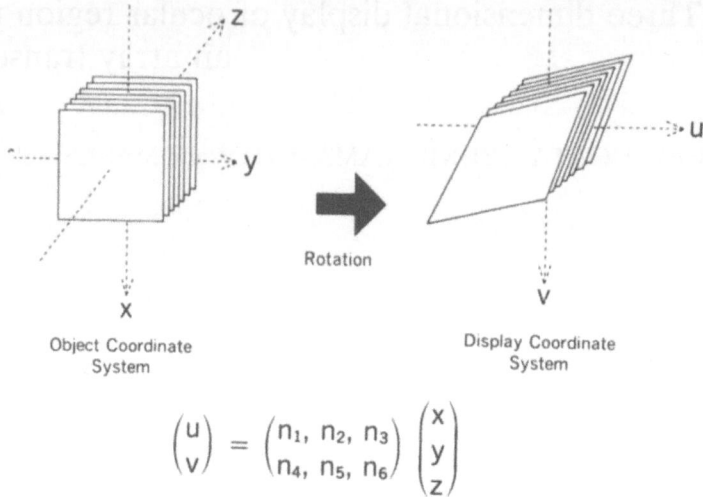

$$\begin{pmatrix} u \\ v \end{pmatrix} = \begin{pmatrix} n_1, & n_2, & n_3 \\ n_4, & n_5, & n_6 \end{pmatrix} \begin{pmatrix} x \\ y \\ z \end{pmatrix}$$

Fig. 1. Concept of rotation process.

Principles

The shape of the tissue is displayed as a 3D images which consists of gradated cross-sectional plane images, which are overlayed to show the total shape of the tissue. Each cross-sectional image represents the contour and the cross-section, and is obtained from the corresponding ultrasonogram by image processing. We call such a 3D display technique "Intensity Gradated Sectional Image Method" for convenience.

In generating a view of a tissue, the effects of different viewing positions and directions should be considered. The perspective transformation is carried out simply by the rotation process (Fig. 1). The rotation of the 3D image (Rotation display for short) makes it easy to display a hidden lesion behind a tissue. Furthermore the relative locations of a tissue to others are observed using the same stored data, i.e., without scanning the tissue again.

System

The developed system consists of two main subsystems, i.e., the 3D data acquisition system (Data Storage Unit) and the real time 3D display one (Fig. 2). All clinical data is obtained by the immersion method supine.

Data acquisition and contour extraction

Mechanical scan of an array transducer gives three dimensional echo data of ROI of about 57.6 mm as shown in Fig. 3. Total of 128 cross-sections are

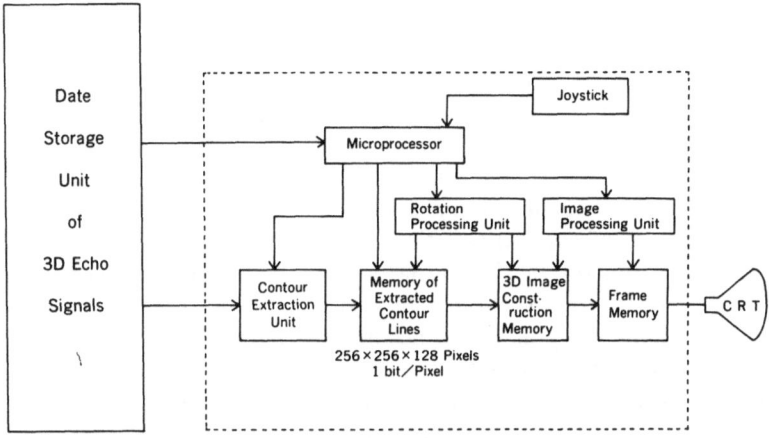

Fig. 2. Block diagram of the 3D display unit.

sampled every 57.6/128 (mm) apart, and each forms the ultrasonotomogram of $256 \times 256 \times 8$ bits.

Realtime 3D display unit

This unit plays an important role in the system and composed of contour extraction unit, rotation process unit, image processing unit, cross-section and contour image store unit, 3D image construction memory, and joystick, which are totally controlled by a microprocessor. This unit has two functions, one is contour extraction, and the other is real time display of the rotation of the 3D image. The cross-sections together with their contours are each

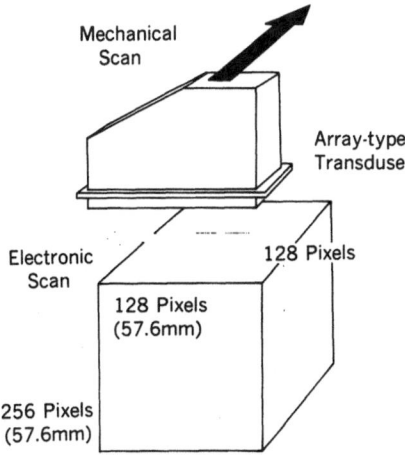

Fig. 3. Electro-mechanical scan for 3D echo storage and sampling points.

extracted from the corresponding tomograms through thresholding after interpolation and smoothing processes. Thus we have 128 frames of cross-sections, part or all of which represent the total shape of the scanned region. Each frame has 256 × 256 pixels with the intensity value of 1 bit.

Necessary parameters concerning viewing direction is set by a joystick and the calculated parameters are fed to the rotation process unit. Fig. 4 shows the functions of the rotation processing unit, which transforms the (x, y, z) coordinates of the cross-sections and contours of the object space to the (u, v) coordinates of the display space. In the figure, each square is supposed to be a cross-section with contour of the lesion and the plane changes its shape as a diamond according to the viewing direction. The transformation, which is usually calculated by product-sum method using a matrix, is carried out here only on the sum base. The sum operation is suitable for the hardware implementation.

Now a maximum of any 32 frames among 128 can be overlayed as intensity gradated images. The maximum possible error of coordinate transformation in eight dots, which is equal to 1.8 mm.

Experimental results

Three dimensional echo data can be collected to store in less than 10 seconds from the tissue of 57.6 mm in size. It takes only 2.5 seconds to transfer the 3D raw data to the rotation process unit including interpolation, smoothing, and binarization. 3D image can be constructed and displayed in 0.3, 0.6, and 1.2, depending on the number of the overlaying cross-sections of 8, 16, and 32 frames, respectively. Fig. 5 shows a 3D image of a sponge

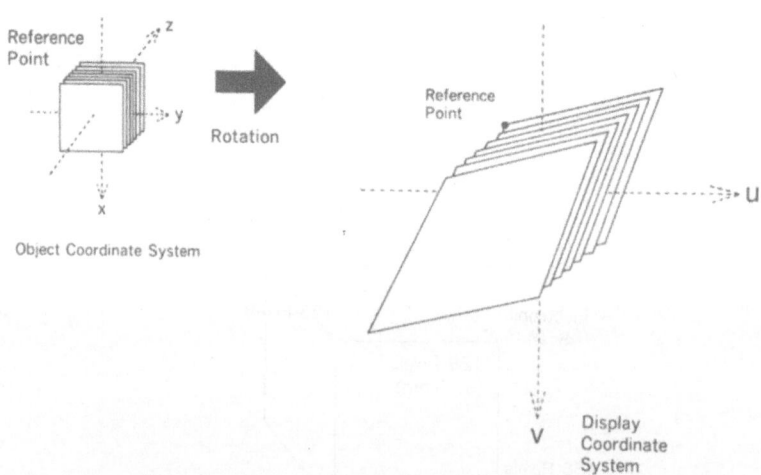

Fig. 4. Function of rotation processing unit.

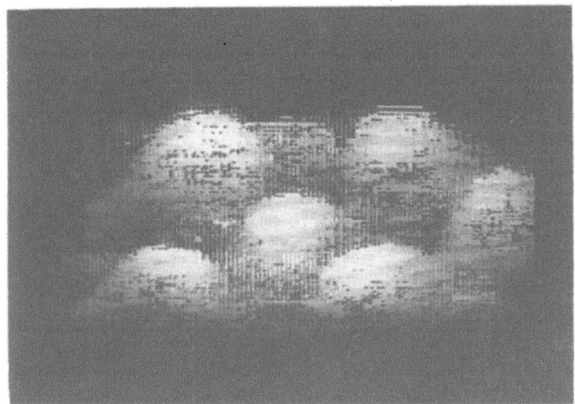

Fig. 5. 3D display of a sponge phantom.

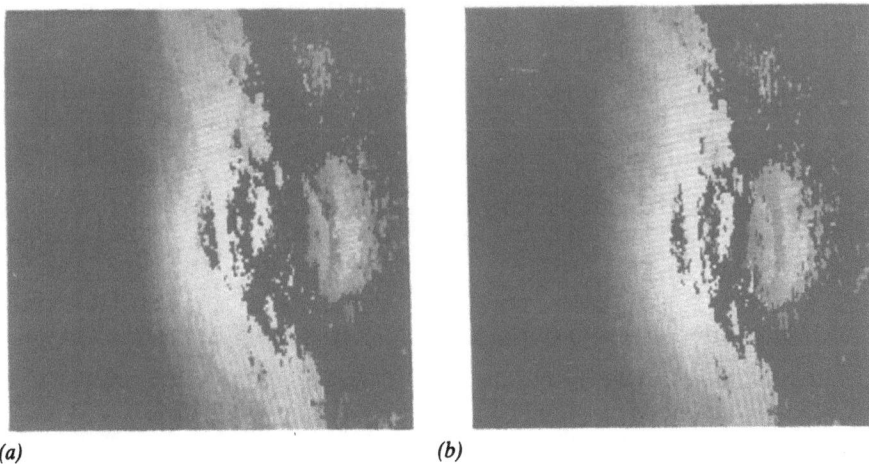

(a)   *(b)*

Fig. 6. Rotational display of retinal detachment. Pictures (a) and (b) together give streographic
view.

phantom. The resultant 3D display of retinal detachment is shown in Fig. 6,
which also show that stereographic images can be obtained by this system.

In practice, rotational displays are continuously made in real time, in
accordance with the viewing direction. Those pictures (a), (b) in Fig. 6, are
taken as parts of real time rotation display.

Concluding remarks

The developed system is useful for observation of the shape of a tissue as
well as for the reconstruction of tomogram of any section. This means that

466

the conventional B-mode ultrasound diagnostic equipment can be replaced by this kind of 3D system owing to its advantages and many functions.

The total shape viewed from any direction can be displayed almost instantly. Memory of positional echo information and fast processing lead to short time examination for ultrasonography of ocular areas, which are mobile due to cardiac pulsation, respiration, emotional movements, and so on.

References

Yamamoto Y, Sugata Y, Tomita M, Yamauchi H. 1986. Image processing of ocular region in ultrasonic diagnosis and clinical significance-Three dimensional display and volume-measurements of intraocular mass based on the spiral scanning, Acta Soc Ophthalmol Jpn 90(1). 131–140.

Yamamoto Y, Sugata Y, Tomita M, Ito M. 1987. Three dimensional display of the ocular region. Improvement of scanning method, In: K C Ossoinig (ed) Ophthalmic Echography pp. 207–214.

60. The development and clinical application of the digital quantitative color scan-converter connected with the ophthalmic contact ultrasonographic apparatus

SADANAO TANE and YOTARO KIMURA

All existing commercially available ophthalmic contact B-scan ultrasonic units produced in- and outside Japan have monochromatic displays. They are not color gray-scale display units.

We developed, on an experimental basis, a color digital simultaneous tomographic ultrasonic display unit that can be connected with a Topscan ophthalmic contact ultrasonic unit developed by us, in order to improve the accuracy of ultrasonic imaging diagnosis. In the present study, we evaluated the clinical application of the new unit.

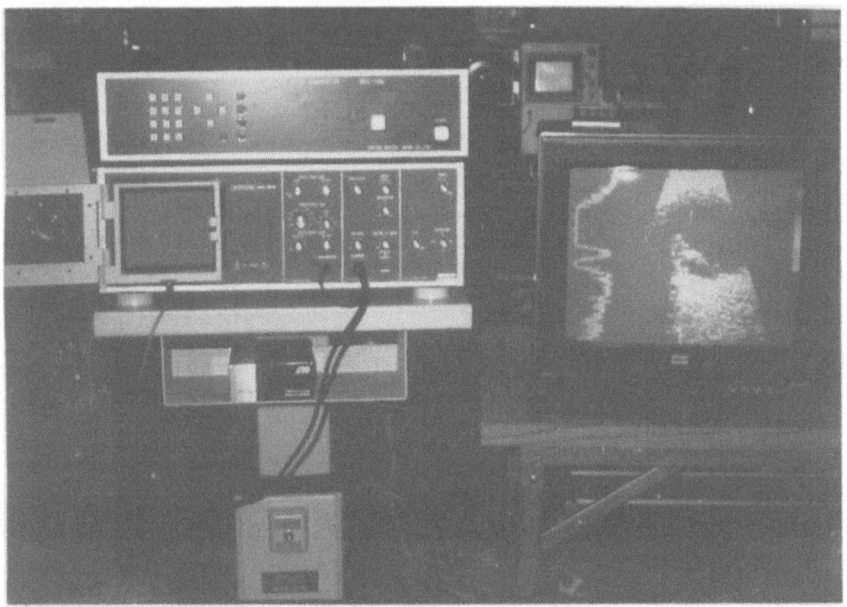

Fig. 1. The digital quantitative color scan-converter unit connected with the Topscan Ophthalmic Contact ultrasonographic apparatus.

Dept. of Ophthalmology, St. Marianna University, School of Medicine, Kawasaki, Japan

R. Sampaolesi (ed.), Ultrasonography in Ophthalmology 12, 467–474.
© *1990. Kluwer Academic Publishers, Dordrecht*

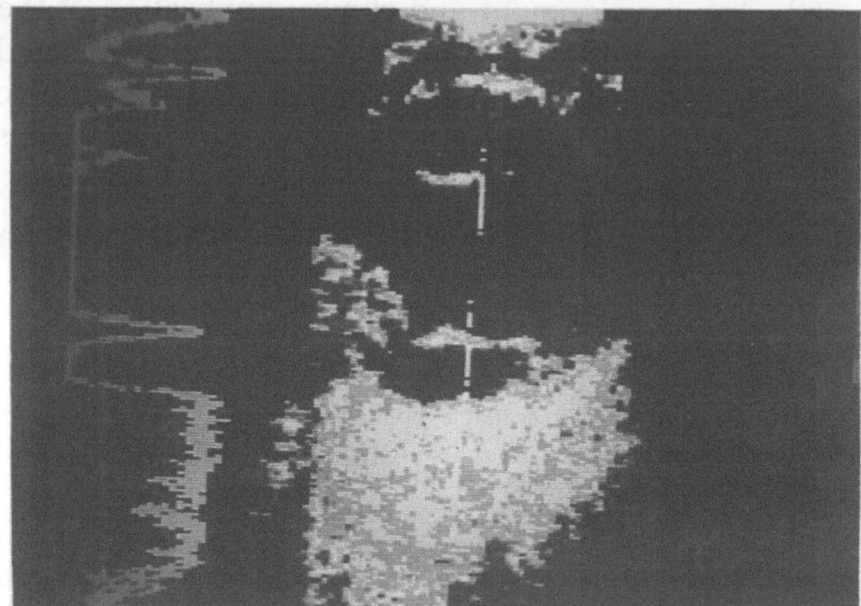

Fig. 2. The digital quantitative color B-mode and vector A-mode images of an eye with retinal detachment in a 40-year-old male shown the unite.

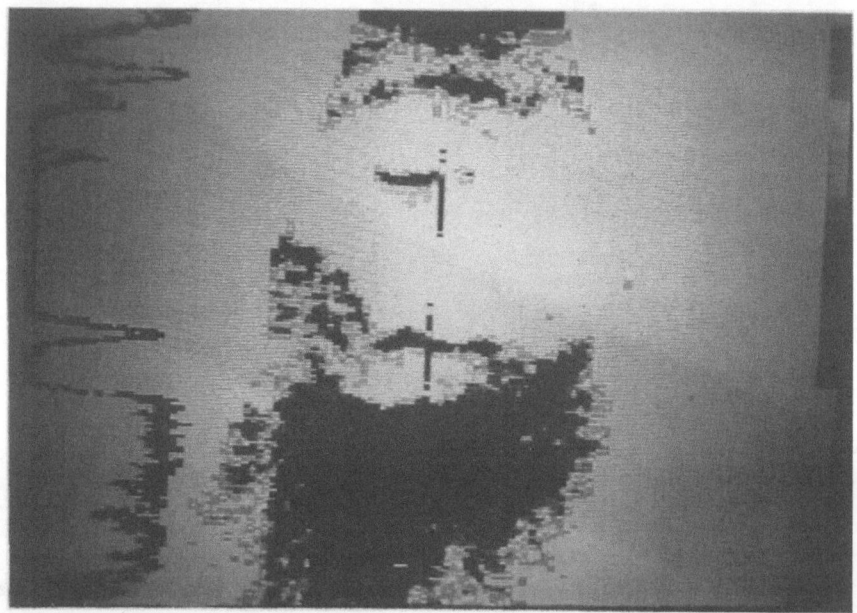

Fig. 3. The negative color imaging display of the retinal detachment in the same case.

The unit we developed for the present experiment is shown in Figure 1.

In Figure 2, the B-mode and vector A-mode images of an eye with retinal detachment are shown on the digital color display of the unit developed for the present experiment. The color display provides clearer differentiation of the echo than the monochromatic display. The color display is also better for quantitative diagnosis. It enables linear display with equivalent sensitivity and the recording of data on video tape. The digitalization thus facilitated much more image processing.

When this unit is used, the image diagnosis input from the Topscan ophthalmic ultrasonic (diagnostic) equipment is converted from analogue to digital signals, stored in memory, output as standard television signals, and displayed as a color or monochromatic digital image on a color or mono-chromatic video monitor. The number of pixels of the digital color display is twice that of the immersion ophthalmic ultrasonic equipment we developed previously; the new unit has 256 pixels in both vertical and horizontal directions. In addition, images are presented by fractionation in a fifteen-grade gray scale, regardless of color or monochromatic display. We can freeze images at any time by using a foot switch, for extended observation.

The subjects were 46 eyes of 46 patients, consisting of 16 eyes with retinal detachment (16 patients), 21 with vitreous hemorrhage (21 patients) and 9 with exophthalmos (9 patients).

I will present some of them.

Figure 2 shows a B-mode image of the old stage of retinal detachment in a 40-year-old male, displayed by this new unit. This is a positive color imaging display, and Figure 3, a negative one. Both images display the gray scale (color-grading) of the echo-enhanced site of retinal detachment well. A vector A-mode image with a sharp rise is simultaneously displayed, providing easy diagnosis and analysis of the lesion.

As shown in Figure 4-A and B, positive and negative monochromatic digital display are available. They can be used according to diagnostic purpose.

Figure 5-A and B shows B-mode images from a 58-year-old female with advanced diabetic retinopathy leading to retinal detachment.

Figure 5-A is a positive digital color image, and Figure 5-B, a negative one. Both show the echo of a hematoma beneath the funnel-shaped echo of retinal detachment, which is supported by the vector A-mode image.

Figure 6-A, and B shows findings of vitreous syneresis in a 66-year-old female. On the Figure 6-A is a positive digital color image, and the Figure 6-B, a negative one. The vector A-mode image shows a solitary spike with a slow rise at the site of vitreous syneresis. This characteristic finding is useful for differentiation from retinal detachment.

Figure 7 shows the B-mode images of the intravitreal membrane observed after vitreous hemorrhage in a 66-year-old female. On these findings are a positive digital color image, a negative digital color image and positive and negative monochromatic images. These images including, the vector A-

470

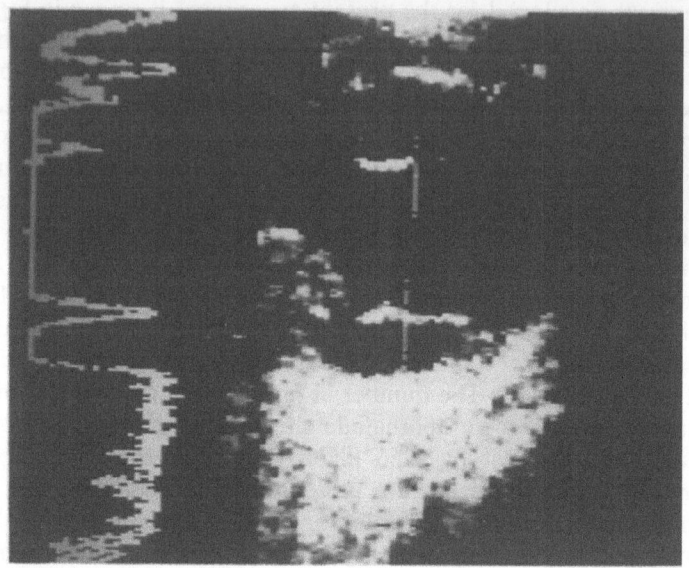

(A) The positive display.

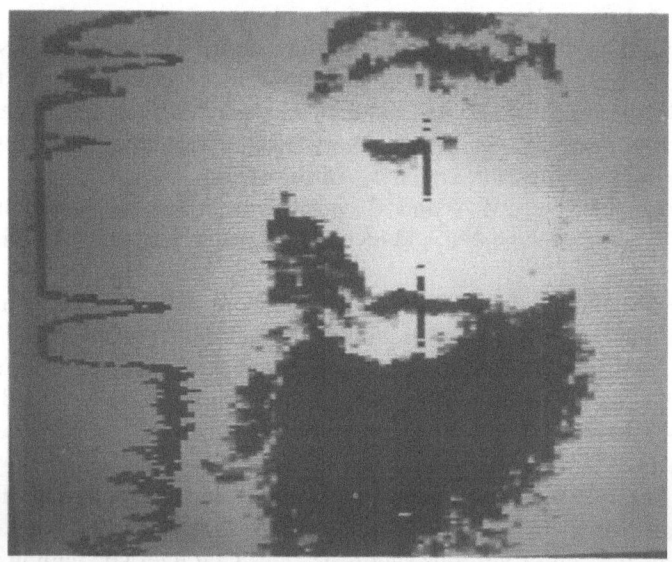

(B) The negative display.

Fig. 4-A and B. The positive and negative monochromatic digital quantitative display of the retinal detachment in the same case.

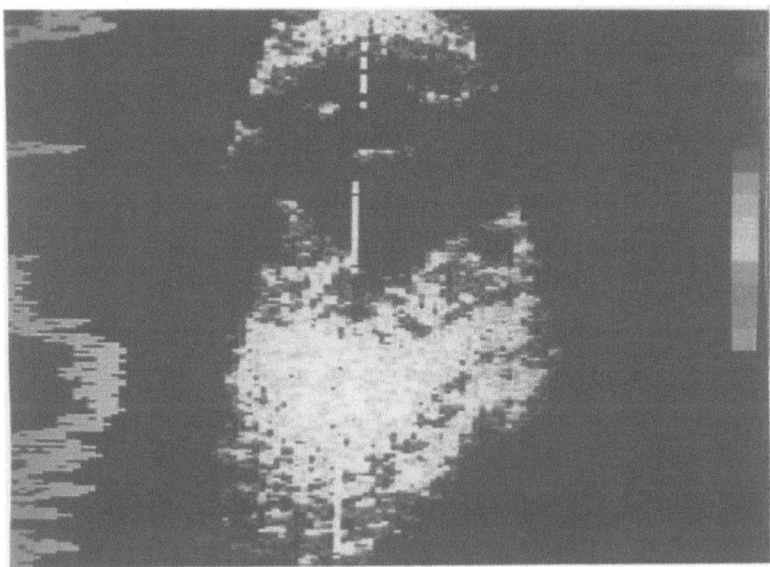

(A) The positive color display.

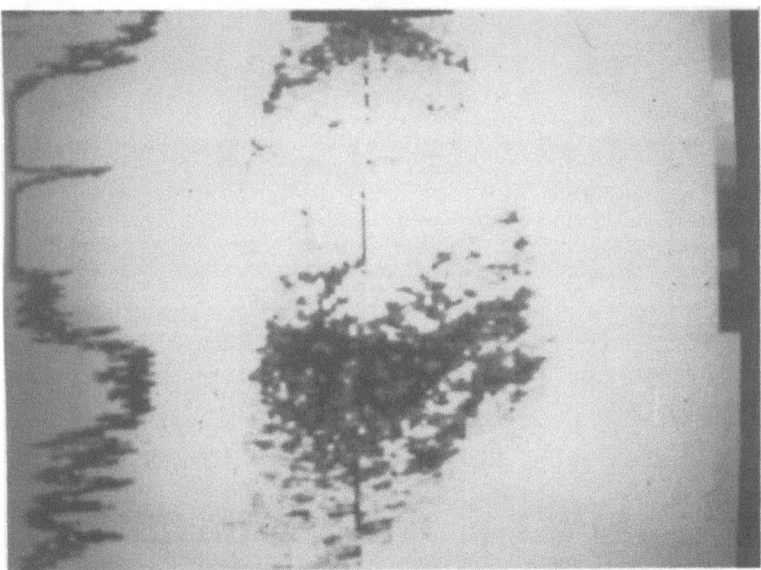

(B) The negative color display.

Fig. 5-A and B. The digital quantitative color B-mode and vector A-mode images of an eye with advanced diabetic retinopathy leading to retinal detachment in a 58-year old female.

472

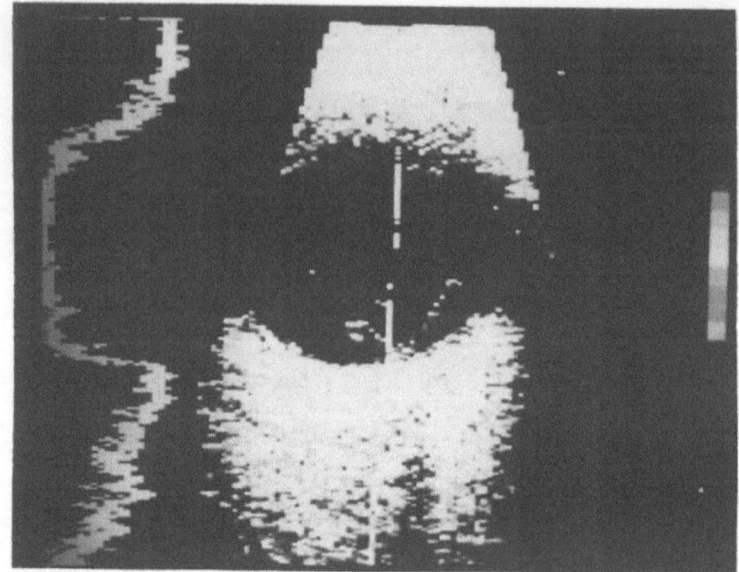

(A) The positive color display.

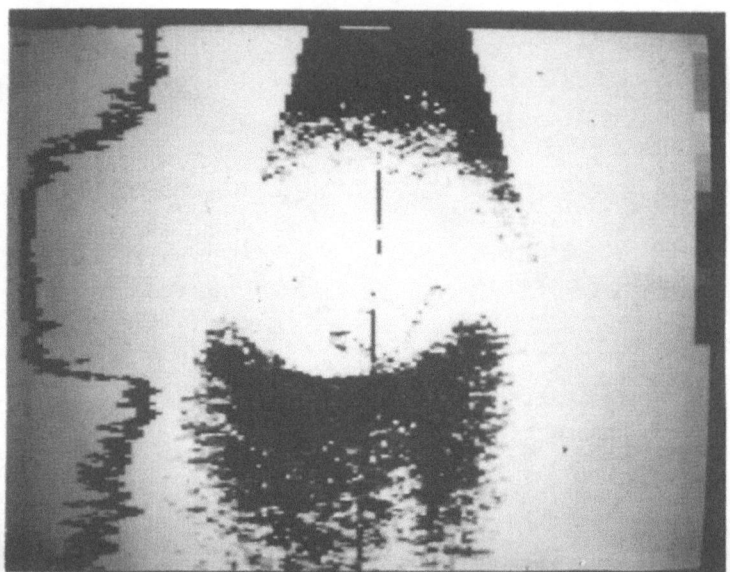

(B) The negative color display.

Fig. 6-A and B. The digital quantitative color B-mode and vector A-mode images of an eye with vitreous syneresis in a 66-year-old female.

473

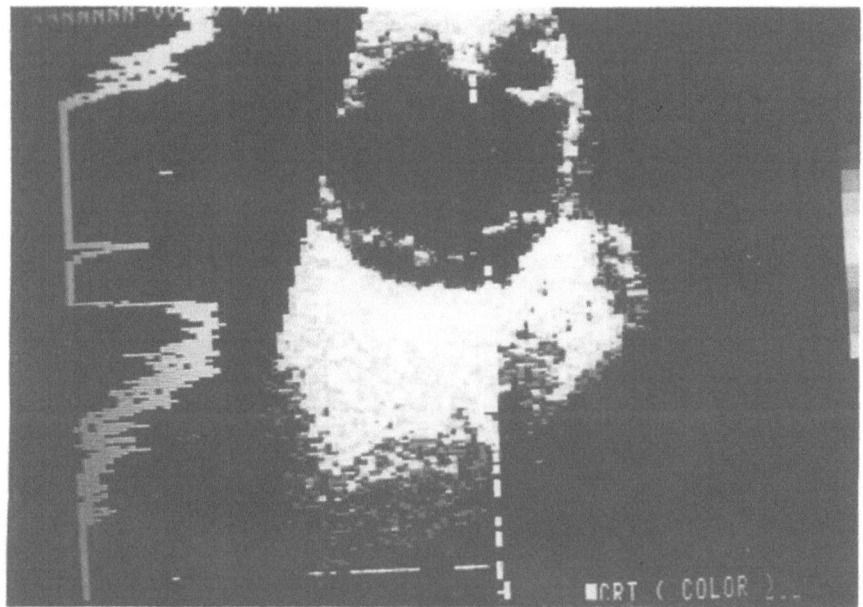

Fig. 7. The digital quantitative color B-mode and vector A-mode images of an eye with the intravitreal membrane in a 66-year-old female.

mode image, allow differentiation from retinal detachment with its definite enhanced gray scale, since they show a moderate gray scale.

In conclusion, the new unit that was developed for the present experiment allows observation of real-time B-mode images in color and monochromatic digital imaging displays by converting the B-mode imaging signal to a standard television signal via a digital image memory through connection with a Topscan ophthalmic ultrasonic diagnostic unit (Type ES-100). The system also enables images to be frozen at random.

In other words, the color display of the new unit provides:
1) more distinct gray-scale differentiation, and 2) better quantitative ultrasonic diagnosis than the monochromatic displays of conventional direct systems. The former also makes topographic display possible. In addition, digital imaging enables image recording on VTR and other electronic imaging management much more available.

References

Baum G. 1974. Color ultrasonography for tissue differential diagnosis, In: D L King (ed) Diagnostic Ultrasound, The C. V. Bosby Co., Saint Louis, pp. 282–289.
Coleman D, Lizzi F L, Jack R L. 1977. Ultrasonography of the Eye and Orbit, Lea & Febiger, Philadelphia. pp. 77–79.

474

Tane S et al. 1975. Studies on ultrasonic diagnosis, (Report 9) Ophthalmic color ultrasono-graphy, Japanese Journal of Clinical Ophthalmology 29: 319–323.

Tane S, Kimura Y, Ito K. 1976. On the evolution of digital color ultrasonography for ocular differential diagnosis., Ultrasonic in Medicine, Vol. 3A, Proceeding of 1st meeting of the world Federation of Ultrasound in Medicine and Biology. pp. 943–953.

61. Analysis of fundus blood flow dynamics by the ultrasonic Doppler method in blocking therapy for the stellar ganglions of cervical sympathetic nerve

SADANAO TANE and TOSHIO KANEKO

Thrombolytic drugs and vasodilators have conventionally been administered in the treatment of occlusive diseases of the retinal arteries, and hyperbaric oxygen therapy has occasionally been attempted. Recently, particular attention has been increasingly paid to the efficacy of stellate ganglion-blocking therapy, aimed at vessel dilation.

In the present study, we confirmed the efficacy of stellate ganglion blocking applied to these diseases and attempted to elucidate the mechanism involved by analysis of the hemodynamics of the fundus oculi before and after blocking by the ultrasonic Doppler method.

The subjects were 26 patients with occlusive diseases of the retinal vessels who were examined during the period between January 1987 and February 1988. They consisted of 11 males and 15 females, and the proportion of elderly patients aged 50 years or more was high. As for complications, hypertension and heart disease were present in 14 (54%) and 8 (31%), respectively.

The patients consisted of 2 with occlusion of the central retinal artery, 3 with occlusion of the central retinal vein and 21 with branch obstruction of the retinal vein. They were assigned to two groups: group A patients who had already undergone treatment including laser photo-coagulation of the retina and drug therapy, and group B patients who had not been treated since the onset of the disease. Stellate ganglion blocking was performed in these groups.

The para-tracheal method, emloying 7 ml of 1% carbocaine and 24-G, 4-cm needles, was used. Within about 5 minutes after injection of a local anesthetic, Horner's syndrome appeared, being recognized as a sign of the nerve block. Blocking was performed 5–24 times, with a mean of 9 times. The course of changes in visual acuity was recorded after blocking. Blood flow wave patterns of the internal carotid artery and the intraocular central retinal artery before and after blocking were determined with a real-time spectrum analyzer ECHO Spectrum and Vaso-Flow-3.

Dept. of Ophthalmology, St. Marianna University, School of Medicine, Kawasaki, Japan

R. Sampaolesi (ed.), Ultrasonography in Ophthalmology 12, 475–481.

476

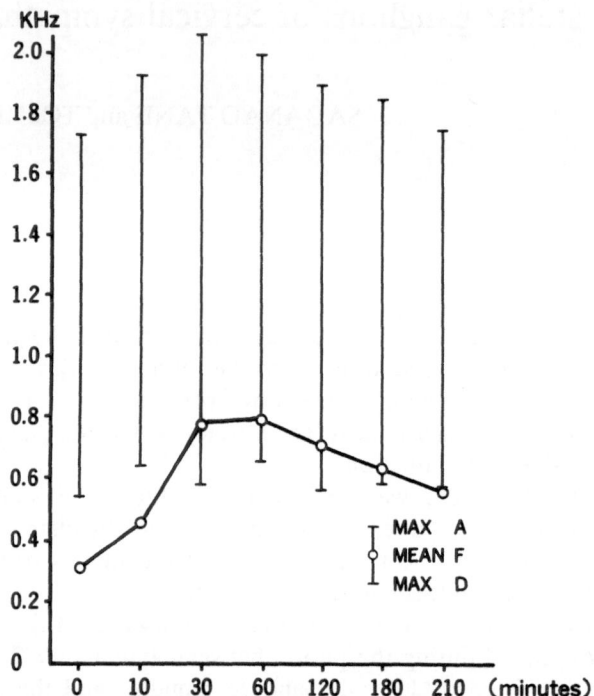

Fig. 1. The blood flow speed values of the internal carotid artery determined before the blocking and 10, 30, 60, 120, 180 and 210 minutes after blocking by the ultrasonic doppler method.

Figure 1 shows the blood flow speed values of the internal carotid artery determined before the blocking and 10, 30, 60, 120, 180, and 210 minutes after blocking by the ultrasonic Doppler method. After 10 to 60 minutes after blocking, the blood flow speed rapidly increased, and then it tended to gradually decrease.

Figure 2 shows the time-course changes in the blood flow speed value of the central retinal artery. In a similar manner to that of the internal carotid artery, the value increased 10 to 30 minutes after blocking and reached a peak 60 minutes after blocking, thereafter showing a tendency toward a gradual decrease.

I would like to present one patient here. She was a 62-year-old woman who visited our hospital 2 weeks after onset of branch obstruction of the retinal vein.

Figure 3 shows the blood flow wave pattern of the internal carotid artery

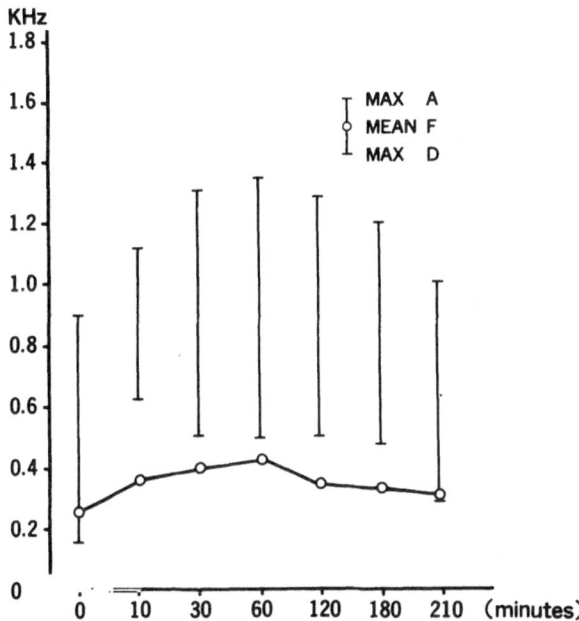

Fig. 2. The time-course changes in the blood flow speed value of the central retinal artery in a similar manner.

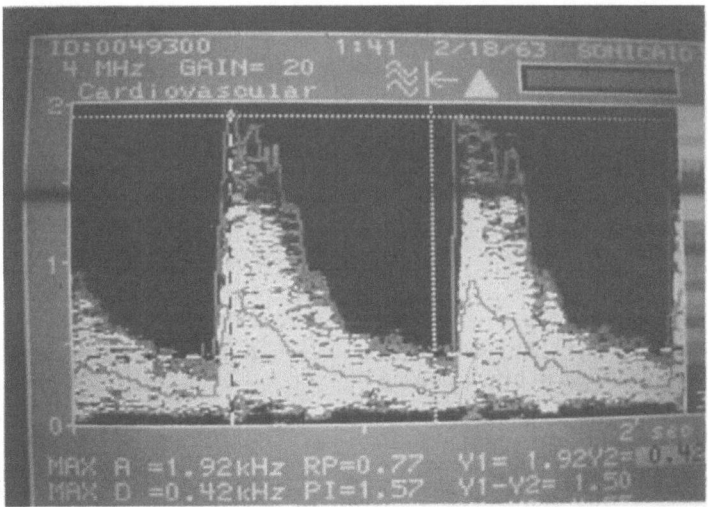

Fig. 3. The blood flow wave pattern of the internal carotid artery determined in a 62-year woman with branch abstruction of the retinal vein by ultrasonic doppler before stellate ganglion blocking.

478

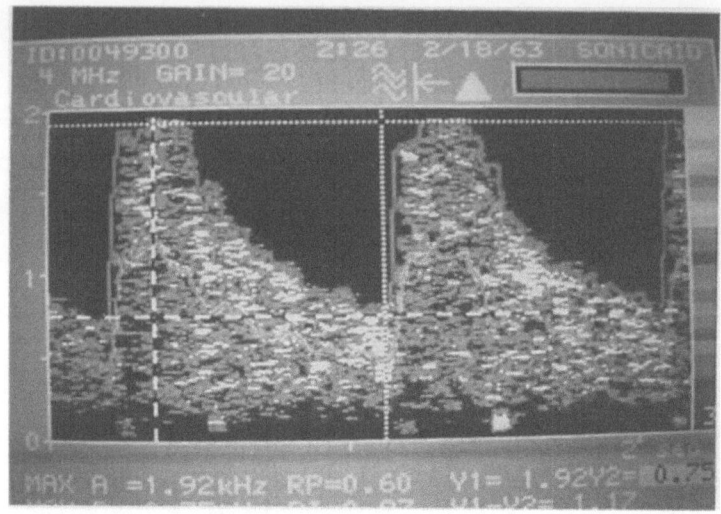

Fig. 4. The blood flow wave pattern of the internal carotid artery determined 10 minutes after blocking.

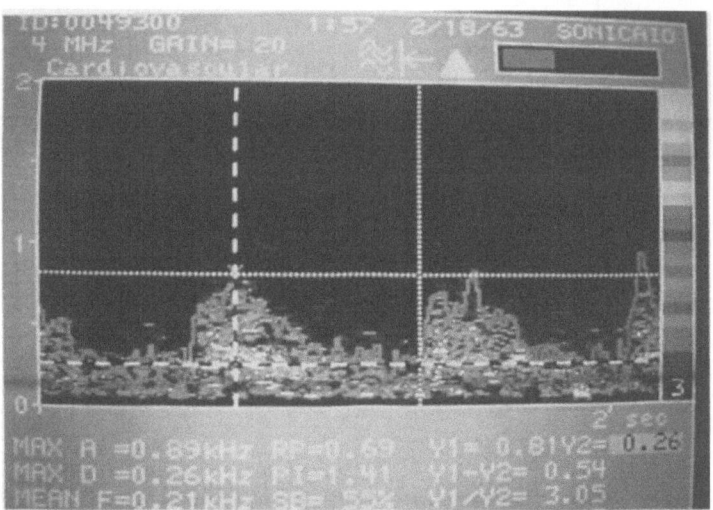

Fig. 5. The blood flow wave pattern of the central retinal artery on the optic disc of the same patient determined before blocking.

determined in this patient by ultrasonic Doppler before stellate ganglion blocking.

Next, Figure 4 shows the blood flow wave pattern of the internal carotid artery determined 10 minutes after blocking. The peak blood flow wave

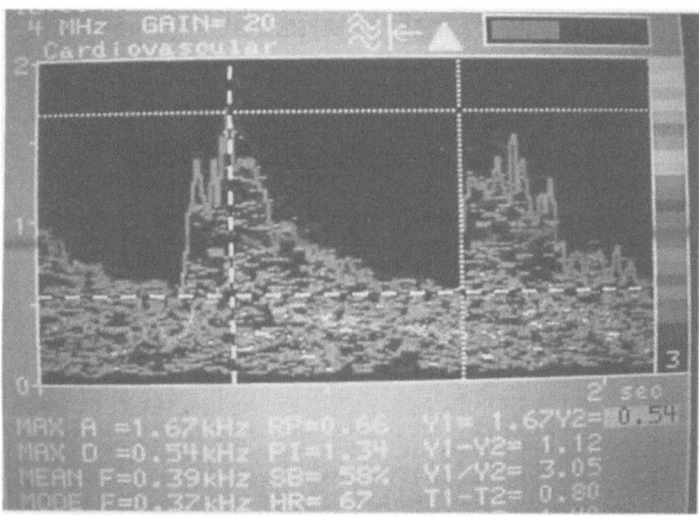

Fig. 6. The blood flow wave pattern of the central retinal artery determined 10 minutes after blocking, revealing a definite 2-fold increase in blood flow speed.

pattern of the internal carotid artery corresponding to the systol period of the heart was 1.92 kHz before and after blocking, whereas the pattern for the maximally dilated blood vessel corresponding to the diastole period of the heart increased from 0.42 kHz before blocking to 0.75 kHz after blocking, with a distinct increase in the mean from 0.37 kHz to 0.75 kHz, indicating a significant increase in the blood flow speed of the carotid artery after blocking.

Figure 5 shows the blood flow wave pattern of the central retinal artery on the optic disc of the same patient determined before blocking.

Figure 6 shows the blood flow wave pattern determined 10 minutes after blocking, revealing a definite 2-fold increase in the blood flow speed.

Figure 7 shows the course of improvement in visual acuity in group A, i.e., the previously treated group, after blocking. Almost all patients showed a tendency toward improvement in visual acuity.

Figure 8 shows the course of improvement in visual acuity in group B, i.e., the untreated group. All the patients visited our hospital within 2 weeks after onset, and an increase or improvement in the visual acuity was observed in almost all patients. No decrease in visual acuity has since occurred even 6 months after the completion of treatment.

The blood flow volume of the internal carotid artery and of the intraocular central retinal artery 30 minutes or 1 hour after blocking was increased by about 1.5- and 2-fold, respectively, relative to the volume before blocking.

Stellate ganglion blocking has been employed for the treatment of Raynaud's disease and Bürger's disease for blocking of the sympathetic

480

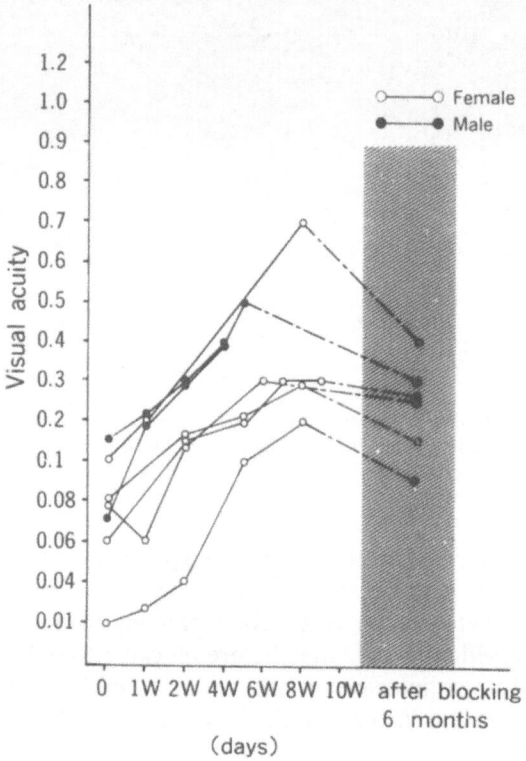

Branch obstruction of the
retinal vein (treated cases)

Fig. 7. The course of improvement in visual acuity in group A, i.e., the previously treated group, after blocking.

nerves to the head, neck, upper arms, heart and lung. In the present cases, this therapy might have facilitated improvement in the blood circulation of the retina and absorption of retinal edema, leading to marked improvement of ocular fundus disease. Several months have passed since the completion of blocking therapy, but none of the patients have shown aggravation of symptoms or hypofunction.

Conclusion

1) Observation of blood flow wave patterns of the internal carotid artery and the intraocular central retinal artery by the ultrasonic Doppler method revealed that stellate ganglion blocking in untreated patients with occlusive

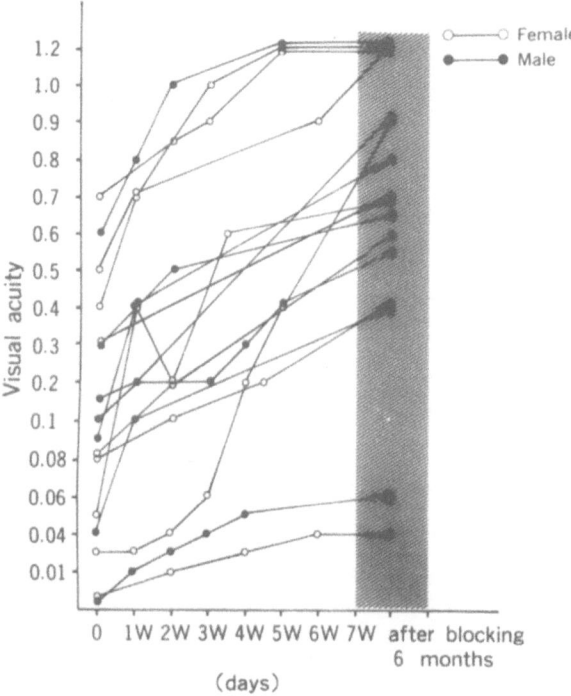

Branch obstruction of the
retinal vein (not treated / fresh cases)

Fig. 8. The course of improvement in visual acuity in group B, i.e., the untreated group, after blocking.

diseases of the retinal arteries was more effective than in previously treated patients with these diseases.

2) Stellate ganglion blocking induced an increase in intraocular blood flow, which lasted for about 4 hours, indicating the possible effectiveness of blocking for occlusive blood vessel diseases.

References

Futenma M et al. 1976. Stellate anglion block therapy in Ophthalmology, Folia Ophthalmol Jpn 27: 260–265.
Ishida M. 1987. Stellate ganglion block therapy on occlusion of the retinal vessels. Ophthalmology 29: 71–76.

62. Computerized analysis of echo signals: multicentric experience

LEONARDO FALCO*, FABIO ANDREUCCETTI*, STEFANO
ESENTE*, NICOLA PASSARELLI*, VINCENZINA MAZZEO**,
PAOLO PERRI**, ALFREDO REIBALDI***
and TERESIO AVITABILE***

Summary

The authors report their multicenter experience on computerized analysis of echo signals, utilizing the same ultrasound machine model, hardware and software. The theoretical note of this study and some clinical aspects are presented and discussed.

Introduction

Over the years, computerized analysis of A- and B-scan echo signals, has aroused the interest of researchers around the world.

As early as 1977 Colemann developed and applied computerized processing in the frequency range of ultrasonographic images. The work done by his research group has a considerable scientific significance. Currently, however, it is a unique item and probably very expensive.

Thijssen in 1981, Cennamo and Mazzeo in 1983, Reibaldi in 1984 and Haigis and Tane 1986 on various occasions presented the results they obtained from computerized analysis of echo signals, in the diagnosis of tumors and in echobiometry of the eye structure. These research groups, with different aims, used more or less complex and costly processing devices which are often beyond the reach of many ultrasonographists.

Most of these groups developed echo signal processing in terms of radio-frequency and only a few used video frequencies.

We have developed (Falco, 1987) a system which, using a RS-232 output of a commercially available ultrasonograph, high level software and a IBM PC-AT or IBM compatible PC, provides a video frequency analysis of the frequency range (FFT) of an A-Scan diagnostic tracing.

* Centro Oculistico, Firenze, Italy
** Clinica Oculistica, Universita' di Ferrara, Ferrara, Italy
*** Clinica Oculistica, Universita' di Catania, Italy

R. Sampaolesi (ed.), Ultrasonography in Ophthalmology 12, 483–486.
© 1990. Kluwer Academic Publishers, Dordrecht

Materials and methods

The multicenter research group was made possible through the uniformity of the equipment used at the centers which participated in the trials.

Basically the equipment consists of:
- Sonomed B 3000 ultrasonograph by Sonomed Technology, Inc. with RS 232 output.
- IBM or IBM compatible AT personal computer with a hard 20 MHz disc.
- A written program for patient management and A-scan trace processing. The processing consists of a fast Fourier Transform (FFT) which analyzes the harmonic contents of a signal in the frequency range.

Specifically

The Sonomed B 3000 is capable of memorizing any A-mode type scan, after having 'sampled' approximately a thousand points. The instrument is also equipped with an adapter circuit for asynchronous communications which provides the possibility of transferring the data recorded during any ultrasonographic test directly to the computer. Thus each frame, comprised of 1040 points is formed and memorized in the Sonomed in real time and processed by the computer on-line.

The programme which manages data transfer and subsequent processing is written in high level language. The interface for asynchronous communications is of the serial type and follows the RS-232C standard.

Once the data transfer from the ultrasonograph to the computer has been completed, the programme memorizes the frame containing the received data on disc 'files'. This results in the creation of a frame file, with one or more 'files' for each patient. A programme (in compiled BASIC language) was prepared for processing the ultrasonographic data. It begins with the reading of any single file in the memory and the selection of the first 1024 points of the acquired graphic selection of the pertinent area of the A-mode tracing on which the subsequent processing will be done.

This processing consists of the calculation of the power spectrum of the selected portion of the signal, after elimination of the average value of the signal itself.

Spectral analysis makes it possible to study the harmonic content of a signal and thus recognize the existence of given frequencies which are not immediately evident from the temporal time signals analysis.

In this specific case, the analyzed temporal time signal is the one supplied directly by the Sonomed B 3000. This will provide data in the frequency range, on the spectral distribution of the envelope of the ultrasonographic signal picked up by the piezoelectric transducer.

Patients with clinically and/or ultrasonographically confirmed pathologies were the primary subjects of the study.

Results

The current state of the art does not differ significantly from papers which one of us (Falco) presented previously. In fact, even if the amount of data is interesting (103) it still does not permit us to define the characteristics of the frequency range of the pathologies examined with any great accuracy.
The pathologies examined can be divided into two main groups:
1) membranous vitreo-retinal pathologies.
2) endobulbar neoplastic pathologies.

The second group is so limited that the results cannot be evaluated critically in any way.

The first, and larger group, shows two FFT tracings which we could empirically define as typical of the pathologies examined (vitreal membranous structures, retinal membranous structures). Regarding the retinal membranous structures, we noted a greater spectral decay which is localized at the lower frequencies. The two pathological situations reveal different spectral components.

The segmented linear interpolation of the tracings can lead to a line with a low angular coefficient or to two or more segments with different angular coefficients.

Discussion

The groundwork has been laid for a multicenter study aimed at evaluating ultrasonographic signals in the frequency domain through FFT processing of an A-Scan tracing. Such a tracing that can easily be used in several modern ultrasound devices with a serial RS 232 port can contain useful diagnostic information.

The fact we used this type of signal for our computerized processing rather than a RF signal is based on the immediate and simple possibility of using it with the ultrasonograph we selected.

The difficulty in identifying a pathological lesion by A-scan, even if it is subsequent to a B-scan image could be overcome in the near future through the direct acquisition of a selected vector on the B-scan, on which Fourier's analysis could be done.

The large number of cases that can be tested through a multicenter study, refinement of the system (readings and analysis done by vectors) and a statistical analysis will be able to confirm the theoretical assumptions and thus the viability of this system for computer assisted analysis of ultrasound signals.

486

References

Cennamo G, Savastano M. 1983. Acquisizione, memorizzazione ed elaborazione di segnali ecografici in oftalmologia. AICA Annual Conference Proceedings p. 263.

Coleman D J, Lizzi F L, Jack R L. 1977. Ultrasonography of the eye and orbit: Lea & Febiger, Philadelphia. pp. 83–87.

Falco L, Andreuccetti A. 1988. Analisi computerizzata del' segnale ecografico: nostra esperienza. II Congresso SIEO 1987. Clin Ocul IX: pp. 257–261.

Haigis W. 1987. Computer-assisted clinical A-Mode analysis in ophthalmic ultrasonography. In: Ossoinig K C (ed) Ophthalmic Echography, Doc Ophthal Proc Series, Vol 48, M. Nijhoff/ Dr. Junk Publishers, Dordrecht.

Mazzeo V. 1983. What the clinician may expect from tissue characterization in the ophthalmological field (state of art). In: Thijssen J M, Irion K (ed) Ultrasonic Tissue Characterization. Proceedings of 3rd EC Workshop, Stuttgart.

Reibaldi A, Guerriero S, Avitabile T, Uva M, Veneziani N, Pasquariello G, Pasquali F. 1987. Texture analysis di immagini ultrasonografiche in oculistica. Clin Ocul 1: 17–25.

Tane S. Kimura Y, Kano M. 1988. Spectral analysis for ultrasonic tissue characterization. In: Thijssen J M (ed) Ultrasonography in Ophthalmology II, Doc Ophthal Proc Series, Vol. 51, Kluwer Acad Publ, Dordrecht, pp. 73–76.

Thijssen J M, Verbeek A M. Computer analysis of A mode echograms from choroidal melanoma. In: Thijssen J M and Verbeek A M (eds.) Ultrasonography in Ophthalmology 8, Doc Ophthal Proc Series, Vol. 29, Junk, The Hague, pp. 123–130.

63. RGB output: our experience

LEONARDO FALCO*, STEFANO ESENTE*, NICOLA PASSARELLI*
and AGOSTINO LATORRE**

Summary

The RGB output of the new ultrasound machines is used to prove again the diagnostic possibilities of the coloured ultrasound images.
The results are presented and discussed.

Introduction

The application of false color techniques in ultrasonography of the eye and orbit was developed by Coleman (1974), Liebesny (1973) and Reibaldi (1983).

By using commercially available ultrasonography instruments and computerized electronic systems, they transformed the scale of greys into different colors and created 'full color' ultrasonograms. The results obtained by these authors opened the way for new, interesting and probably useful diagnostic possibilities in ophthalmic echography. However, this technique, which was limited to these experimental systems, never reached adulthood.

Today, the commercial availability of an echographic instrument which, in addition to a computerized signal processing system, provides an RGB output, has again brought this testing system to the attention of echographists.

Here we present our experience with the RGB system, highlighting its advantages and drawbacks, as well as some diagnostic impressions.

Materials and methods

We used a Sonomed B 3000 ultrasonograph by Sonomed Technology Inc. Without delving into the instrument's technical features we just want to

* Centro Oculistico, Firenze, Italy
** I Clinica Oculistica, Universita'di Firenze, Firenze, Italy

R. Sampaolesi (ed.), Ultrasonography in Ophthalmology 12, 487–489.

point out that a false color ultrasonogram, in real time or on frozen images, can only be obtained via an RGB output connected to an RGB monitor.

The false color technique replaces a given shade of grey on the ultrasonogram with a false color that is attributed to that specific shade of grey.

The term 'false color' is derived from the fact that the color itself is 'fictitious'. It is merely the result of a convention that assigns a different color to the various threshold levels of grey tones (from 1 to 15 LVL). Thus, LVL 1 of the grey threshold (the darkest grey on an ultrasonogram) corresponds to the false color dark blue (in all the amplification). As the shades of grey become lighter, the false colors take on different shadings of blue, green, yellow, orange and finally red, so that LVL 15 of the grey threshold is a deep red (the lightest grey on the ultrasonogram).

We subjected the patients who came under our observation, first to a traditional A/B-scan ultrasonography and then to a B-scan test using the false color technique. In some cases (differential diagnosis of vitreo-retinal structures) we processed the diagnostic A-scan, also, using an FFT program we developed.

Results

The percentage breakdown of diagnosed pathologies is the following:
- hemovitreous   13.33%
- posterior hyaloid detachment   20.00%
- detachment of the retina   20.00%
- foreign bodies   1.66%
- myopic staphyloma (during echobiometry for IOL)   36.66%
- coloboma   3.03%
- malignant melanoma of the choroid   3.03%
- choroidal metastasis   1.66%

The ultrasonographic diagnoses were made using the 'classic' method as described above. The false color technique was, with few exceptions, used after the diagnosis; we only used the false color technique first in case of suspected or ascertained myopic staphyloma.

Discussion

We believe that the false color technique, which has been reproposed thanks to the development of this new instrument, is worthy of careful study.

It is not a question of the visual appeal of the false color, the behaviour or each normal and/or pathological structure in the false color technique.

Initially we believed that this artificial processing would only create confusion and complicate even simple diagnoses. Subsequently, after careful study and a comparison of the responses obtained from normal and/or pathological structures in the grey scale and in the false color scale, we began to understand and to become familiar with these colored ultrasonograms. The experience we have acquired up to this time is not sufficient to allow 'standardization' of a false color technique. However, we believe that this ultrasonographic method could be a useful tool in vitreo-retinal pathologies, in the differentiation of vascular structures, in uncovering some types of F. B. and even for a better definition of common profiles in contiguous pathologies. At the current point in our study, comparing photographic material rather than real-time images, we have been able to ascertain the following:

– Vitreal pathologies are defined more accurately than with the grey scale.
– In cases of association of vitreo-retinal membranous structures, we have noted that the false color resolves the subtle differences of greys in a higher percentage than an observer can when using a black and white monitor.
– In defining a neoplasm, a coloboma, a myopic staphyloma, false color seems to provide better results than the grey scale method also with image processing (smooth image).

We believe that a study protocol should be drafted in order to 'standardize' the criteria for the most feasible study possible.

Notwithstanding the limits of our studies to date, we believe that we have demonstrated that this technique is not so easy. Furthermore, we are just as firmly convinced that the initial impact with US, in the current state of the art, cannot and should not be with the false color technique.

References

Coleman D J, and Katz L. 1974. Color coding of B Scan ultrasonograms. Arch Ophthalmol 91: 429–431.
Colemann D J, Lizzi F L, Jack R L. 1977. Ultrasonography of the eye and orbit. Lea & Febiger, Philadelphia.
Liebesny J P, Lele P P. 1973. Enhancement of ultrasonic B scans by chromatic encoding. Proceedings IEEE Ultrasonics Symposium, pp. 37–38.
Reibaldi A, Avitabile T, Guerriero S, Uva M G. 1987. Possibility of ocular tissue differentiation by means of false-color assisted echography. In: Ossoinig K C (ed) Ophthalmic Echography, Proc of the 10th SIDUO Congress, Florida, 1984. Doc Ophthal Proc Series, Vol. 48, M. Nijhoff/Dr. Junk Publishers, Dordrecht.

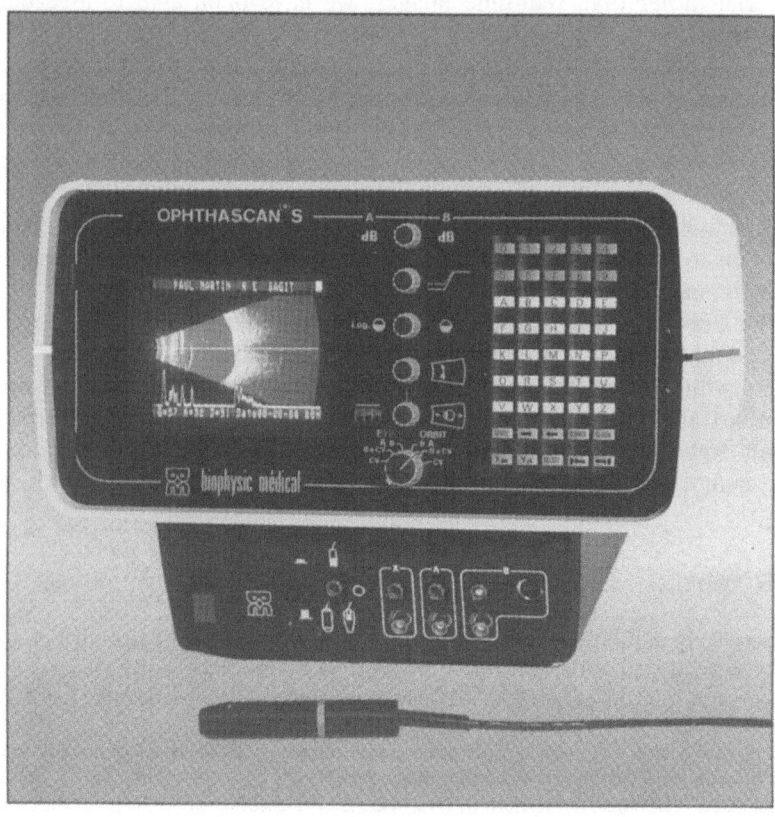
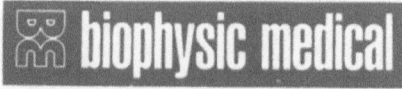

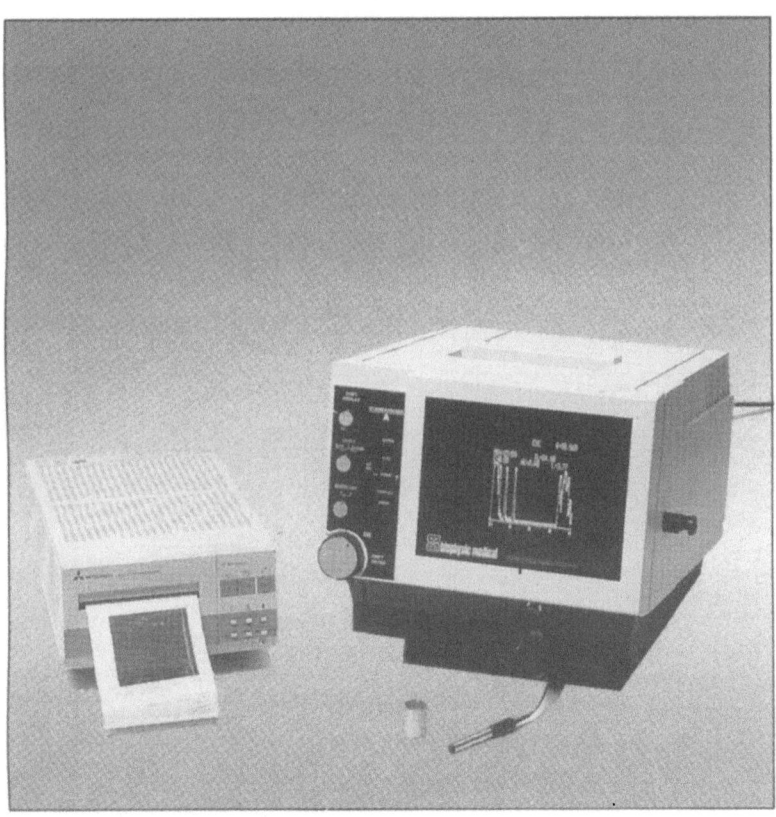
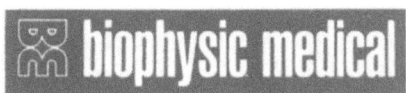

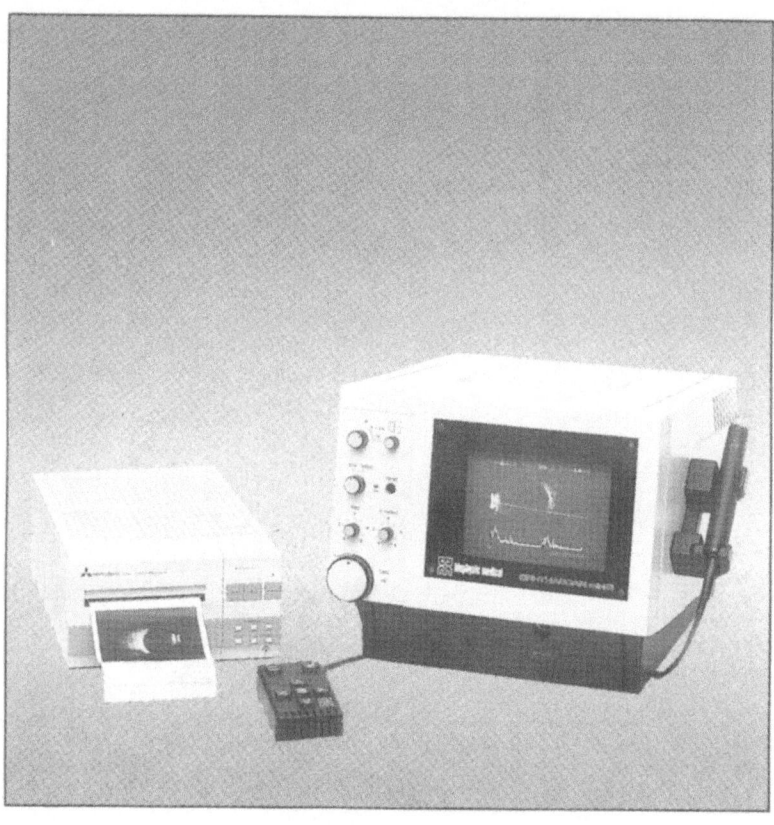
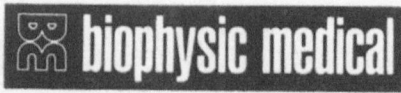

Authors index

494

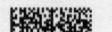

International Perspectives in Values-Based Mental Health Practice